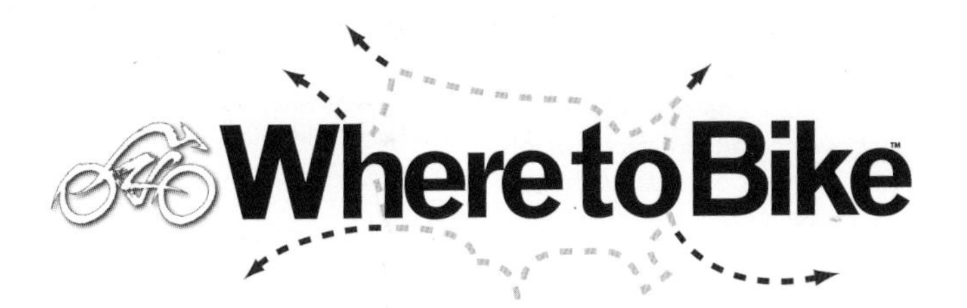


# Los Angeles

- San Fernando Valley
- San Gabriel Valley
- The Westside
- Downtown to Beverly Hills
- Long Beach
- Kids' Rides

By Jon Riddle & Sarah Amelar

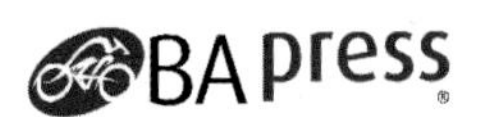

Where to Bike LLC

Email: mail@wheretobikeguides.com
Tel: +61 2 4274 4884 - Fax: +61 2 4274 0988
www.wheretobikeguides.com

First published in the USA in 2012 by Where to Bike LLC.



Design and Layout - Justine Powell
Advertising - Phil Latz
Photography - All photos taken by Sarah Amelar or Jon Riddle unless otherwise specified
Mapping - Justine Powell
Printed in China by RR Donnelley
Cover: Photo by Sarah Amelar

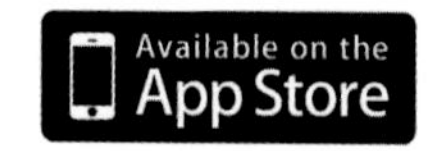


Library of Congress Control Number: 2011943180
Author: Jon Riddle & Sarah Amelar
Title: Where to Bike Los Angeles
ISBN: 978-0-9808587-6-1 (paperback)
978-0-9808587-7-8 (box set)

*The Cycling Kangaroo logo is a trademark of Lake Wangary Publishing Company Pty Ltd.*

*Where to Bike is a proud sponsor of World Bicycle Relief.*

*Where to Bike is a proud member of the Bikes Belong Coalition, organisers of the People for Bikes campaign.*

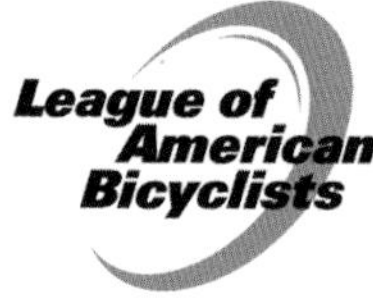


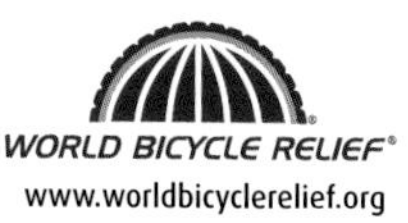


***Also in this series:***

Where to Ride Melbourne
Where to Ride Adelaide
Where to Ride Perth
Where to Ride Sydney
Where to Ride Canberra
Where to Ride South East Queensland
Where to Ride Tasmania
Where to Ride Western & Northern Victoria
Where to Ride Eastern Victoria
Where to Ride Sydney MTB
Where to Ride London
Where to Bike Chicago
Where to Bike Washington, D.C.
Where to Bike Philadelphia

***Coming Soon:***

Where to Bike New York City
Where to Ride Auckland
Where to Ride Melbourne MTB
Where to Bike Portland
Where to Bike Orange County
Where to Bike Los Angeles MTB
Where to Bike Orange County MTB

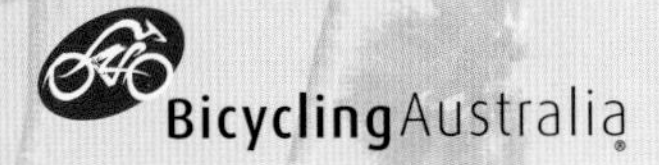


# About us...

Cycling has many health and environmental benefits, but apart from these it's a fun leisure time activity for all ages. Most of our small team are active cyclists; we love to ride and hope that we can, through interesting, exciting and timely information, make your cycling experience more enjoyable.

Founded more than 20 years ago by Phil and Catie Latz, Lake Wangary Publishing Company began with a single black and white road cycling magazine. We now publish four cycling magazines as well as the growing series of Where to Ride guides in Australia, New Zealand, the UK and now Where to Bike in the United States.

We're committed to our vision of enhancing all aspects of cycling by providing information for all our customers. Whether through our magazines or books, we hope to make your riding experience as enjoyable as possible.

Look out for BA Press books and the 'cycling kangaroo' logos in newsstands and bookstores; it's your key to great cycling publications.

We have made every effort to ensure the accuracy of the content of this book, but please feel free to contact us at mail@wheretobikeguides.com to report any changes to routes or inconsistencies you may find.

For more information about *Where to Bike Los Angeles* and other books in this series, go to **www.wheretobikeguides.com**.

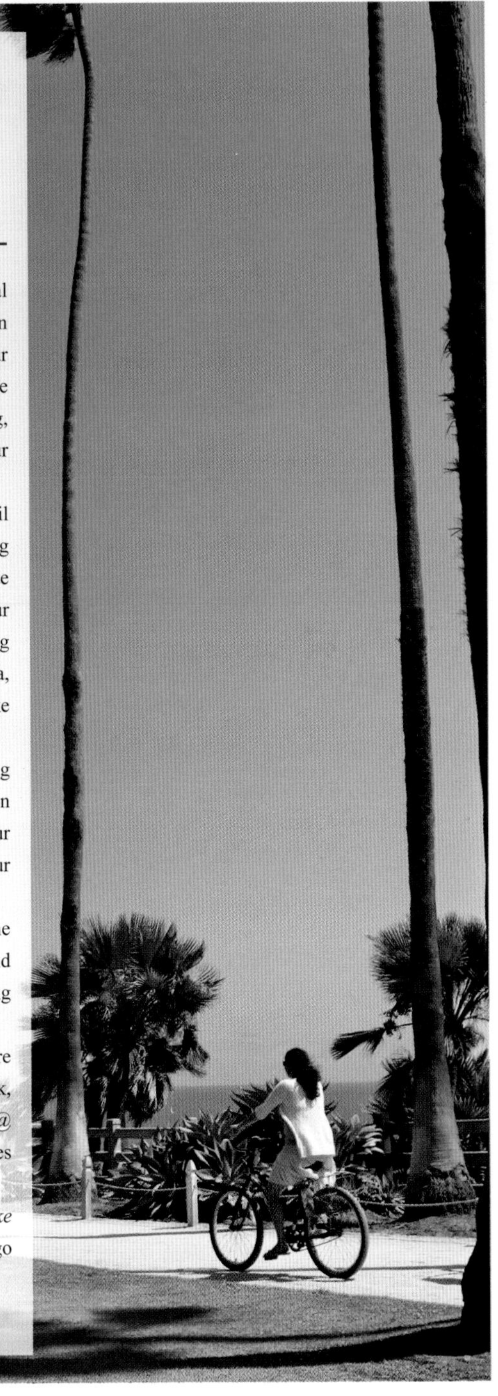

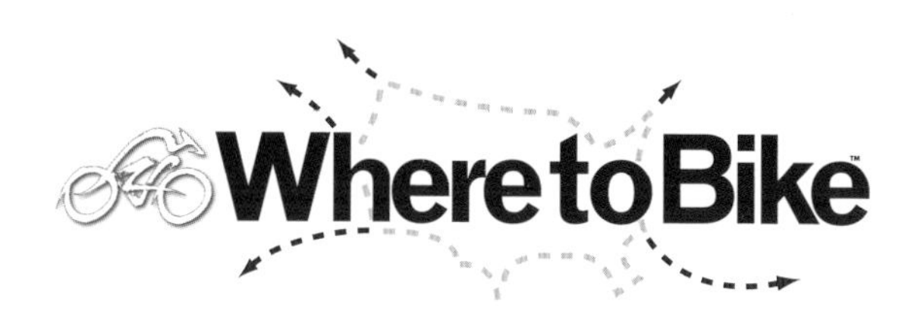


**Los Angeles**

## Contents


About Us ........ 3
Authors' Note ........ 8
About the Authors ........ 9
Introduction ........ 10
Ride Overview ........ 12-15
How to Use This Book ........ 16
Before You Go / What to Take ........ 18
World Bicycle Relief ........ 20
On the Road in L.A. ........ 22
Communal Cookery: L.A.'s Bicycle Co-Op Movement ........ 24
You, Your Bike and Public Transportation in L.A. ........ 26
Public Transport Maps ........ 28-29

**San Fernando Valley (with the Santa Clarita Valley)**

Introduction ........ 34
Ride 1 - Griffith Park ........ 36
Ride 2 - Los Angeles River ........ 40
Ride 3 - Chandler Bikeway ........ 44
Ride 4 - Orange Line Bikeway ........ 48
Ride 5 - Sepulveda Basin ........ 52
Ride 6 - Encino Velodrome ........ 56
Ride 7 - San Fernando to Santa Susana Pass ........ 60
Ride 8 - The Rock Store ........ 64
Ride 9 - Vasquez Rocks ........ 68
Ride 10 - Santa Clarita: The Cloverleaf ........ 72
Ride 11 - Little Tujunga Canyon Road ........ 76
Ride 12 - Hansen Dam ........ 80

**San Gabriel Valley**

Introduction ........ 86
Ride 13 - Rose Bowl Circuit ........ 88
Ride 14 - Descanso Gardens ........ 92
Ride 15 - A Tour of Pasadena ........ 96
Ride 16 - Three Rivers: Rio Hondo, San Gabriel & Los Angeles ........ 100

Ride 17 - Whittier Greenway Trail ........ 104
Ride 18 - Rio Hondo ........ 108
Ride 19 - San Gabriel River: Whittier Narrows to the Mountains ........ 112
Ride 20 - West Fork of the San Gabriel River ........ 116
Ride 21 - Glendora Mountain Road ........ 120
Ride 22 - Royal Oaks Bike Path ........ 124

**The Westside**

Introduction ........ 130
Ride 23 - Topanga Canyon ........ 132
Ride 24 - Pacific Coast Highway ........ 136
Ride 25 - A Tour of Santa Monica ........ 140
Ride 26 - San Vicente and Mandeville Canyon ........ 144
Ride 27 - Santa Monica Bike Path ........ 148
Ride 28 - Marina del Rey Loop ........ 152
Ride 29 - South Bay Bike Path ........ 156
Ride 30 - Ballona Creek ........ 160
Ride 31 - The Donut: Palos Verdes Peninsula ........ 164
Ride 32 - Double Donut Holes: Palos Verdes Peninsula ........ 168

**Downtown to Beverly Hills**

Introduction ........ 174
Ride 33 - Mulholland Drive ........ 176
Ride 34 - Lake Hollywood Reservoir ........ 180
Ride 35 - Mount Hollywood Drive ........ 184
Ride 36 - Silver Lake ........ 188
Ride 37 - Elysian Park ........ 192
Ride 38 - California Cycleway ........ 196
Ride 39 - Beverly Hills: Starlets, Heroes & Villains ........ 200
Ride 40 - The UCLA Connection ........ 204
Ride 41 - A Tour of Downtown L.A. ........ 208
Ride 42 - L.A. River: Downtown to Long Beach ........ 212
Ride 43 - Cross-Town Shuffle: Skyscrapers to Surf ........ 216

**Long Beach**

Introduction ........ 220
Ride 44 - Surf City USA ........ 222
Ride 45 - Long Beach Arts & Craftsmen ........ 226
Ride 46 - Long Beach Bicycle Periferico: The Perimeter Route ........ 230
Ride 47 - El Dorado Park ........ 234
Ride 48 - Coastal Long Beach: Long and the Shore of It ........ 238
Ride 49 - Marine Stadium to Cal State Long Beach ........ 242
Ride 50 - San Pedro's Waterfront ........ 246
Ride 51 - Experiencing Watts Towers ........ 250

## Kids' Rides

Introduction .......... 254

**San Fernando Valley**

Ride K1 - Santa Clara River Banks **Santa Clarita** .......... 256
Ride K2 - Summit Park **Valencia** .......... 257
Ride K3 - Lake Balboa **Van Nuys** .......... 258
Ride K4 - El Cariso Park **Sylmar** .......... 259
Ride K5 - Rio de Los Angeles State Park **Cypress Park** .......... 260

**San Gabriel Valley**

Ride K6 - Arroyo Seco **Montecito Heights** .......... 261
Ride K7 - Lacy Park **San Marino** .......... 262
Ride K8 - Belvedere Park **East Los Angeles** .......... 263
Ride K9 - Legg Lake **South El Monte** .......... 264
Ride K10 - Santa Fe Dam Recreation Area **Irwindale** .......... 265
Ride K11 - Ralph C. Dills Park **Paramount** .......... 266
Ride K12 - Wilderness Park **Downey** .......... 267

**The Westside**

Ride K13 - Santa Monica Pier **Santa Monica** .......... 268
Ride K14 - Burton W. Chase Park **Marina del Rey** .......... 269
Ride K15 - Clover Park **Santa Monica** .......... 270
Ride K16 - Westwood Park **Los Angeles/Westwood** .......... 271
Ride K17 - Hermosa Beach Strand **Hermosa Beach** .......... 272
Ride K18 - Highridge Park **Rolling Hills Estates** .......... 273

**Downtown to Beverly Hills**

Ride K19 - The Cornfield **Downtown Los Angeles** .......... 274
Ride K20 - Kenneth Hahn State Recreation Area **Baldwin Hills** .......... 275
Ride K21 - Ladera Park **Ladera Heights** .......... 276
Ride K22 - "Magic" Johnson Recreation Area **Willowbrook** .......... 277
Ride K23 - John Anson Ford Park **Bell Gardens** .......... 278

**Long Beach**

Ride K24 - Columbia Park **Torrance** .......... 279
Ride K25 - Ken Malloy Harbor Regional Park **Harbor City** .......... 280
Ride K26 - Scherer Park **Long Beach** .......... 281
Ride K27 - Shoreline Aquatic Park **Long Beach** .......... 282
Ride K28 - Recreation Park **Long Beach** .......... 283
Ride K29 - Cabrillo Beach **San Pedro** .......... 284
Ride K30 - Wilmington Waterfront Park **Wilmington** .......... 285

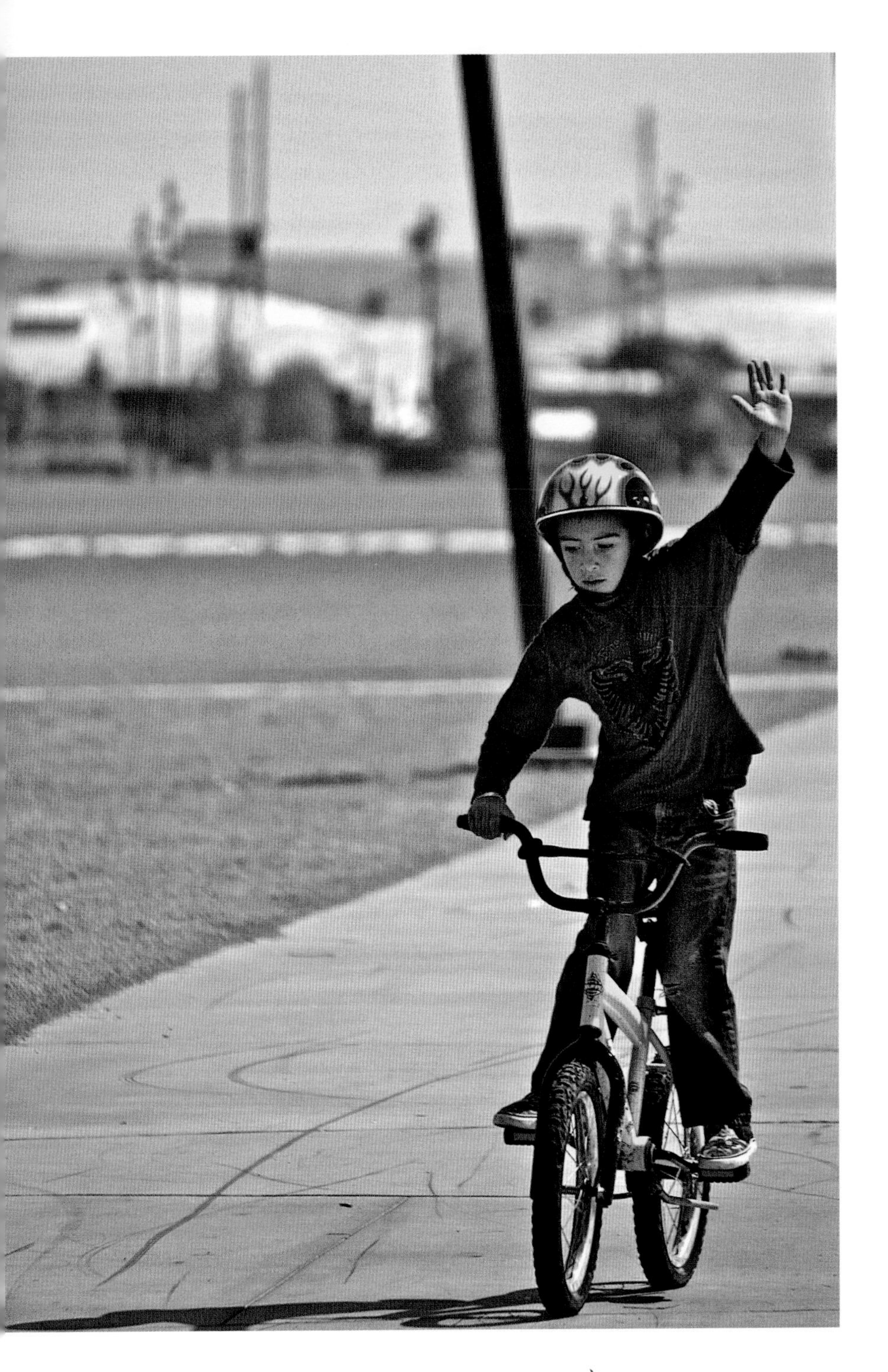

# Authors' Note

As we put the finishing touches on the pages before you—and take a moment to catch our breath—we are amazed by the long journey across and around Los Angeles we've just completed. Over the past year, we've each pedaled more than 4,800 miles to locate and shape this book's 81 rides: from Vasquez Rocks, in the northern high desert, to the shores of Santa Monica, Palos Verdes and Long Beach; from rural passes in the San Gabriel Mountains to Downtown city streets. Though we set out as seasoned locals, the challenge of creating *Where to Bike Los Angeles* turned us into voyagers in our own city. We got to hunt down new paths, re-experience journeys we hadn't done in ages, coast along favorites and nix the ones we didn't consider worthy of you. We rode about four miles for every one we're recommending to you—just to make sure we'd be leading you down the most enticing and safest routes. Along the way, we must have looked like star-struck tourists as we snapped thousands of photos, ultimately to zero in on the few hundred that appear here. Sometimes we wondered if we'd ever finish.

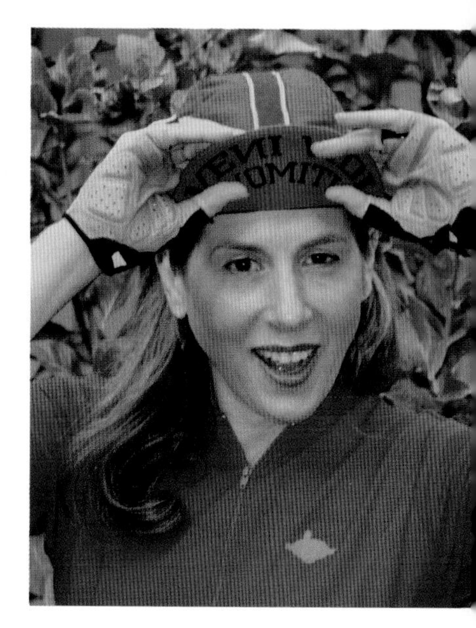

But, yes, a light is beaming at the end of the tunnel. Now you can press your feet to the pedals and simply savor these diverse rides, without taking the wrong turns we took. With a GPS strapped on, we've mapped each route for you accurately turn by turn—peppered with great info about eating spots, historical lore and fun detours.

While our book evolved, we saw L.A.'s bicycling scene undergo its own positive transformations. New bike lanes now line Seventh Street past MacArthur Park, Spring Street through the Downtown core and Metro's Expo Line corridor. Long Beach gained the county's first physically separated, protected bike lanes, or cycletracks. And the Wilmington Waterfront Park, opened in 2011, offers great cycling for young kids. If the bike master plans that have received recent approval on county, city and community levels are future indicators, L.A. will add many more miles of bike lanes and paths in the next five years (progress thanks in large part to advocacy by the Los Angeles County Bicycle Coalition and others).

We hope this book inspires you to explore Greater Los Angeles—its remarkably diverse landscapes, cultures, microclimates, urban life and wayside attractions. If you venture off route, into inviting neighborhood corners, down a country lane or up a mountain road, or if you modify rides or devise your own, please share your adventures and discoveries via wheretobikela@gmail, our Facebook page, Twitter or at **www.wheretobikelosangeles.com**. We welcome your feedback.

Meanwhile, buckle on your helmets … and enjoy the rides.

**Jon Riddle and Sarah Amelar**
Authors and Photographers

# About the Authors

Jon Riddle is a native Californian, born in Needles, along the state's eastern edge, and raised among lizards and blowing sand. When he was six, his family moved to L.A.'s fringes, where Jon learned to ride a red Schwinn Stingray with a banana seat. Following graduate school, he settled in Los Angeles, where he's been cycling for more than 15 years. He has also biked Spain's Camino de Santiago pilgrimage route and Peru's Sacred Valley and ridden in Burma, Thailand, Vietnam (from north to south), Mexico and France. Jon, who holds a doctorate in economics, runs a consulting practice and has taught at the University of California in Los Angeles and Santa Barbara.

Sarah Amelar has a passion for urban cycling that dates back to her girlhood in New York City, where she logged hundreds of miles on a Raleigh three-speed with a chirpy bell and wicker basket. Her daily cycling gained momentum and her curiosity about cities grew as she completed a Masters of Architecture at Yale, practiced architecture and became an editor at *Architectural Record* magazine. Her writing has appeared in venues including *The New York Times, Dwell, Metropolis, New York Newsday,* and *The Phaidon Atlas of 21st Century World Architecture*.

Jon and Sarah met bicycling in Southeast Asia. They soon began exploring L. A. together by bike. In 2008, Jon convinced her to join him on his fourth AIDS/LifeCycle: a seven-day, 545-mile fundraising ride from San Francisco to L.A.

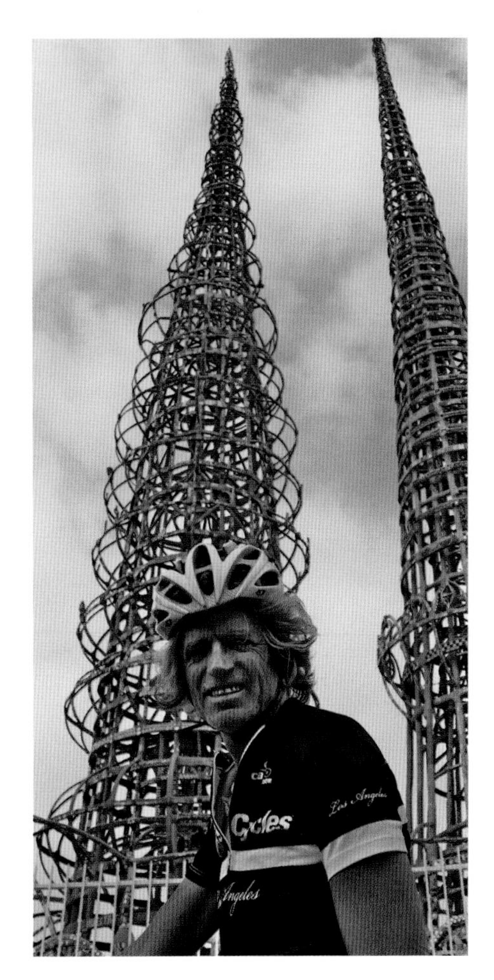


## Acknowledgements

We would like to thank our friends who rode with us through the creation of this book, especially Jennifer Klausner, Greg Laemmle, Martin Lopez-Lu, Kelli Bachmann and Bobby Gadda of the Los Angeles County Bicycle Coalition and our neighbor, Peter Stowell. Our gratitude also goes to the Pasadena History Museum; to Teresa Halliday, Dmitry Shapiro, Barry Elliott, his Mapei gang and cyclists of all ages who patiently posed for our photos; to riders who stopped to offer assistance as we puzzled over maps; to bike shop staffers who generously shared secret routes; and to Helen's Cycles for keeping our vélos roadworthy.

## Dedication

We dedicate this book to our parents: to Alice Amelar, who biked across the U.S. as a young teen, in an era when such a trip was unthinkable; to Richard Amelar, who's never stinted on encouragement and provided his young daughters with wonderful bicycles; to June Riddle, an outdoor adventurer, who has always believed her children could bike up any mountain; and to the memory of Jack Riddle.

# Introduction—Let's Roll

"Nothing compares to the simple pleasure of a bike ride."

—John F. Kennedy

As we write, bicycling is gaining ground in Los Angeles—moving forward with momentum. Over 1,265 miles of bicycle paths, lanes and routes lace through the county's 4,752 square miles, with more infrastructure in the works. Compared with gasoline's 31,500 calories per gallon, it's stunningly efficient—and certainly appealing for the health of your body and the planet—to fuel up with a snack bar instead and power some of your journeys with your own two legs.

Free from automotive shells of steel and glass, you'll experience more directly the area's cultural diversity and microclimates—from beaches with palms to golden high desert and gritty Downtown streets, in the shadow of winter's snow-capped peaks. L.A. sprawls across a virtually flat, 35-by-45-mile basin with mountains to the north and the Pacific Ocean along the south and west. This geography allows for gentle bike paths along its shores, rivers and parks—and spectacularly challenging mountain ascents. Within this vast county, there are even places where you can easily bike in and camp by a stream in the wilderness.

So, where to begin? Whether you're just steadying yourself on wheels or already flying on your bike; whether you're a leisurely weekend cyclist or a daily commuter; a visitor or a local, we have recommendations for you. Following geographic and constructed dividing lines, we've parceled L.A. County into five areas—and linked our ride starts with mass transit, wherever possible. This book starts with the two northernmost regions: the San Fernando and San Gabriel valleys, enfolding a total of 22 rides, some into the San Gabriel Mountains and several into Santa Clarita's desert communities. For the Westside, we propose 10 rides, including jaunts along beaches from Malibu to the Palos Verdes Peninsula. Our Downtown to Beverly Hills section offers 11 routes, many extending out like spokes (well, bent and twisting ones) from the urban hub. In Long Beach, our eight rides wind through and around this harbor-side city, a place outstanding for its energy and resources committed to bicycling innovation. The sixth section, dedicated to children, describes 30 routes across the five regions—designed with fun and safety in mind—for everyone from tots learning to ride to confident young cyclists, ready to turn their cranks and explore.

We're all, in our own ways, learners in La La Land, so onward!

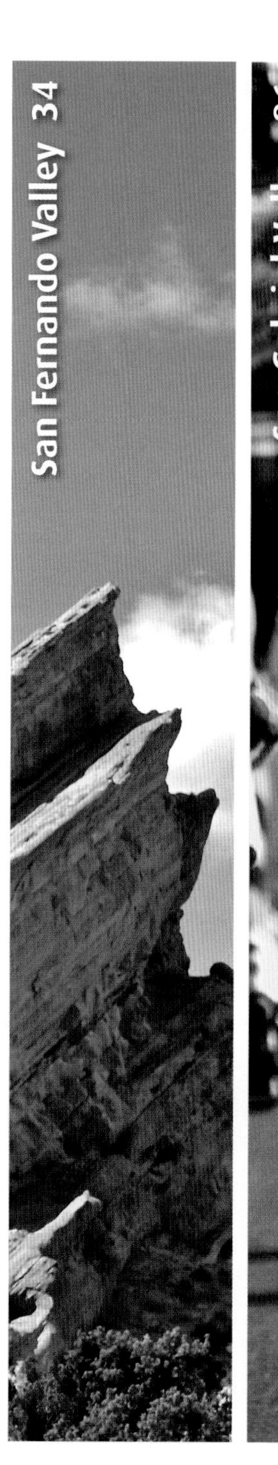

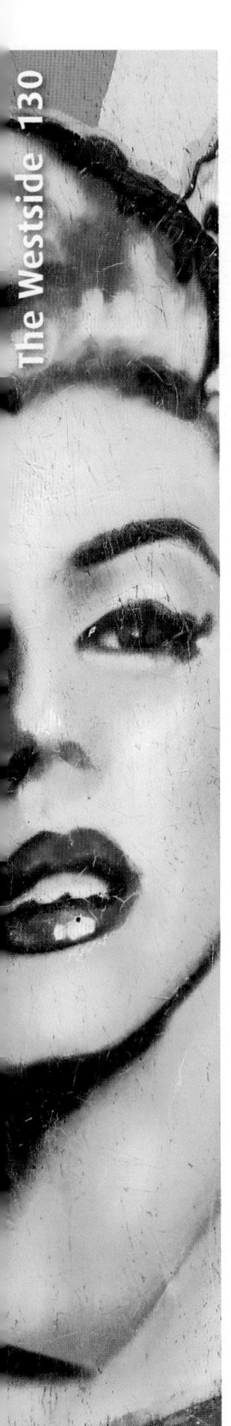
The Westside 130
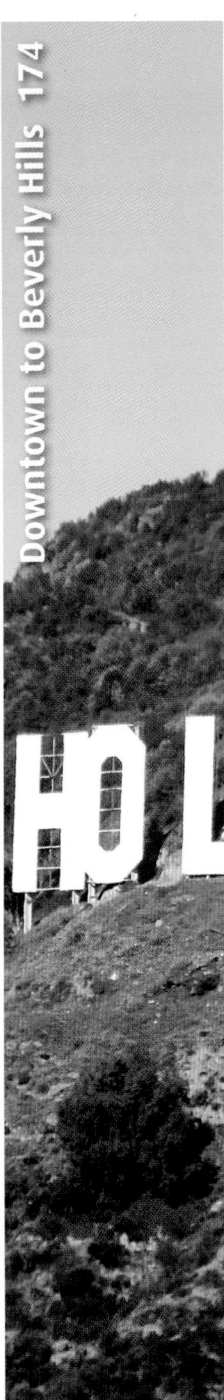
Downtown to Beverly Hills 174
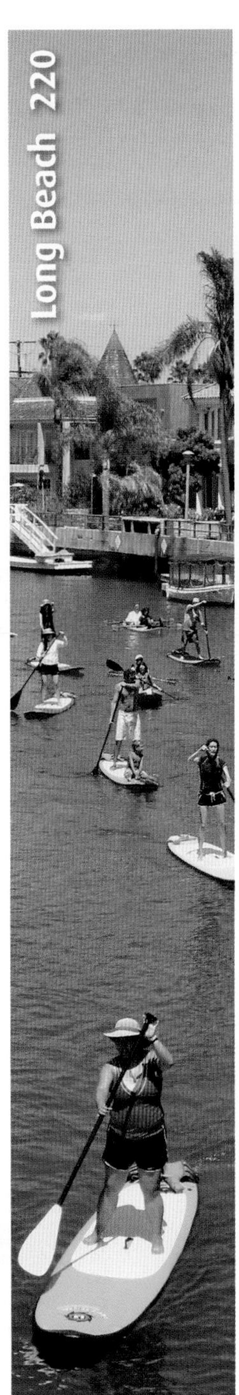
Long Beach 220
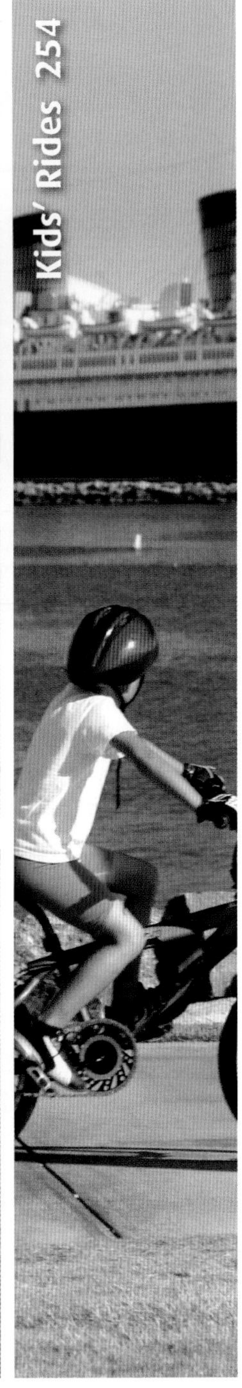
Kids' Rides 254

# Ride Overview

## San Fernando Valley (with the Santa Clarita Valley)



| Page | Ride | Ride Name | Start Location |
|---|---|---|---|
| 36 | 1 | Griffith Park | Los Angeles Zoo, Los Angeles |
| 40 | 2 | Los Angeles River | Los Angeles Zoo, Los Angeles |
| 44 | 3 | Chandler Bikeway | North Hollywood Metro Station, North Hollywood |
| 48 | 4 | Orange Line Bikeway | North Hollywood Metro Station, North Hollywood |
| 52 | 5 | Sepulveda Basin | Lake Balboa, Encino |
| 56 | 6 | Encino Velodrome | Encino Velodrome on Oxnard Street, Encino |
| 60 | 7 | San Fernando to Santa Susana Pass | Sylmar/San Fernando Metrolink Station, San Fernando |
| 64 | 8 | The Rock Store | Las Virgines Road & Mulholland Hwy, Agoura Hills |
| 68 | 9 | Vasquez Rocks | Vaquez Rocks Park, Agua Dulce |
| 72 | 10 | Santa Clarita: The Cloverleaf | Promenade trailhead on McBean Pkwy, Santa Clarita |
| 76 | 11 | Little Tujunga Canyon Road | Sylmar/San Fernando Metrolink Station, San Fernando |
| 80 | 12 | Hansen Dam | Hansen Dam Recreation Area, Lakeview Terrace |



## San Gabriel Valley



| Page | Ride | Ride Name | Start Location |
|---|---|---|---|
| 88 | 13 | Rose Bowl Circuit | Rose Bowl, Pasadena |
| 92 | 14 | Descanso Gardens | Rose Bowl, Pasadena |
| 96 | 15 | A Tour of Pasadena | Mission Metro Station, South Pasadena |
| 100 | 16 | Three Rivers: Rio Hondo, San Gabriel & Los Angeles | John Anson Ford Park, Bell Gardens |
| 104 | 17 | Whittier Greenway Trail | Guirado Park, Whittier |
| 108 | 18 | Rio Hondo | Whitter Narrows, South El Monte |
| 112 | 19 | San Gabriel River: Whittier Narrows to the Mountains | Whitter Narrows, South El Monte |
| 116 | 20 | West Fork of the San Gabriel River | Highway 38, at West Fork, North of Azusa |
| 120 | 21 | Glendora Mountain Road | Veterans Freedom Park, Azusa |
| 124 | 22 | Royal Oaks Bike Path | Encanto Park, Duarte |



## The Westside



| Page | Ride | Ride Name | Start Location |
|---|---|---|---|
| 132 | 23 | Topanga Canyon | Topango Canyon & Old Topanga Rds, Topanga |
| 136 | 24 | Pacific Coast Highway | Santa Monica Pier, Santa Monica |

| Terrain | Kid-Friendly | Distance (miles) | Elev. Gain (feet) | WTB Rating |
|---|---|---|---|---|
| On Road / On Road Lane | | 8.7 | 750 | |
| Path | | 14.2 | 250 | |
| On Road Lane / Path | | 6.6 | 200 | |
| On Road Lane / Path | | 29.1 | 600 | |
| On Road Lane / Path | partial | 7.9 | 300 | |
| Path | | 0.2 | 0 | |
| On Road / On Road Lane | | 27.0 | 1,700 | |
| On Road | | 27.2 | 3,300 | |
| On Road | | 23.3 | 1,800 | |
| On Road / Path / Off Road | partial | 24.9 | 1,300 | |
| On Road / On Road Lane / Path | | 45.9 | 3,750 | |
| On Road / Path | | 6.3 | 200 | |

| Terrain | Kid-Friendly | Distance (miles) | Elev. Gain (feet) | WTB Rating |
|---|---|---|---|---|
| On Road | | 3.1 | 160 | |
| On Road / On Road Lane | | 12.2 | 900 | |
| On Road / Path | | 13.4 | 800 | |
| On Road / On Road Lane / Path | partial | 43.3 | 1,900 | |
| On Road / On Road Lane / Path | partial | 10.3 | 400 | |
| On Road / Path | partial | 21.6 | 900 | |
| Path | partial | 33.6 | 1,100 | |
| Path | | 14.8 | 1,000 | |
| On Road | | 35.6 | 3,600 | |
| On Road / Path | partial | 5.4 | 200 | |

| Terrain | Kid-Friendly | Distance (miles) | Elev. Gain (feet) | WTB Rating |
|---|---|---|---|---|
| On Road | | 26.8 | 3,800 | |
| On Road / Path | | 23.8 | 400 | |

# Ride Overview continued

| | | | |
|---|---|---|---|
| 140 | 25 | A Tour of Santa Monica | Santa Monica City Hall, Santa Monica |
| 144 | 26 | San Vicente and Mandeville Canyon | Westwood Recreation Center, West Los Angeles |
| 148 | 27 | Santa Monica Bike Path | Venice Fishing Pier, Venice |
| 152 | 28 | Marina del Rey Loop | Venice Fishing Pier, Venice |
| 156 | 29 | South Bay Bike Path | del Rey Lagoon Park, Playa del Rey |
| 160 | 30 | Ballona Creek | Syd Kronenthal Park, Culver City |
| 164 | 31 | The Donut: Palos Verdes Peninsula | Veterans Park, Redondo Beach |
| 168 | 32 | Double Donut Holes: Palos Verdes Peninsula | Palos Verdes Drive West at Paseo Del Mar, Palos Verdes |

## Downtown to Beverly Hills

| Page | Ride | Ride Name | Start Location |
|---|---|---|---|
| 176 | 33 | Mulholland Drive | West Hollywood Park, West Hollywood |
| 180 | 34 | Lake Hollywood Reservoir | Lake Hollywood Drive, Hollywood |
| 184 | 35 | Mount Hollywood Drive | Ferndell Park, Los Feliz |
| 188 | 36 | Silver Lake | Silverlake Meadow, Silver Lake |
| 192 | 37 | Elysian Park | Grace E. Simons Lodge , Elysian Park |
| 196 | 38 | California Cycleway | Chinatown/Union Station area, Los Angeles |
| 200 | 39 | Beverly Hills: Starlets, Heroes & Villains | Roxbury Memorial Park, Beverly Hills |
| 204 | 40 | The UCLA Connection | Culver City Expo Line station, Culver City |
| 208 | 41 | A Tour of Downtown L.A. | Chinatown, Los Angeles |
| 212 | 42 | L.A. River: Downtown to Long Beach | 7th Street Metro/Center Station, Los Angeles |
| 216 | 43 | Cross-Town Shuffle: Skyscrapers to Surf | 7th Street Metro/Center Station, Los Angeles |

## Long Beach

| Page | Ride | Ride Name | Start Location |
|---|---|---|---|
| 222 | 44 | Surf City USA | Joe's Crab Shack at Alamitos Marina, Long Beach |
| 226 | 45 | Long Beach Arts & Craftsmen | Bixby Park, Long Beach |
| 230 | 46 | Long Beach Bicycle Periferico: The Perimeter Route | Metro Blue Line Wardlow Station, Long Beach |
| 234 | 47 | El Dorado Park | El Dorado Park, Long Beach |
| 238 | 48 | Coastal Long Beach: Long and the Shore of It | Bixby Park, Long Beach |
| 242 | 49 | Marine Stadium to Cal State Long Beach | Mothers Beach at Marine Park, Belmont Shores |
| 246 | 50 | San Pedro's Waterfront | SS Lane Victory Maritime Museum, N. Front St, San Ped |
| 250 | 51 | Experiencing Watts Towers | Metro's Blue Line Del Amo Station, Long Beach |

| Terrain | Kid-Friendly | Distance (miles) | Elev. Gain (feet) | WTB Rating |
|---|---|---|---|---|
| On Road / On Road Lane | | 18.8 | 900 | |
| On Road / On Road Lane | | 23.7 | 1,700 | |
| Path | | 12.4 | 400 | |
| On Road / On Road Lane / Path | | 11.0 | 100 | |
| On Road / On Road Lane / Path | partial | 23.5 | 500 | |
| Path | | 13.2 | 300 | |
| On Road / On Road Lane | | 27.1 | 2,300 | |
| On Road / On Road Lane | | 13.0 | 1,400 | |

| Terrain | Kid-Friendly | Distance (miles) | Elev. Gain (feet) | WTB Rating |
|---|---|---|---|---|
| On Road / On Road Lane | | 26.1 | 2,300 | |
| On Road / Path | partial | 4.8 | 150 | |
| On Road / On Road Lane / Path / Off Road | | 19.3 | 2,100 | |
| On Road / On Road Lane | | 6.9 | 800 | |
| On Road / Path | | 7.5 | 750 | |
| On Road / Path | | 20.0 | 1,100 | |
| On Road | | 12.1 | 1,000 | |
| On Road / On Road Lane | | 16.1 | 800 | |
| On Road | | 12.3 | 1,200 | |
| On Road / Path | | 25.1 | 1,000 | |
| On Road / On Road Lane / Path | | 31.7 | 1,300 | |

| Terrain | Kid-Friendly | Distance (miles) | Elev. Gain (feet) | WTB Rating |
|---|---|---|---|---|
| On Road / On Road Lane / Path | partial | 21.1 | 300 | |
| On Road / On Road Lane | | 10.9 | 400 | |
| On Road / On Road Lane / Path | partial | 25.6 | 1,000 | |
| On Road / Path | partial | 3.9 | 100 | |
| On Road / Path | partial | 15.0 | 500 | |
| On Road / On Road Lane / Path | | 12.4 | 400 | |
| On Road / On Road Lane / Path | partial | 11.0 | 700 | |
| On Road / On Road Lane / Path | | 15.0 | 650 | |

# How to Use This Book

From Santa Clarita to Long Beach, Glendora to Malibu, this book's adult rides are organized into five color-coded geographic sections. Our sixth and final section profiles 30 car-free kids' rides, sprinkled across the entire territory.

The routes are as diverse, rich and textured as Los Angeles itself—from short spins on leisurely surf-side bike paths to Downtown tours on city streets to mountain journeys on sparsely traveled, winding country roads. *Where to Bike Los Angeles* has tools to help you pick the ride to suit your mood and occasion. The inside cover's Key Map and Ride Overview table are good starting places, helping narrow your choices by region and terrain.

Within the five regional sections, we devote four pages to each ride, beginning with our "At A Glance" thumbnail sketch, providing directions to the route's start and info on total distance, amount of climbing, terrain, typical traffic conditions, refreshment locations, links to other rides and cool side trips. On the next page, our "About" section presents a ride narrative, describing features, highlights and sometimes morsels of local lore. The final two pages contain navigational aids for your use while cycling: a detailed, GPS-generated map and ride elevation profile, supplemented by a ride log with turn-by-turn directions.

## Ride Scale

To sum up a ride's level of difficulty, we assign it a *Where to Bike* rating, indicated by the number of cycling kangaroos on red ovals at the bottom of At A Glance:

This rating system is the standard scale developed by the publisher, Bicycling Australia, (yes, Down Under even kangaroos ride bikes) for all its guidebooks. The ratings derive from each ride's accumulated points for distance, elevation gain and predominant road surface conditions, as outlined in the tables below.

| | 1 pt | 2 pts | 3 pts | 4 pts | 5 pts |
|---|---|---|---|---|---|
| **Distance – Road (miles)** | <12 | 12-19 | 19-25 | 25-37 | >37 |
| **Distance – MTB (miles)** | <6 | 6-9 | 9-16 | 16-25 | >25 |
| **Climbing (feet)** | <500 | 500 - 1,000 | 1,000 - 1,500 | 1,500 - 2,000 | >2,000 |
| **Surface** | Paved smooth | Paved rough | Unpaved smooth | Unpaved moderate | Unpaved rough |

| Accumulated Points | Riding Level/Grade | Suggested Suitability |
|---|---|---|
| 3 | 1 | Beginner |
| 4-5 | 2 | |
| 6-7 | 3 | Moderately fit |
| 8-9 | 4 | |
| 10+ | 5 | Experienced cyclist |

## Ride Classifications

Ride Classifications are used to represent the distinct character of the ride itself and are usually a reflection of the environment or landscape the cyclist will enjoy as they travel the route.

In *Where to Bike Los Angeles*, there are six classifications to look for on the ride At a Glance page:

**Kid Friendly (100% Car-Free)**

**Park Ride**

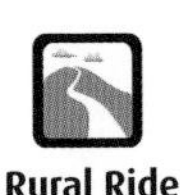

**Rural Ride**

**Mountain Ride**

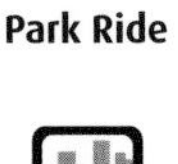

**Urban Ride**

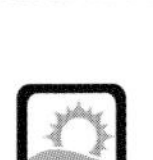

**Coastal Ride**

## Ride Links

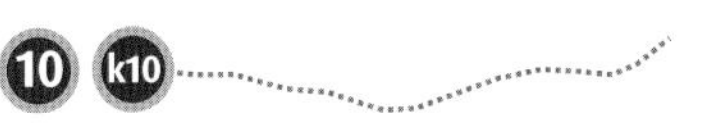


If you're partial to adding to your ride, or simply interested in other routes nearby, information on ride links can be found on both the ride At a Glance page, and on the maps.

*At a Glance:* Ride numbers included in the 'Links to' panel on the At a Glance page are considered direct links—rides that intersect with, or can be accessed with ease from the current route.

*Maps:* Each map includes easy to identify ride link icons at either the location of junction, or at the closest point the linked ride can be accessed from the current ride. The maps show all links, both direct and non-direct—and each link route is highlighted with an easy to identify orange dashed line.

## Terrain Guide

To help you understand what to expect on the route, terrain types are described on both the At a Glance page, and directly on the maps with easy to follow colored ride lines, as follows:

### On Road:

A *red ride line* depicts sections of the ride that are on road. The cyclist shares the road with vehicular traffic, and is expected to abide by road rules and laws. These routes are either Class III Bike Routes, or are considered comparably safe for recommendation by the author.

### On Road Bike Lane:

A *blue ride line* depicts sections of the ride where exclusive on road bike lanes are provided. Here the cyclist is clearly separated from vehicular traffic by either a traffic lane marked on an existing roadway that is restricted to cycle traffic, or by a physical barrier. These routes are Class II Bike Routes, and are only indicated if such infrastructure is in place.

### Path:

A *yellow ride line* depicts sections of the ride that are on smooth bike paths where the cyclist is completely separated from roads. The path can either be a sidepath (designated for use by cyclists) or a shared-use footway (for use by both cyclists and pedestrians). These routes are either Class I Bike Routes, or are considered comparably safe for recommendation by the author.

### Off Road:

A *brown ride line* depicts sections of the ride that are on wide, unpaved dirt trails, that are smooth enough for navigation by any type of bike.

# Before You Go

Your health and safety are most important—and very much tied in with your enjoyment of bicycling. So, if you're returning to cycling after time off, or if you plan to ride more intensively than in the past, consult your physician first. If you experience any lasting pain after riding, also see your doctor. And finally, take advantage of short- and medium-distance rides to build up endurance before taking a crack at longer expeditions.

A well-functioning bike that fits you, with the seat height properly adjusted, is essential. Consult a good bike shop for fit and adjustment — your knees deserve it. Then, before you roll out on a ride, do a quick equipment check. **An easy-to-remember checklist is ABC:**

**Air** — Inflate tires to the manufacturer's specs. Inspect them for excessive wear, cracking or damage; remove foreign matter from the treads. Confirm that the quick releases (or axle nuts) are tight.

**Brakes** — Test the levers to make sure your brakes are in top working order. Inspect the cables, pads and rims (or disks) for wear.

**Chain and Cranks** — Clean them (at least with a good wipe-down) and then, apply a drop of oil to each link. Check that the crank, pedals and cogs are all in working order.

If you're unsure about any of these pre-ride checks – or of your bike's mechanical worthiness – **visit your favorite bike shop or co-operative workshop for advice and service**. And, finally, let someone know where you are going and the estimated time of your return. Then, *stick to the plan.*

# What to Take

With a few exceptions, these Los Angeles rides are near modern conveniences or bike shops. Even so, it's smart to uphold the Boy Scout motto **Be Prepared**. Here's a list of what to take, nearly all of which will fit on your body, comfortably into your pockets and/or into a small under-saddle bag.

- A bicycle helmet: properly fitting and safety-approved.
- Gloves (with or without fingers).
- Eyewear (ideally with UV-filtering lenses — tinted if it's a sunny day).
- A fully-charged cell phone, a credit card, ID and important health information.
- Cash (at least $1.50 for the bus — Metro drivers can't make change).
- Plenty of water.
- Snacks.
- A couple of individually wrapped hand wipes.
- Spare inner tubes, tire levers, patches and a small air pump.
- A compact multi-tool that will work on your bike.
- Sunscreen.
- A strong lock.
- Front and rear lights (if you're riding after dark).
- A little first aid kit (or, at least, a few individually packaged alcohol pads and band-aids, plus anti-bacterial ointment and tissues).
- Rain/wind jacket or outer layer.
- Salt or electrolyte tablets (if it's a hot day).
- Camera (optional).
- This book.

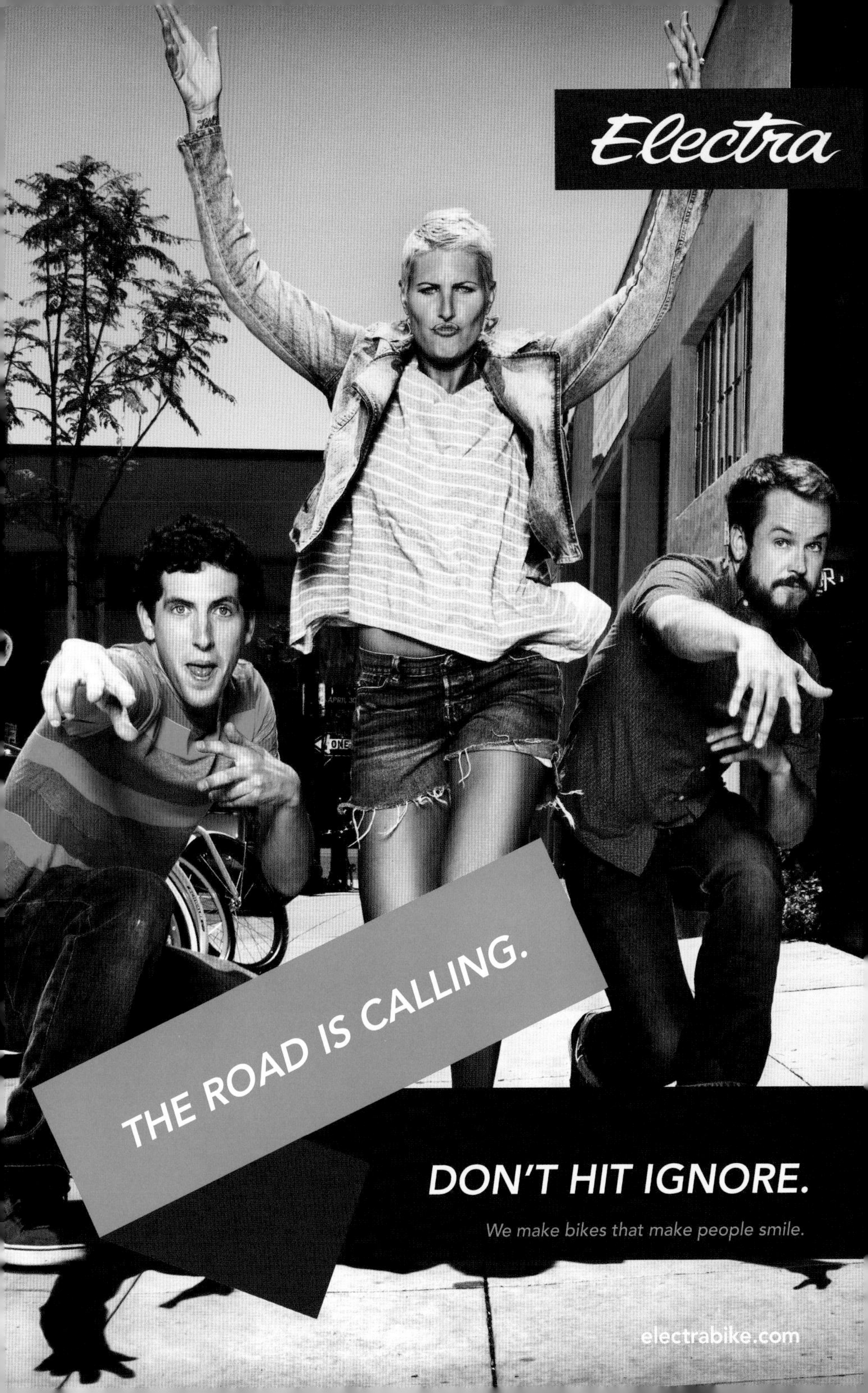
Electra
THE ROAD IS CALLING.
DON'T HIT IGNORE.
We make bikes that make people smile.
electrabike.com

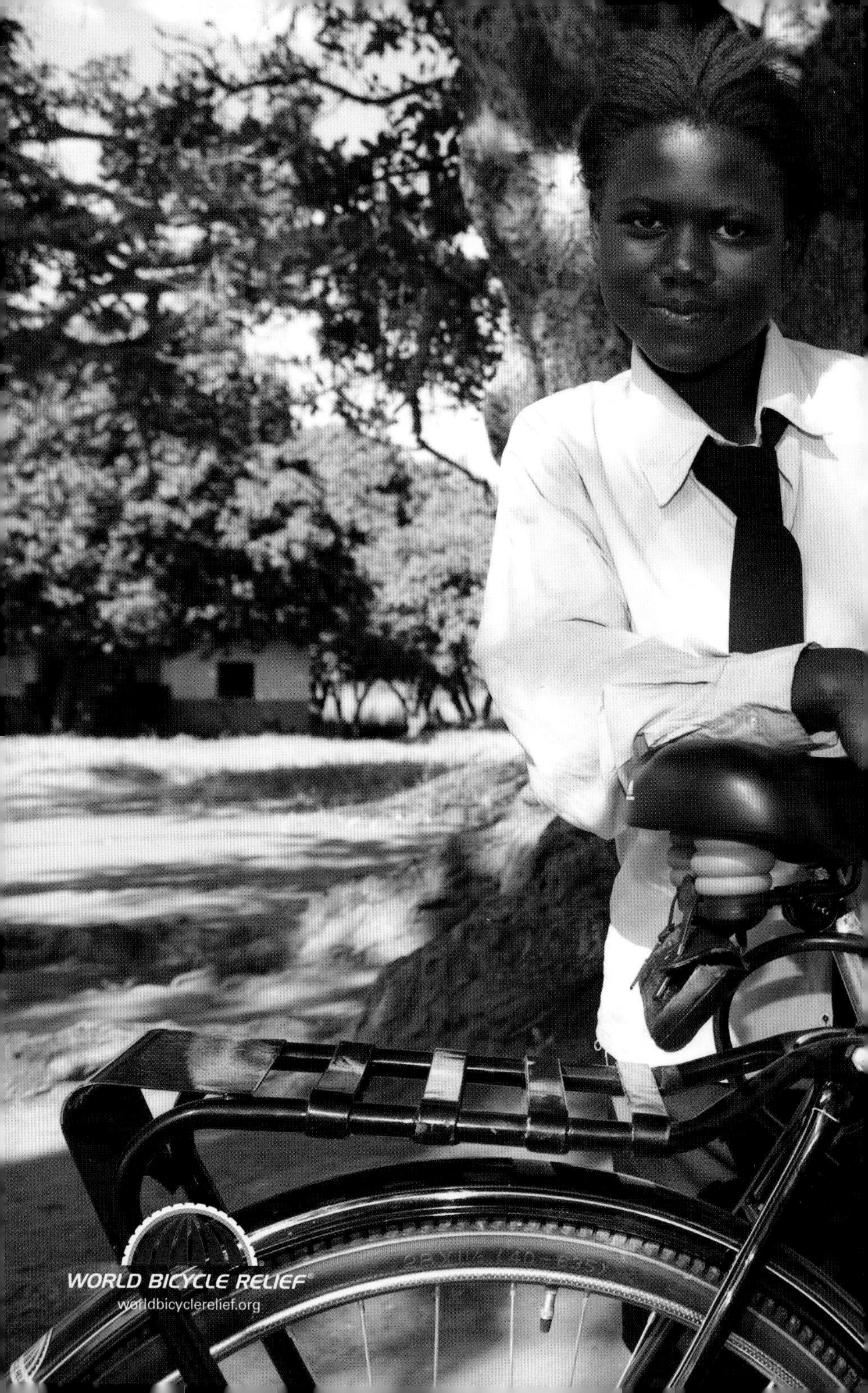

WORLD BICYCLE RELIEF®
worldbicyclerelief.org

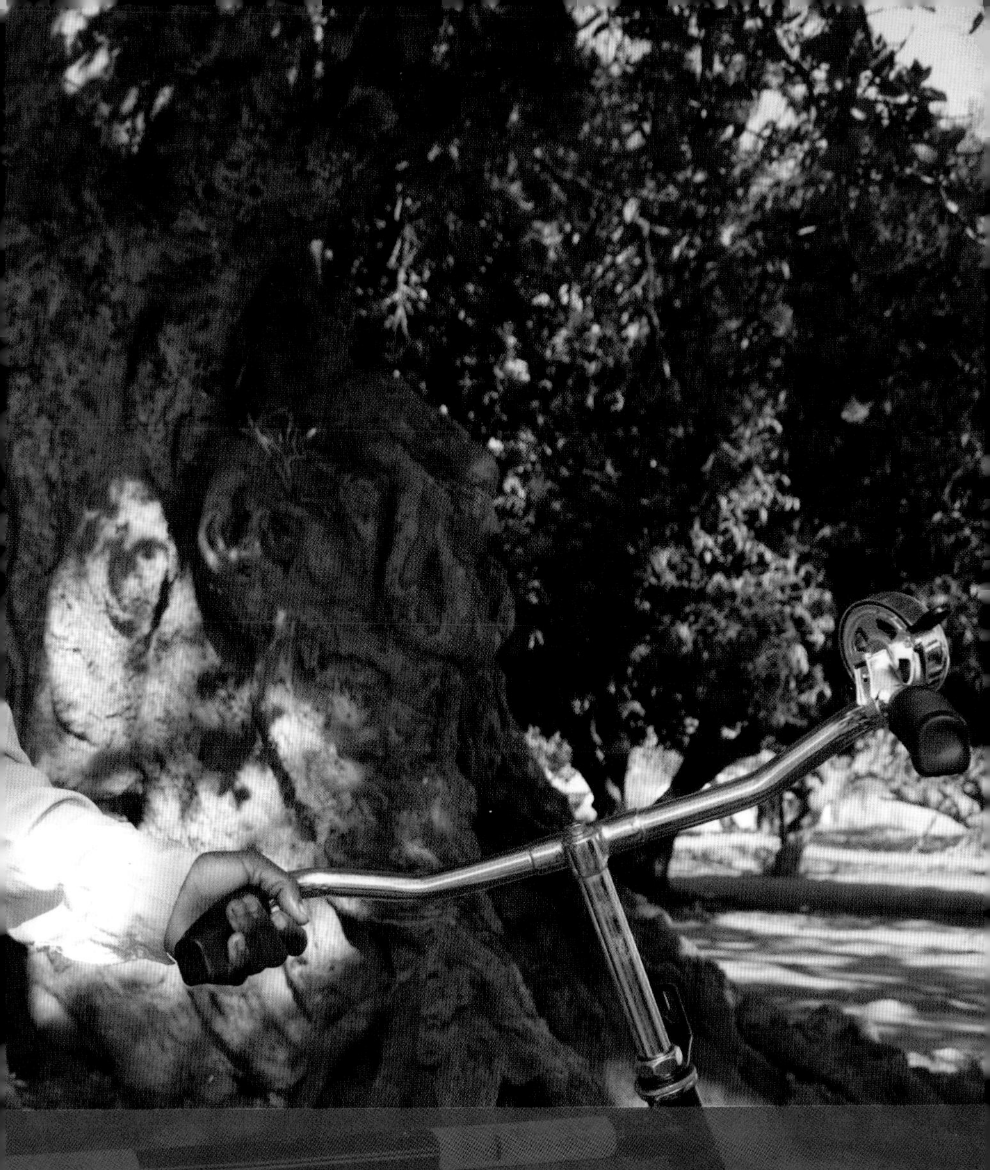

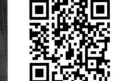

# On the Road in L.A.

It's hardly uplifting to think about the dangers of cycling, particularly when you're contemplating a fun ride, navigating dense urban traffic or flying down a remote, twisting, steep mountain pass. Though the purpose of this section is not to frighten you, the reality is that each year riders get killed or seriously injured, sometimes even on empty bike paths. Accidents happen. The good news is that you can do much to avoid mishaps or worse while riding the bike paths, streets and back roads of Los Angeles.

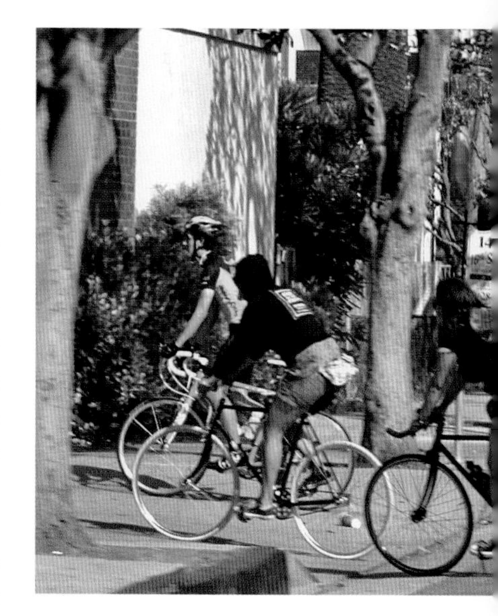

Safety begins with your equipment, and the single smartest decision you can make is to wear an approved, properly fitted helmet—*with* the chin strap securely buckled, please. Wear your helmet whenever you "saddle up" because you never know…. It's also wise to wear gloves to buffer road vibrations and protect your hands from nasty scrapes should you fall. We also recommend good eyewear (with UV-filtering lenses) to shield your eyes from sun and wind, as well as road grime and loose debris. Brightly colored clothing increases your visibility to drivers and others. A properly fitted and well-maintained bicycle will make any outing safer, healthier and more fulfilling.

Road manners and riding attitude/style contribute to your safety, as well. Bear in mind that you are in traffic, whether you're on a bike path or a city street, and in California cyclists must obey all traffic laws. Ride predictably: Keep as far to the right as is reasonable, heed stop signs or lights and follow all other traffic controls, just as you would driving a car. Assume that drivers do not see you and try to establish eye contact before maneuvering around them.

Be aware of your moment-by-moment surroundings, remaining simultaneously relaxed and alert—this should become second nature. Engage all your senses, as keen situational awareness can help avoid troublesome encounters. This means keeping your eyes moving and registering hazards near and far, such as inattentive pedestrians or car occupants poised to swing open vehicular doors. Develop an on-the-road sense of hearing—sounds can tip you off to what's happening around you. Staying attuned also means minimizing distractions: Don't text, tweet, email, conduct cellphone conversations, or use earphones or earbuds while riding.

### Some Bullet Points on Safe Riding:

- Ride in the direction of traffic, not against it. (Salmon don't survive.)
- Stay in your lane.
- Only pass other riders and roller-bladers on the left. Call out "on your left" two bike lengths before passing.
- Ride single file with at least one bike length between riders.
- Use hand signals to alert others when you're turning, slowing or stopping.
- Call out turns and stops and, espcially for cyclists behind you, point out road hazards—such as vehicles pulling out, shattered glass, nasty potholes, bike-unfriendly grates and loose rocks.
- Pull entirely off the road or bike path when stopping for breaks (even if only to consult a map

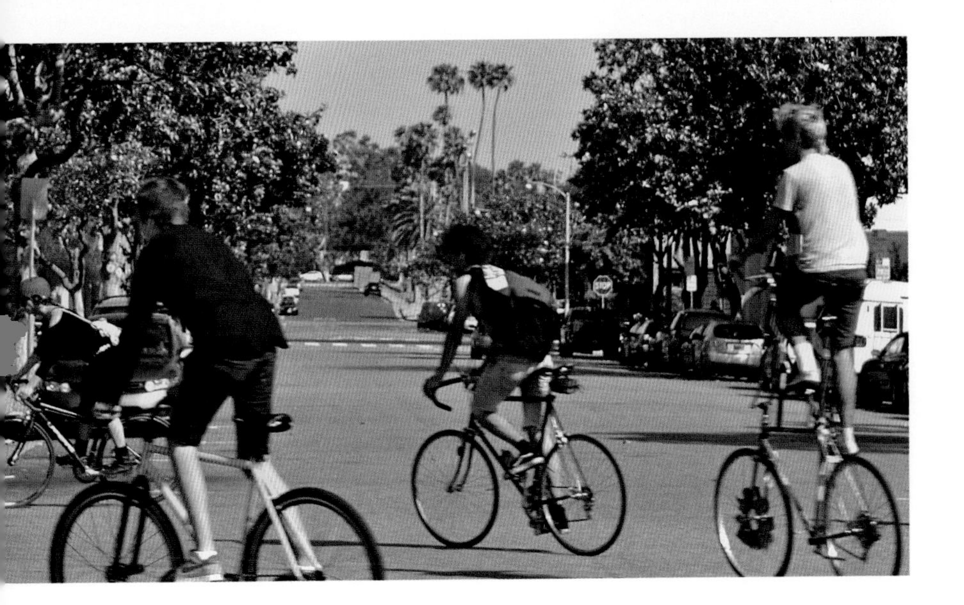


or chat with a friend).

- Yield to pedestrians and equestrians.
- Ride over rail tracks at an angle as close to 90 degrees as possible.
- Cross busy intersections via pedestrian crosswalks.
- Be vigilant for "right hooks" (right-turning drivers cutting across your trajectory), "left hooks" (drivers turning from the left across your line of travel) and "door prizes" (drivers opening parked car doors).
- Fasten extra gear or bungees securely, making sure nothing comes loose and gets caught in your spokes, chain or controls.
- Activate a headlight (white) and taillight (red) after dark. The flashing mode increases visibility.
- Consider using a bell and a rear view mirror (the latter affixed either to your handlebars, helmet or eyeglasses).

## Ride With a Proper Attitude

Streets and bike paths belong to us all—we need to share them responsibly. Cyclists have every right to use roads and expect safety. Always obey the rules of the road—and ride with confidence, determination, and purpose: Asserting your rightful place can be as important as defensive riding tactics.

At the same time, always remember: Riders must respect the rights of fellow bicyclists, pedestrians, drivers and animals. Show courtesy and patience, particularly to slower or less experienced riders and non-cyclists. Stopping to aid a fellow bicyclist in need is always the right thing to do. Good actions help build positive cycling and a sterling image for us all.

## Your Bike's Safety

Sorry, but bicycles do get stolen sometimes, particularly in big cities—and L.A. is no exception. We recommend you bring along a sturdy bike lock (so you can confidently check out some of the cool side attractions we'll be suggesting). The best bet is a U-lock and heavy-duty cable or chain. Find an appropriately immovable hitching post—a bike rack, approved railing or lamppost—and lock your bike's frame to it with the U-lock. It's also a good idea to lace the chain or cable through the front and rear wheel (especially if they have quick-release levers) and secure the ends to the U-lock. Take any removable gear with you, such as quick-release saddles, saddlebags, water bottles, lights and odometers. Then, for heaven's sake, enjoy yourselves!

# Communal Cookery: L.A.'s Bicycle Co-op Movement

While community bike workshops, or bicycle repair collectives, have been around for nearly 30 years, currently in dozens of countries around the globe and almost every state in the U.S., this grassroots movement has unmistakably tapped into the urban-survival ethos of Greater Los Angeles—and really taken root here. Some co-ops throughout the U.S. were born out of specific needs: to provide, for example, refurbished bicycles to the homeless or inner city youth. Others got launched from a broader springboard of bicycle and environmental advocacy. Typically founded in humble ad hoc quarters—in home garages; kitchens; office buildings; a church basement; free or dirt-cheap, unrented or unrentable storefronts—the collectives have emerged independently, each with a distinct personality. Yet they all share the common goal of supporting community cycling by making bike repair, maintenance and education—the skills, tools, resources and collegial support—accessible to people from young to old, in all walks of life, for little (or no) money. Whether you want to learn how to fix a simple flat, refurbish an entire bike or devise ways to build the funky, tricked-out, "multi-story" tall-bike of your dreams, you can probably do it with your own two hands at one of Los Angeles' bike co-ops.

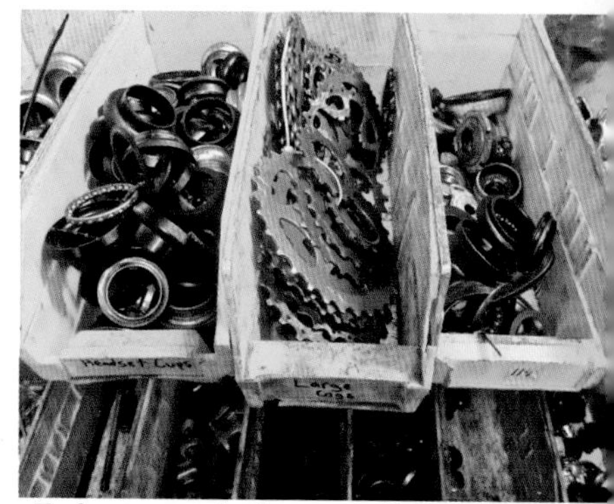
*Used parts—cogs, headset cups and bearings—fill the bins.*

L.A.'s first—and still thriving—bicycle collective is the Bicycle Kitchen, also called Bici Cocina ("bike kitchen," in vélo-chic Italian). Founded in Eco Village, a Downtown sustainable community, it took form literally in the kitchen of an apartment then used as village bike storage. What started with a few people meeting occasionally to share pizza and work on bikes grew into a not-for-profit, volunteer-run, donation-supported bicycle repair and educational organization in Koreatown. It inspired the creation of others across L.A. County, many adopting the "cooking" theme: the Bike Oven, in Highland Park; Bikerowave, on the Westside; and the Valley Bikery, in the San Fernando Valley (dealing in "freshly biked goods"). The HUB Community Bike Center, in Long Beach, is another rising bike co-op, as is the more recent Bike Angels, in Burbank. By some estimates, L.A. has as many as 16 collectives, including campus-based ones and others in various stages of development, such as Bici Libre, near MacArthur Park, and, believe it or not, the Ovarian Psyco-Cycles for women, in East Los Angeles.

As do-it-yourself (DIY) and do-it-together (DIT) bike shops, co-ops provide bike-repair and maintenance essentials: work space, repair stands and tools (from simple screwdrivers to far more expensive and specialized headset presses, chain whips and cable clippers). They do charge for shop time, typically only \$5.00 to \$7.50 per hour—with no one turned away for lack of money. Give what you can. They'll also sell you parts (at low prices, too), mostly scavenged from unfixable bikes, as well as some new items, mainly tires, tubes and accessories.

The most important asset of a co-op may be its collective wisdom about bike repair. Many of the volunteer mechanics started with little understanding of it and, through hours of turning wrenches side-by-side with mentors, have learned the techniques and tricks they're ready to pass on. As Bikerowave founder Alex Thompson points out, "If you wanted to understand everything about your own car, so you

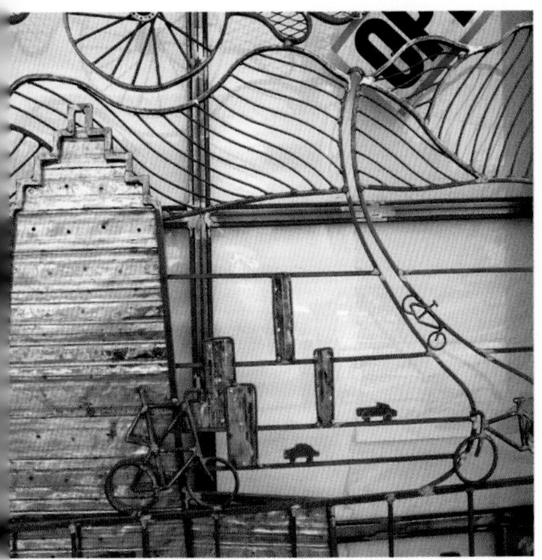

*Artist and welder Steve Campos created the Bike Oven's front grille.*

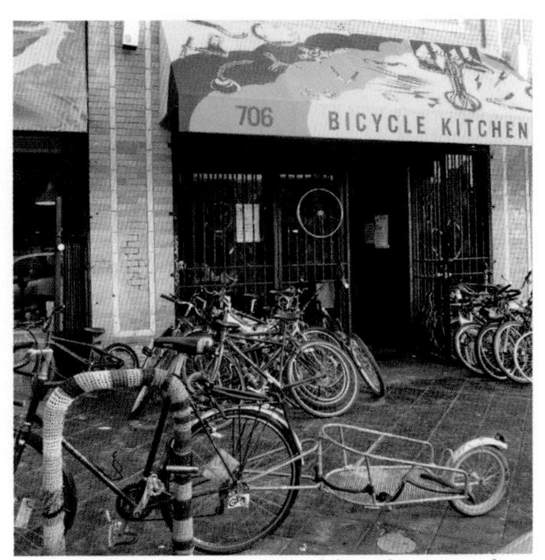


*Outside the Bicycle Kitchen, a bike rack is wrapped in a hand-crocheted "cozy."*

could fix it yourself, it would take you at least 300 hours; but if you want to understand everything about your bike (not all bikes, but just yours), you're going to understand everything you need to know in just nine hours of study." Collectives regularly teach people with no mechanical background to become totally self-sufficient with bike care.

The ultimate recyclers—diverting bikes and parts from land fills—co-ops give new life to old bicycles and independence to those riding them. You can donate bikes, buy the refurbished ones or "adopt" a bicycle and restore it for a collective to sell or give to someone in need. You can also get involved in co-op outreach programs, such as mobile bike-repair-and-service clinics at farmers' markets, or efforts supporting underserved communities, including day laborers, reliant on bikes as their sole means of transportation.

The social aspect of the co-ops is a big draw, providing relaxed working-congregating spaces, many with worn sofas, old fridges, music and cyclists of all persuasions—from single-speed hipsters to commuters and athletic types. Many collectives exhibit art and host parties, movie nights or art tours and are, naturally, starting places for rides—both organized and impromptu.

Many collectives also have earn-a-bike programs, where teens can work for a bicycle—while learning repair and safe street riding—at the co-op. "One day," recalls a Bike Oven volunteer mechanic named Chicken Leather, "there was a shooting nearby, and we suddenly realized all the teens were in here, safely working on their bikes."

**Where to Cook:**

*Bicycle Kitchen*

706 N. Heliotrope Drive, Los Angeles (Koreatown)

Tel: 323-662-2776, **www.bicyclekitchen.com**

*Bike Oven*

3706 Figueroa Street, Los Angeles (Highland Park)

Tel: 323-223-8020, **bikeoven.com**

*Bikerowave*

12255 Venice Boulevard, Los Angeles (Mar Vista)

Tel: 310-230-5236, **www.bikerowave.org**

*Valley Bikery*

14416 Victory Boulevard #104, Van Nuys (San Fernando Valley)

Tel: 818-921-6522, **valleybikery.com**

*The HUB*

1730 Long Beach Boulevard, Long Beach

**hublb.com**

**Note:** *Co-ops (relying on volunteer schedules) have far more limited hours than regular bike shops. Call ahead or check the website for hours.*

# You, Your Bike and Public Transportation in L.A.

When you consider how to get around Greater Los Angeles, it's hard to overlook the automobile's dominance. And, yes, one reason car culture and the spaghetti of freeways developed here is that distances can be vast—the Los Angeles Basin measures roughly 45-by-35 miles. But there are definitely other ways to tackle this sprawling county. And the good news is that healthier and more environmentally inspired means of mobility are becoming increasingly viable and desirable here. Just as L.A.'s bicycling infrastructure continues to grow, our mass transit system has gotten better and more extensive. Abandoned rights of way are being reclaimed and adapted to the 21st century, with swift new routes, evolving even as we write. It's easy to reach the start of many of our rides via public transportation—and we encourage you to do so (if you're not planning to pedal there, instead). Some of our routes even offer the option of combining bicycling with public transportation, allowing you, for example, to head out by bike and return by train. And we've written this guide in anticipation of upcoming system improvements—a new light rail line and the extension of two others.

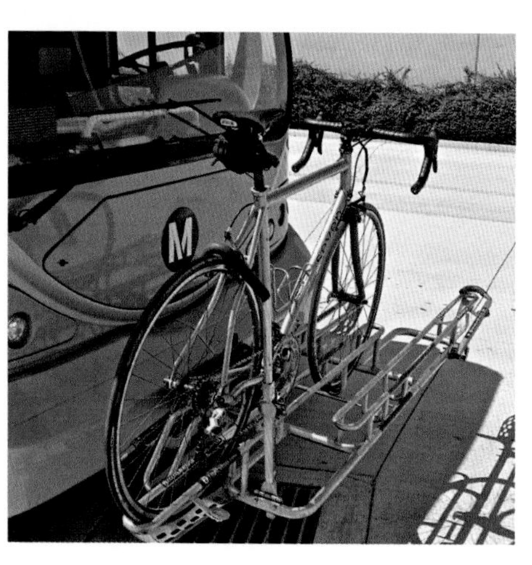


### The Basics (with a few impressive stats) About Transit in L.A.

The Los Angeles County Metropolitan Transportation Agency (Metro) oversees L.A.'s three branches of public transportation: [1] buses, operated in partnership with 16 municipalities; [2] light rail, with over 80 miles of track and more than 120 stations; and [3] Metrolink, the regional commuter rail system, with seven lines, 55 stations and over 500 miles of track across Los Angeles, Orange, Riverside, San Bernardino and Ventura counties. With a few exceptions, bicycles are allowed on all three.

### Metro and Municipal Bus Systems

Collectively with such cities as Santa Monica, Culver City and Santa Clarita, Metro operates one of the nation's largest bus fleets, much of it powered by clean-burning CNG (compressed national gas). Local buses, painted California Poppy orange, have routes numbered 1 to 599. Metro rapid buses, painted red, travel along major arterial streets; they make fewer stops and are numbered 701 to 799.

Each bus's front-mounted rack has space for two bikes. Here's the drill: As a bus approaches and you prepare to load the rack, be sure the driver sees and acknowledges you and you've removed or secured any loose items. To operate the rack: (1) Pull up on the D-shaped handle at the rack's center and lower it into the horizontal position; (2) Load your bike in the rear-most empty slot, making sure the wheels drop firmly into the cradles; (3) Raise the upside-down, J-shaped support arm over your bike's front tire (this spring-tensioned arm should clamp snugly over the wheel); and then, (4) Board the bus and pay your fare. Sit near the front, so you can watch your bicycle. As you reach your destination: (1) Inform the driver that you'll be removing your bike; (2) Exit through the front door; (3) Pull the J-shaped support arm off the tire; (4) Lift your bike off the rack; and (5) If yours is the last one off, return the rack to its upright position.

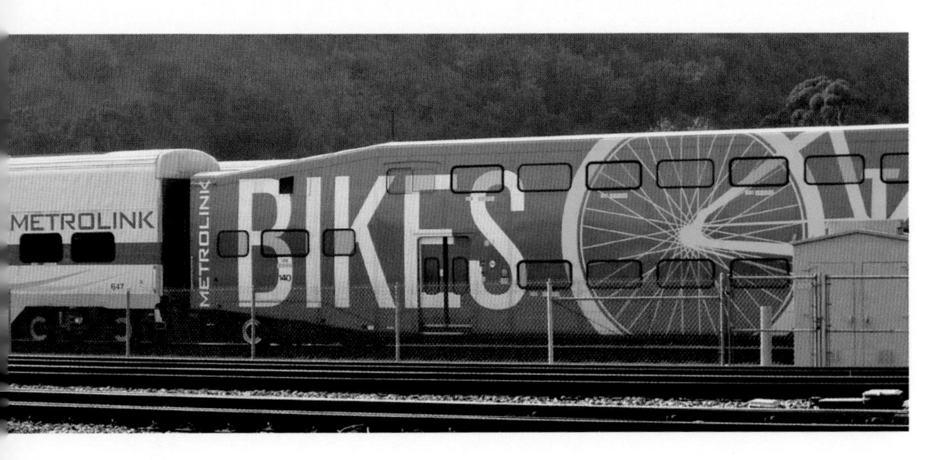


## Metro Light Rail Lines

Throughout Greater Los Angeles, Metro operates eight color-coded lines: Orange, Red, Purple, Gold, Silver, Blue, Green and Expo (aqua), as shown on the map on the following pages. Some are light rail or subways; two others are Metro Liners (long, articulated express buses that, like trains, have their own separate corridors, or "transitways," shared with no other vehicles). The newest light rail—the Expo Line—begins its Downtown-to-Culver City operations in early 2012. The Expo, Orange and Gold lines will be adding stations to Santa Monica, Chatsworth and past Azusa and Glendora, respectively. The Orange and Silver Metro Liners have the same front-mounted bike racks as conventional buses.

Bicycles are allowed on all Metro trains, as long as space is available. Allow other passengers on or off before you board. On Red and Purple subway lines, board cars through doors marked with bicycle symbols. On all lines, once on board, stand with your bike in the designated zone (usually open areas at either end of a car). Bicyclists should use elevators or stairs, not escalators, when entering stations and accessing platforms.

Metro's base bus or train fare is $1.50, with $0.35 transfers to municipal bus lines (no extra charge for bicycles). Metro rail and Orange Line stations have self-service ticket-vending machines, so pay your fare (via cash, or credit or debit card) before boarding. Bus drivers cannot make change—be sure to carry exact fare. As you use Metro more, consider a Transit Access Pass (TAP) stored-value card, which you can simply swipe past a bus fare box or station platform validator box. You can add value to a TAP at any ticket vending machine. For up-to-date fares, schedules, service disruptions, and information on TAP or taking bicycles on Metro, visit **www.metro.net**.

## Metrolink

Metrolink runs approximately 144 regional commuter trains on weekdays, but only 40 on Saturdays and 26 on Sundays. All lines through L.A. County radiate like spokes from Union Station, with very few transfer points between lines, so plan your riding to coincide with Metrolink's lines and schedule, particularly on weekends.

Each Metrolink train car allows up to three bicycles. Some trains also run special "bike cars" carrying up to 18 bikes in lower-level stalls. Bikes must be safely secured there. As you board or leave the train, comply with conductor instructions.

Fares are distance based: For example, Union Station to Chatsworth is currently $8.50 each way. Tickets are available from self-service vending machines in every station. A "Weekend Pass" lets you ride anytime system-wide from 7 p.m. Friday through 11:59 p.m. Sunday for only $10—a great deal for crossing L.A. to weekend rides in the Santa Clarita and San Fernando valleys. For more Metrolink info, including station locations, schedules, fares and service disruptions, visit **www.metrolinktrains.com**.

# Go Metro

metro.net

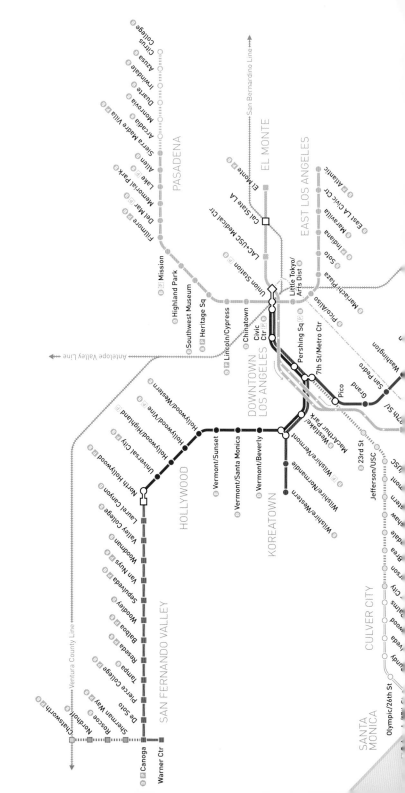

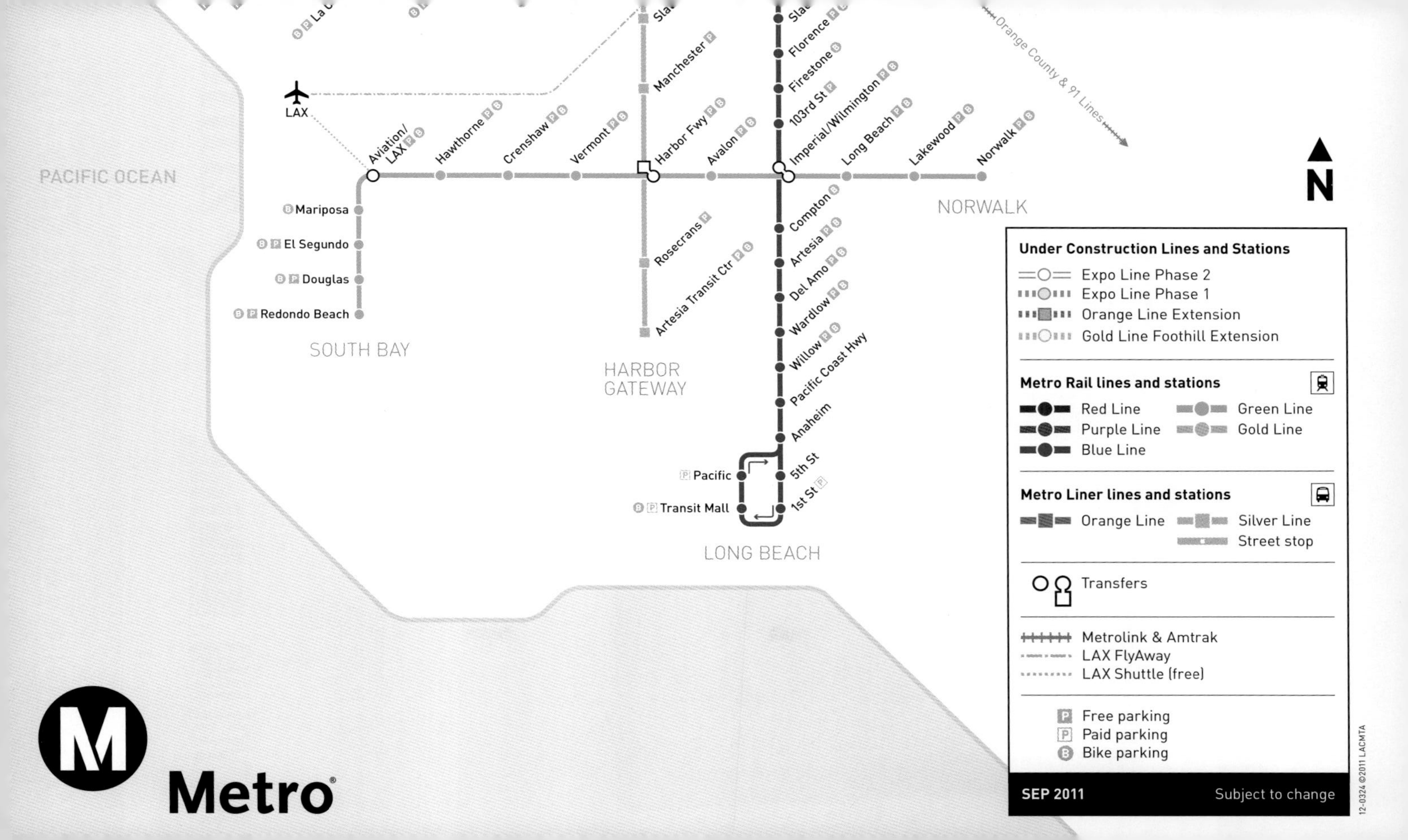

PACIFIC OCEAN

LAX

Aviation/LAX
Hawthorne
Crenshaw
Vermont
Harbor Fwy
Avalon
Imperial/Wilmington
Long Beach
Lakewood
Norwalk

Manchester
Rosecrans
Artesia Transit Ctr

Florence
Firestone
103rd St
Compton
Artesia
Del Amo
Wardlow
Willow
Pacific Coast Hwy
Anaheim
5th St
1st St
Pacific
Transit Mall

Mariposa
El Segundo
Douglas
Redondo Beach

SOUTH BAY

HARBOR GATEWAY

LONG BEACH

NORWALK

Orange County & 91 Lines

N

**Under Construction Lines and Stations**

Expo Line Phase 2
Expo Line Phase 1
Orange Line Extension
Gold Line Foothill Extension

**Metro Rail lines and stations**

Red Line
Purple Line
Blue Line
Green Line
Gold Line

**Metro Liner lines and stations**

Orange Line
Silver Line
Street stop

Transfers

Metrolink & Amtrak
LAX FlyAway
LAX Shuttle (free)

P Free parking
P Paid parking
B Bike parking

**SEP 2011** Subject to change



Metro®

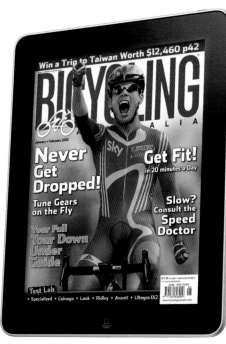

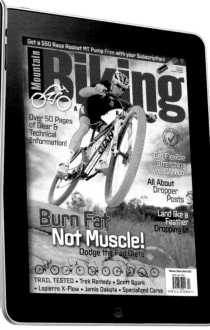

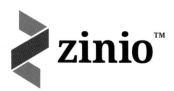

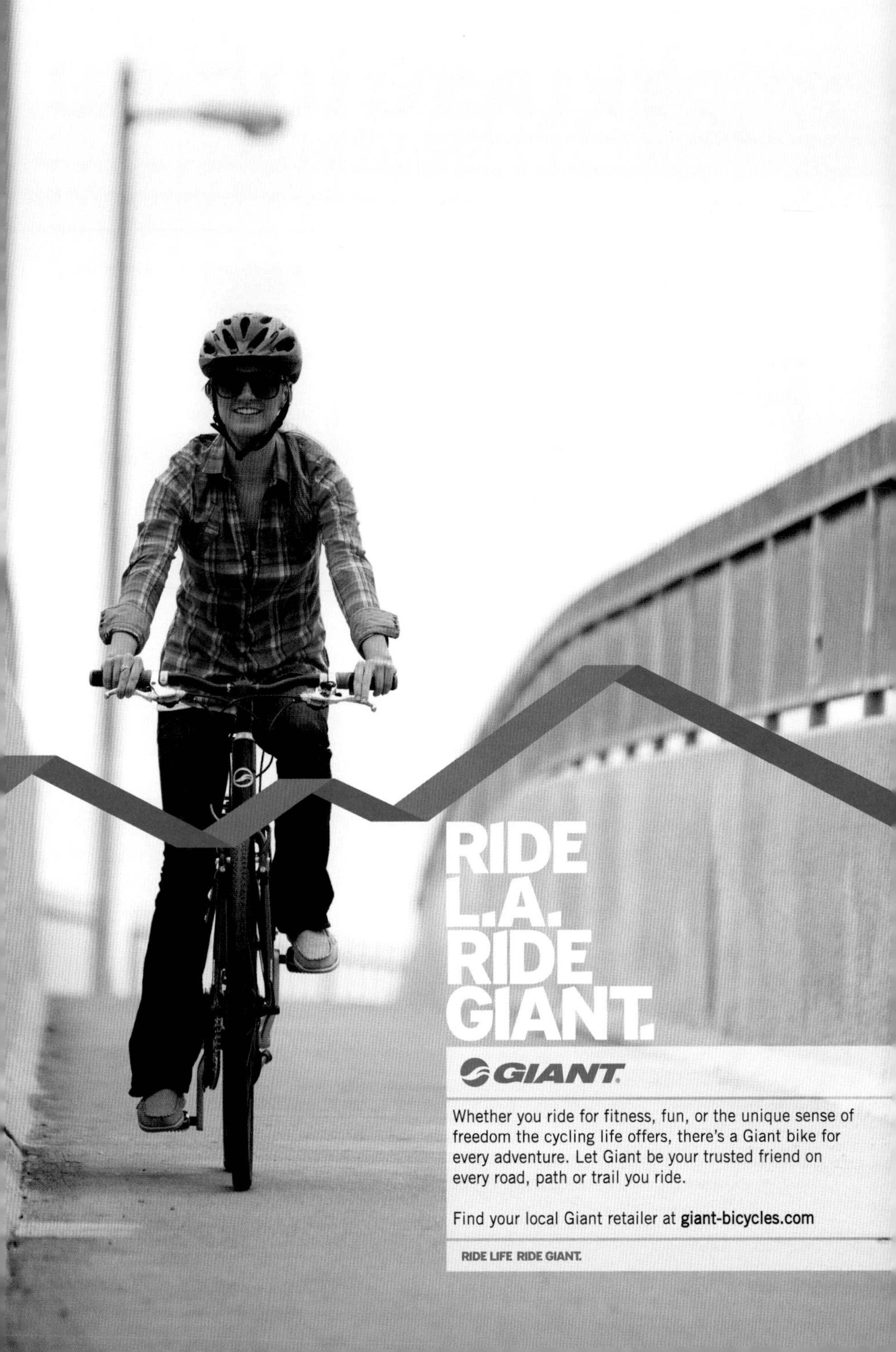

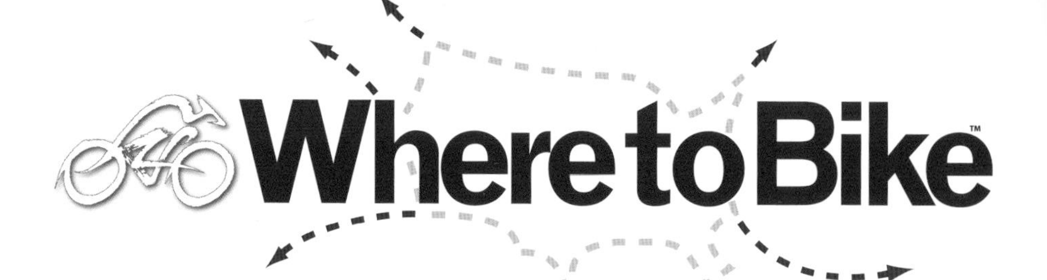


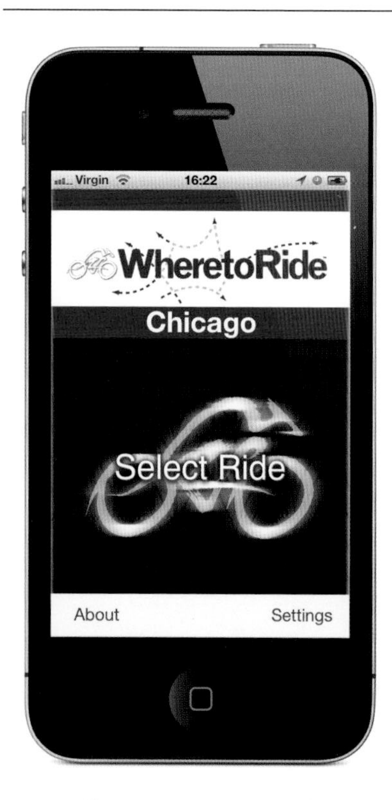


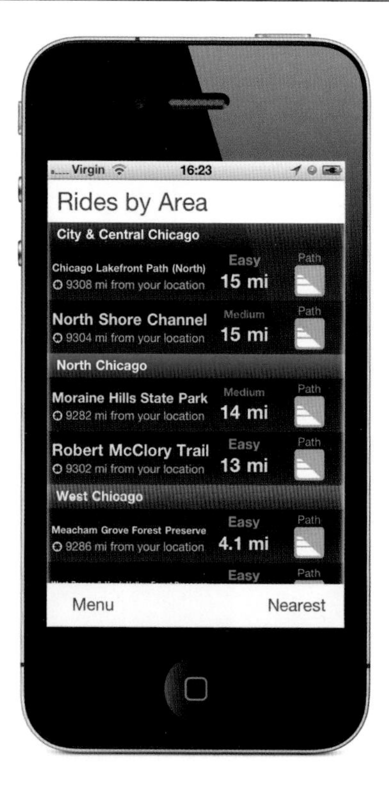


## Getting Started

**Step 1.** Download the *Where to Bike* app for your city on the iTunes App Store. Once you load the app, you'll see this main page where you can select your ride, learn more about us, or configure settings. In the settings menu you can choose between miles and km, whether you want to display your speed, and whether you'd like a fixed or rotating map.

## Select Your Ride

**Step 2.** Tap 'select ride' from the main screen and you will arrive at this page, where you will see a list of great rides organized into sections. These are the same as you will find in your *Where to Bike* book guide. In the bottom right-hand corner you will also see an option to arrange the rides based on their proximity to your current location.

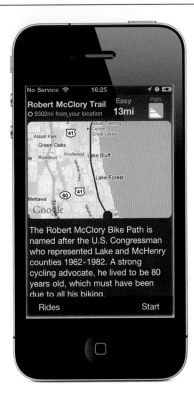

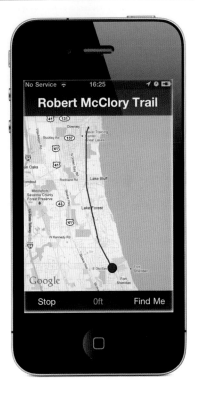

# San Fernando Valley
## (with the Santa Clarita Valley)

Vast swaths of the San Fernando Valley—or simply "The Valley" as locals call it—form a matrix of urban boulevards and residential streets, bedroom communities giving the landscape a seemingly boundless texture of rooftops. The region's best cycling tends to be along its periphery, in and near the Transverse Ranges that encircle it or along its river edge, and in its big city parks. The rides are strikingly varied: from jaunts within the flat valley floor (encompassing 260 square miles) to winding climbs; from semi-industrial urban passages to surprisingly rural terrain.

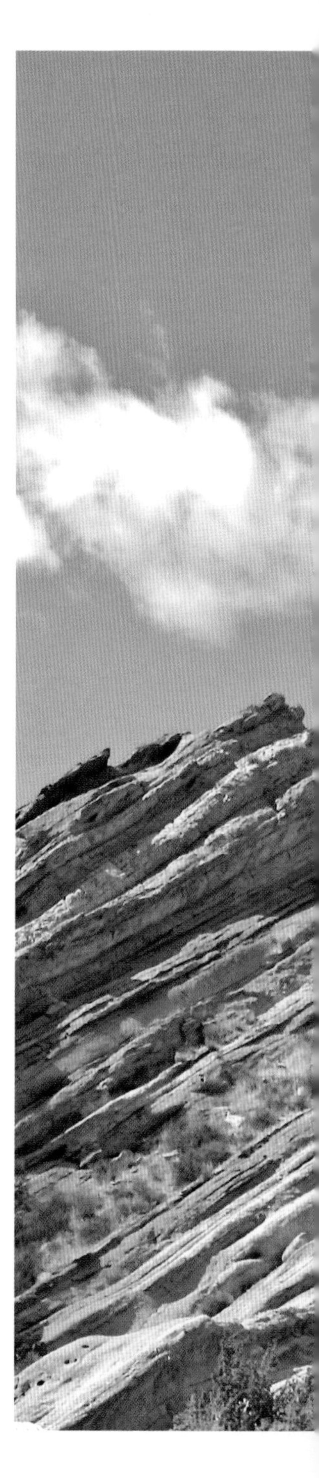

Along the valley's rim, The Rock Store and Tujunga Canyon Road offer challenging, serpentine ascents into stunning mountain landscapes. Further east, the route from San Fernando to Santa Susana Pass leads past a historic Spanish mission to parklands with wilderness hiking. And northward—sneaking into the neighboring Santa Clarita Valley—our Cloverleaf and Vasquez Rocks rides venture into high desert, the latter amid dramatically tilted stone formations.

At Griffith Park, Sepulveda Basin and Hansen Dam, we explore three markedly different urban parks. In part a former ostrich farm, Griffith's 4,210 acres straddle two regions: the San Fernando Valley and Downtown. Part of the fun is these rides' "extracurricular" activities: hiking trails, a zoo, the Autry National Center of the American West and Travel Town's vintage trains. The 2,000-acre Sepulveda Basin Recreation Area (a vast storm catchment for extreme downpours) includes a Japanese garden, athletic fields and a wildlife preserve. For an entirely different cycling experience (which is a blast), we recommend the Encino Velodrome, next to Sepulveda Basin. And at Hansen Dam, you can pedal across the dam's top or plunge (*sans* bike) into a mondo pool—acres of water with a towering, corkscrew slide against a mountain backdrop.

Like much of L.A., The Valley has gained blissfully car-free bicycling stretches through inventive repurposing of existing infrastructure. Just as Hansen Dam now carries a bike and pedestrian path, so too do the L.A. River's concrete levees, where this chapter's easy, semi-industrial ride is punctuated by a medley of pocket parks with local artist interventions. Rails-to-trails also thrive here—in the Chandler Bikeway and Orange Line ride. The joy of transforming hard urban edges emerges vividly in populist murals along the Chandler Bikeway and the Great Wall of Los Angeles, near the Orange Line, a remarkable community project and one of the world's longest murals.

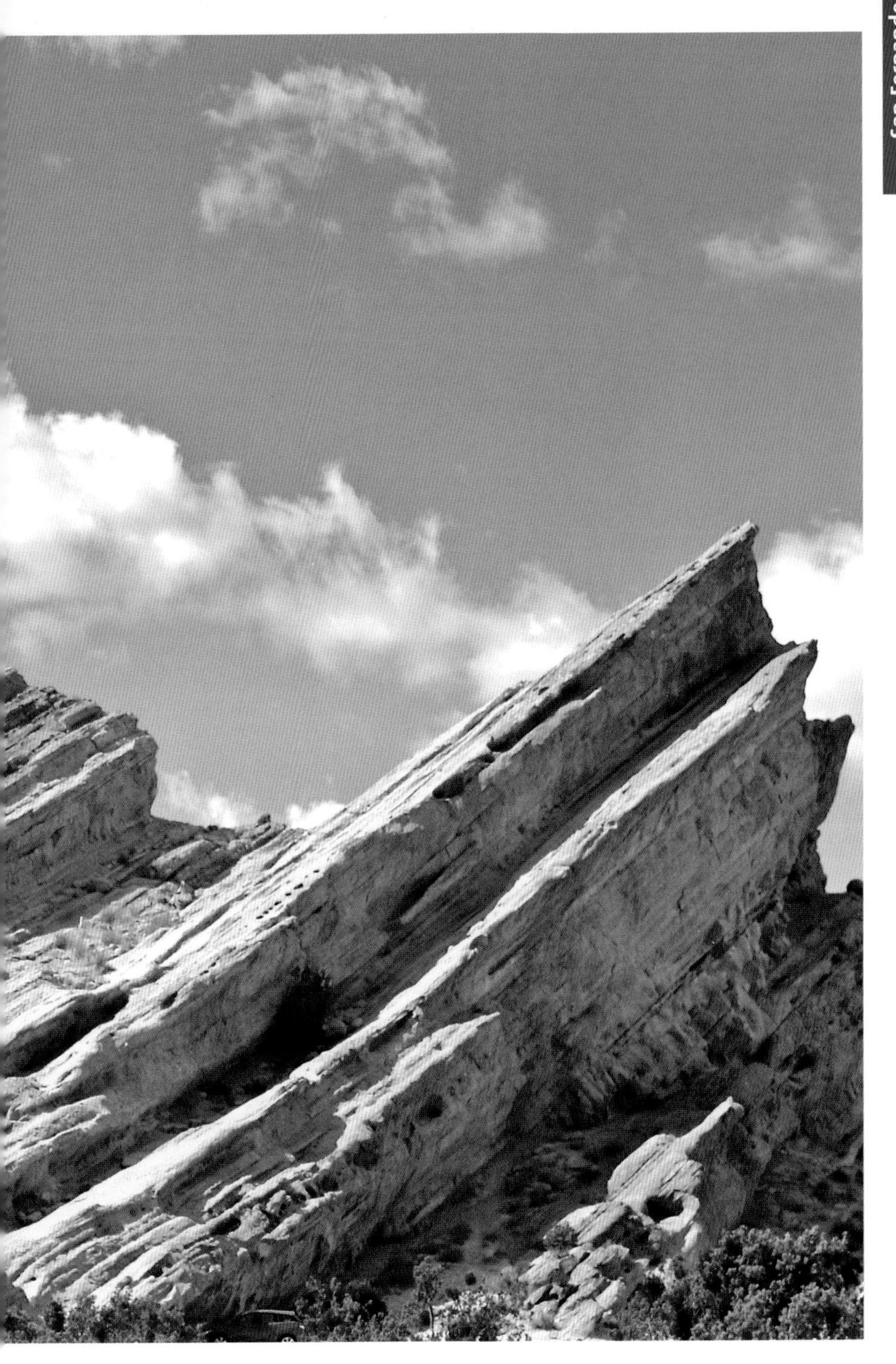

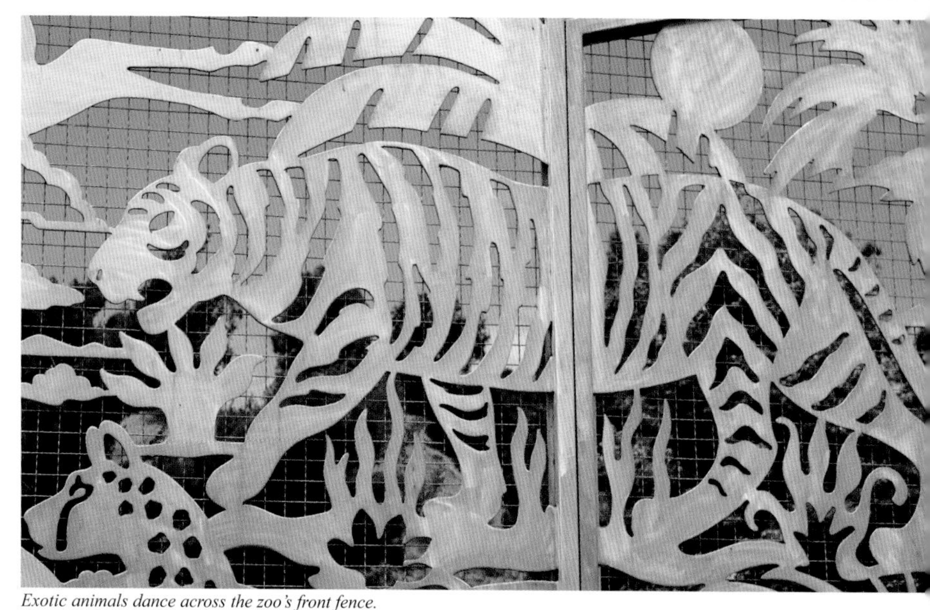

*Exotic animals dance across the zoo's front fence.*

## At a Glance

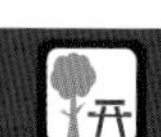

**Distance** 8.7 miles **Elevation Gain** 750 feet

### Terrain

This ride is a mix: flat and easy, punctuated by one moderate climb, with average quality asphalt roads throughout.

### Traffic

Bike lanes and wide shoulders performing as bike lanes comprise this loop. The route narrows from Trash Truck Hill down to the park's golf courses. Bicycle and car traffic typically gets heavier on weekends.

### How to Get There

From the 5 or 134 freeways, exit at Los Angeles Zoo. Follow the signs for zoo parking. If it's full, head south on Crystal Springs Drive to the merry-go-round parking.

### Food and Drink

The Autry National Center's Golden Spur Café—offering eats, a patio and bike racks—is open Tuesday through Sunday. Museum admission not required.

### Side Trip

Consider an excursion to the Griffith Observatory, the glamorous Art Deco landmark that famously appeared with James Dean in *Rebel Without a Cause*. Perched high above sweeping city views, this palace to the stars (and heavens above) houses a superb planetarium, telescopes and exhibitions. To reach the observatory, ride west on the chain of residential streets just north of (roughly parallel to) Los Feliz Boulevard, turn right on North Vermont Avenue and follow the signs.

**Links to** 

**Where to Bike Rating** 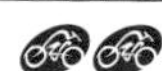

   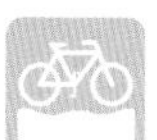

# About...

This route offers something for riders of every stripe (and shape). A leisurely, not-too-taxing journey along the fringes of Los Angeles' urban wilderness, amid vast grassy picnic areas, the path links Griffith Park's most popular destinations: the zoo, Autry National Center, Travel Town, and historic merry-go-round. For the spandex crowd, the ride also provides an excellent training circuit, mixing fast flat sections with the one moderate climb. We've seen many gung-ho cyclists riding this scenic loop over and over in succession.

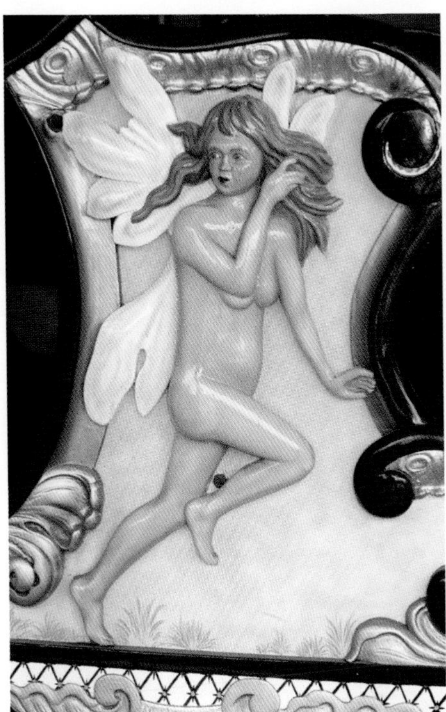

*The 1927 Griffith Park merry-go-round's chariots feature mythical and historic figures.*

Griffith Park is to Los Angeles what Central Park is to New York: the reigning urban park. With roughly 4,210 acres including chaparral-cloaked hills and landscaped parkland, Griffith is the largest municipal park with urban wilderness in the United States. Named after Colonel Griffith J. Griffith, the successful miner, ostrich farmer and later convicted felon, who purchased much of the acreage in the late 1880s. When his plans to develop the land fizzled, he gave the park to Los Angeles as a Christmas gift in 1896.

Taking in scenery along the park's north and east sides, the route meanders past the Los Angeles Zoo, home to the Campo Gorilla Preserve and such rarities as the Sumatran tiger, Visayan warty pigs and yellow-footed rock wallaby; the zoo's integral botanical garden, lush with more than 7,400 plants; the Autry National Center, focused on the American West, the culture and stories of native peoples, cowboys and other frontier folk; and Travel Town, a museum featuring historic trains, locomotives and other relics of L.A.'s rail heritage.

Just past Travel Town, the ride enters a wilder realm. Along the next mile, don't be surprised if deer occasionally emerge from the roadside scrub oak and brush. On one ride, we encountered two different lone coyotes right ahead of us. This section of the route rises, cresting atop "Trash Truck Hill"—ingloriously nicknamed for the garbage trucks that used to haul refuse to a city-operated landfill, just off this road. An unfortunate moniker for a stunning bit of terrain.

From the summit, the loop makes a serpentine descent, past picnic and BBQ areas, two golf courses, and Shane's Inspiration, a fully accessible disabled children's playground. A short distance after the right turn onto Crystal Springs Drive, an access road leads to Griffith Park's merry-go-round, an historic gem, with weathered, vividly painted horses, "prancing" to carnival-like pipe-organ music. As you hang a U-turn at Los Feliz Boulevard and head back towards the start, be sure to tip your helmet to the bronze statue of Col. Griffith and thank him for this wonderful gift.

*Note: Our Mount Hollywood Drive ride (Ride 35) enters Griffith Park from its Downtown side, over the ridge.*

## Ride Log

**0.0** From in front of the Autry National Center, with the Los Angeles Zoo behind you, turn left (north) on the bike lane along Western Heritage Way/Zoo Dr.
**1.9** Zoo Dr bends uphill to the left. The route continues on Griffith Park Dr, ascending past Travel Town Museum on the left. The bike lane ends here.
**2.6** Arrive at the summit of "Trash Truck Hill."
**3.3** Pass the Mineral Wells picnic area.
**3.6** Pass the Wilson/Harding golf course clubhouse.
**4.5** Turn right and join the bike lane running along Crystal Springs Dr.
**6.1** Make a U-turn at Los Feliz Blvd using the crosswalk.
**8.7** Arrive at the Autry National Center. Cross Zoo Dr to the parking lot via the cross walk. End of ride.

*P1* Autry National Center
*P2* Los Angeles Zoo
*P3* Bette Davis Picnic Area
*P4* Travel Town Museum
*P5* Griffith Park Merry-go-round
*P6* Griffith Observatory
*P7* Greek Theatre

(R) *R1* Spokes 'n Stuff
4730 Crystal Springs Drive, Griffith Park

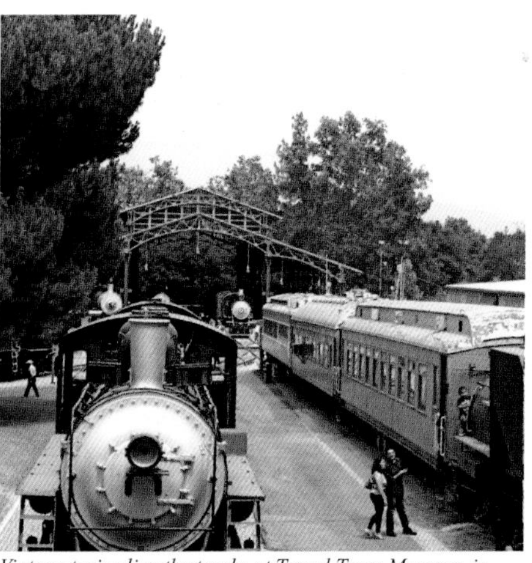

*Vintage trains line the tracks at Travel Town Museum, in Griffith Park.*

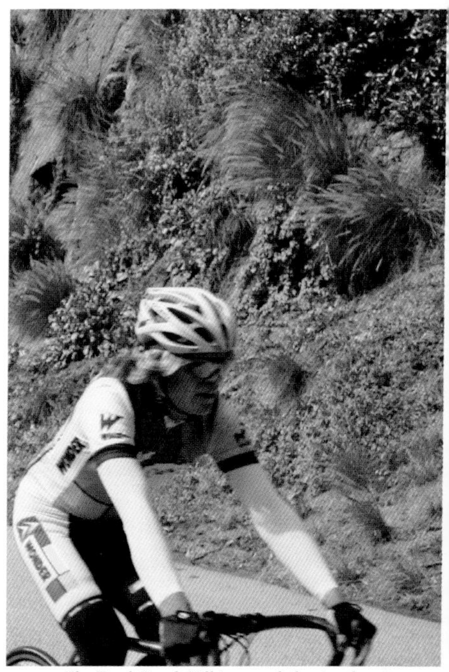

*The Trash Truck Hill is a road classier than its name suggests.*

**Griffith Park**

Altitude ft: 800, 700, 600, 500, 400
Distance miles: 0, 2, 4, 6, 8, 8.7

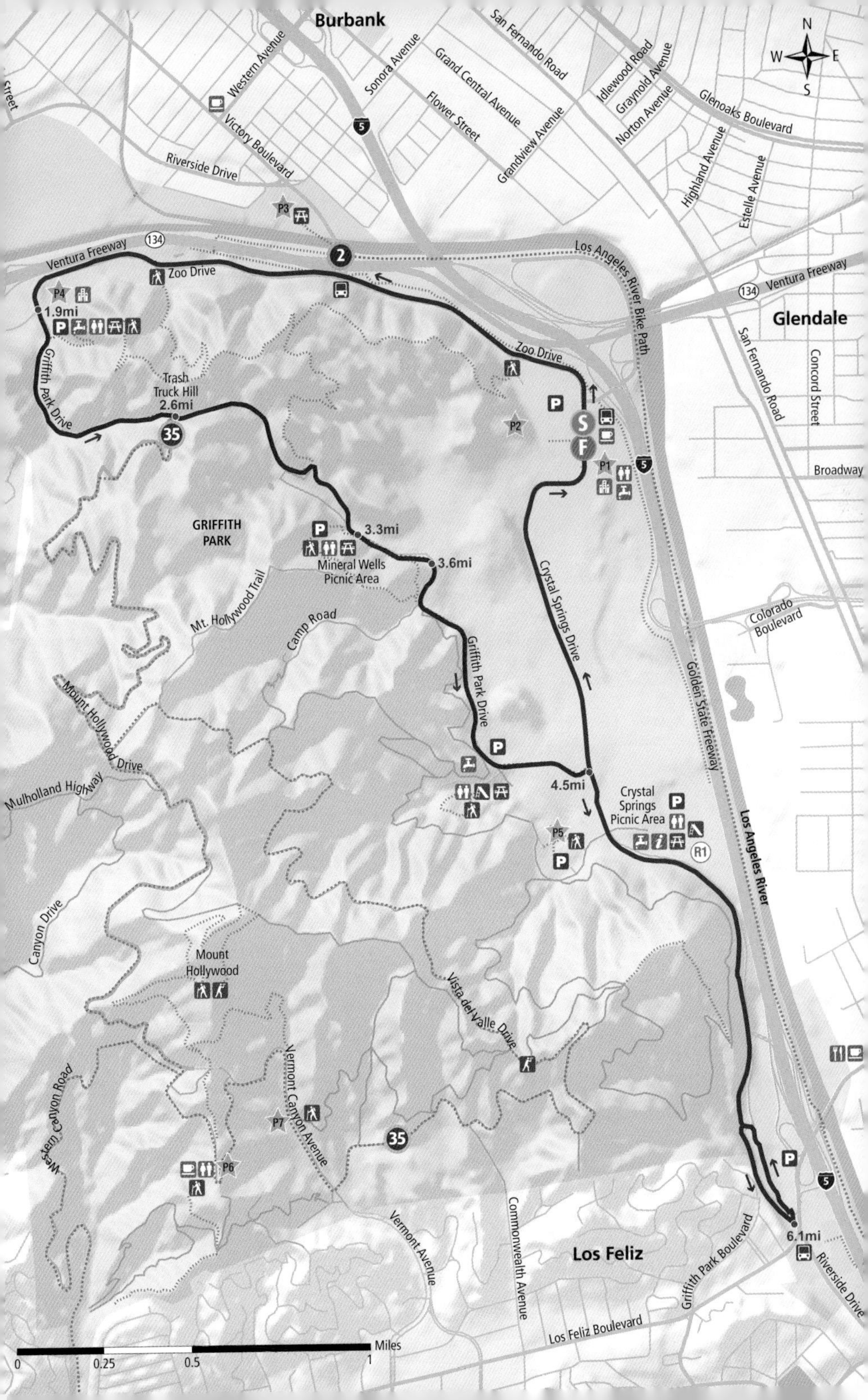

Burbank
Glendale
Los Feliz
GRIFFITH PARK
Western Avenue
Victory Boulevard
Riverside Drive
Sonora Avenue
Grand Central Avenue
Flower Street
San Fernando Road
Grandview Avenue
Idlewood Road
Graynold Avenue
Norton Avenue
Glenoaks Boulevard
Highland Avenue
Estelle Avenue
Ventura Freeway
Los Angeles River Bike Path
Zoo Drive
Griffith Park Drive
Trash Truck Hill
2.6mi
1.9mi
3.3mi
3.6mi
4.5mi
6.1mi
Mineral Wells Picnic Area
Mt. Hollywood Trail
Camp Road
Mount Hollywood Drive
Mulholland Highway
Canyon Drive
Crystal Springs Drive
Crystal Springs Picnic Area
Golden State Freeway
Los Angeles River
San Fernando Road
Concord Street
Broadway
Colorado Boulevard
Mount Hollywood
Vista del Valle Drive
Vermont Canyon Avenue
Western Canyon Road
Vermont Avenue
Commonwealth Avenue
Griffith Park Boulevard
Riverside Drive
Los Feliz Boulevard
Miles
0
0.25
0.5
1

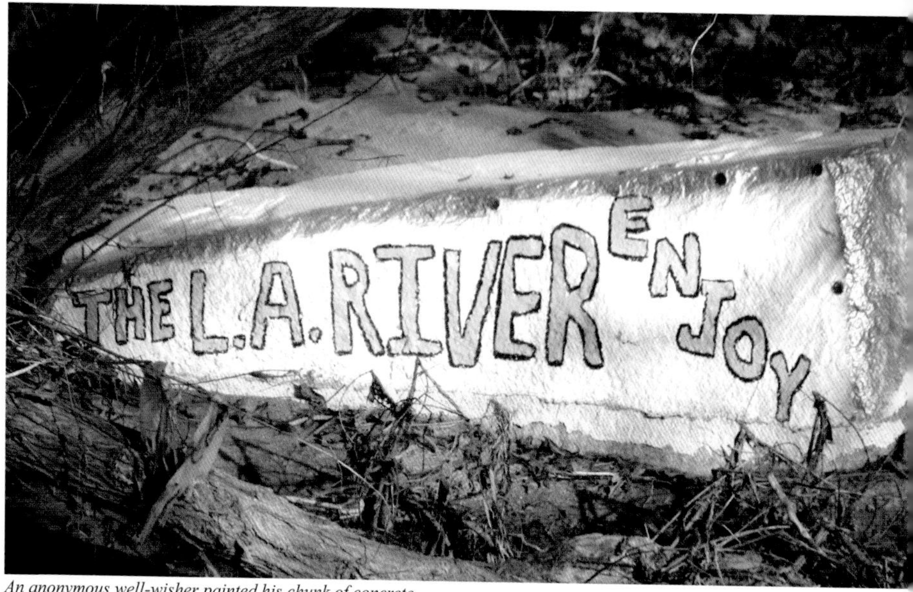


*An anonymous well-wisher painted his chunk of concrete.*

## At a Glance

**Distance** 14.2 miles **Elevation Gain** 250 feet

### Terrain

The ride along the river is flat end-to-end with a relatively smooth asphalt surface. The two-mile segment from Fletcher to Riverside Drive was repaved in 2010 and enhanced with new lighting and landscaping.

### Traffic

This entire riverside route is car-free bike path. From parking to the trailhead, you'll be on Zoo Drive, a well-traveled park road with a bike lane.

### How to Get There

From the 5 or 134 freeways, exit at the Los Angeles Zoo and follow signs to zoo parking. If it's full, look for parking along Zoo Drive west of Riverside Drive.

### Food and Drink

You'll find interesting eateries along Los Feliz Boulevard in Atwater Village, across the river from the bike path. Try the Village Bakery & Café at 3119 Los Feliz Boulevard. To get there, cross the Sunnynook Footbridge over the river, continue straight to Valleybrink Road and make a left on Los Feliz. The bakery is about a block away on the right.

### Side Trip

To explore the river theme further, visit the Los Angeles River Center and Gardens where you can roam the courtyards of this Spanish-style estate, now home to riparian conservation groups and exhibits on the history and ecology of this much-altered river.

**Links to** 1 35 36 37 38 KS

**Where to Bike Rating** 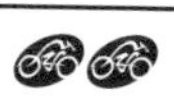

 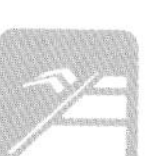 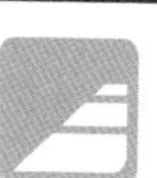 

# About...

In contrast to the boxy, concrete-lined L.A. River that cuts through much of the city, this seven-mile stretch suggests a natural waterway gradually reasserting itself. Though the banks here are still concrete, this soft-bottomed section has been partially reclaimed by wild "islands" of cottonwood, willow, cattail, and brambles, sprouting and flourishing amid river rocks, sandbars and turbulent flowing waters. Along the path's landside is a sprinkling of small parks. Historic bridges over the river add to the experience of this popular ride.

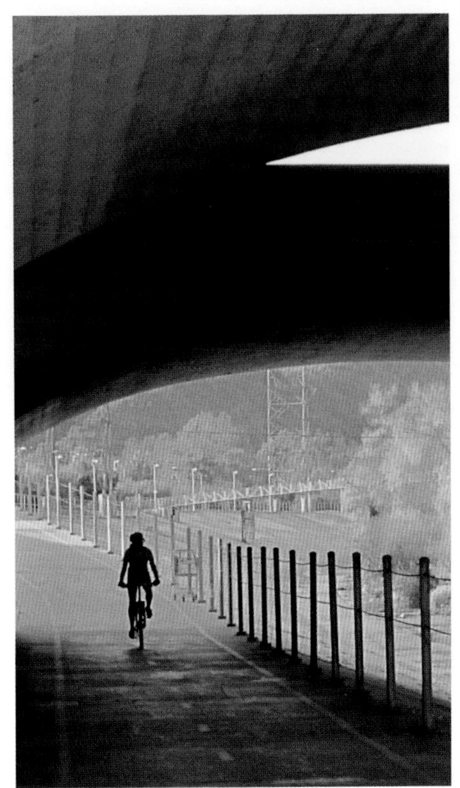

*In a few places, a complex collage of bridges and roadways spans the river.*

More than 50 miles long, the Los Angeles River flows from its headwaters in the northwestern San Fernando Valley all the way to Long Beach, where it empties into the ocean. For years, the cycling community has worked to create bikeways along its banks, so that — someday! — we'll be able to pedal the entire length of the city's namesake river. This short ride through the Glendale Narrows is the best section to date.

Apart from the river itself, the ride highlights include the diminutive path-side parks. Landscaped with native plantings and featuring public art, each one is unique, yet they all comment on the river's once-wild or current condition.

The first park you'll encounter is the L.A. River Bicycle Park, envisioned as a meeting place for cyclists. Artist Leo Limon (known for his graffiti-style "L.A. River Catz," feline faces on the river's storm-drain lids) designed the benches with bicycle-scene cut-outs. Past Fletcher Drive is Rattlesnake Park with its Great Heron Gates by New Zealand artist Brett Goldstone. A pair of beak-to-beak herons, rendered in rust-colored steel, clinch this portal. Across the river on the north side of Fletcher is another Goldstone gate. Entitled "Water with Rocks," it depicts boulders amid wild river surges, flooding skyscraper-spiked downtown Los Angeles.

Past Marsh and Elysian Valley Gateway parks, you'll reach the ride's southern cluster of pocket parks: Steelhead, Egret, and Oso. From Egret's shady benches, you can look across the river to artist Frank Romero's red-and-white "Anza Mural," engaging Native American Tongva tribal symbols to commemorate explorer Juan Bautista de Anza's Las Californias expedition. On the way back, consider stopping at Steelhead Park, with its fence and gate by Goldstone silhouetting steelhead trout. If you leave the park on Oros Street and ride south a short distance to Blake Avenue, you'll reach Oso Park, where artist Michael Amescua's steel-plate sculptures invoke the shadows of grizzly bears and deer, native species that once roamed this land.

## Ride Log

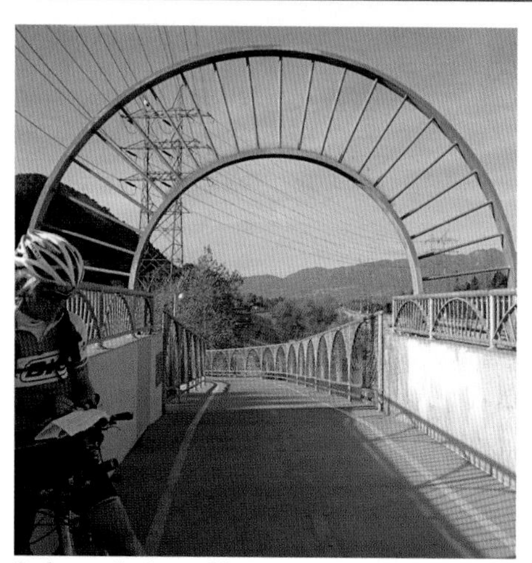

*Spokes are the theme of the Baum Bicycle Bridge.*

*P1* Los Angeles Zoo
*P2* Autry National Center
*P3* Griffith Park Merry-go-round
*P4* Griffith Observatory
*P5* Silver Lake Reservoir
*P6* Great Heron Gates at Rattlesnake Park
*P7* Marsh Park
*P8* Elysian Valley Gateway Park
*P9* Steelhead Park
*P10* Oso Park
*P11* Egret Park
*P12* Elysian Park
*P13* Los Angeles River Center and Gardens

*B1* Glendale Cyclery
1250 Glenoaks Blvd, Glendale
*B2* The Bicycle Mart
1601 S. Brand Blvd, Glendale
*B3* Coco's Variety Store
2427 Riverside Dr, Los Angeles
*B4* Echo Park Cycles
1932 Echo Park Blvd, Echo Park
*R1* Spokes 'n Stuff
4730 Crystal Springs Drive, Griffith Park

**0.0** From the zoo's parking area, ride west along Zoo Dr (toward Travel Town) using the bike lane for roughly one mile. The river ride starts at Riverside Dr, the current terminus of the Los Angeles River Bike Path. Turn right at the stop sign and then, right again onto the river path (you'll need to pass through the security gate's side opening) and begin riding downstream.
**0.7** Pass the Griffith Dog Park and John Ferraro Athletic Fields.
**3.2** Cross the Alex Baum Bicycle Bridge over Los Feliz Blvd.
**3.6** Sunnynook Bridge (leads into Atwater Village).
**4.5** Pass by L.A. River Bicycle Park (up the ramp leading to the north side of Fletcher Dr) and Rattlesnake Park (to reach it cross under Fletcher, make a U-turn and ascend the ramp to Fletcher's south side).
**5.45** Pass Marsh Park (just south of the Glendale Freeway at the end of Marsh Street).
**6.0** Pass Elysian Valley Gateway Park (at the end of Knox Avenue).
**7.0** Pass Steelhead Park (at the end of Oros St).
**7.1** Arrive at Egret Park. Where the bike path meets Riverside Dr: end of river ride. Retrace the same route back to the L.A. Zoo.
**14.2** Zoo parking lot and end of ride.

**Los Angeles River**

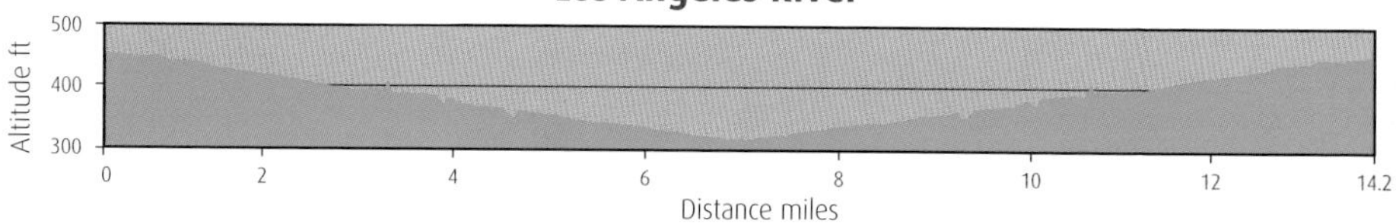

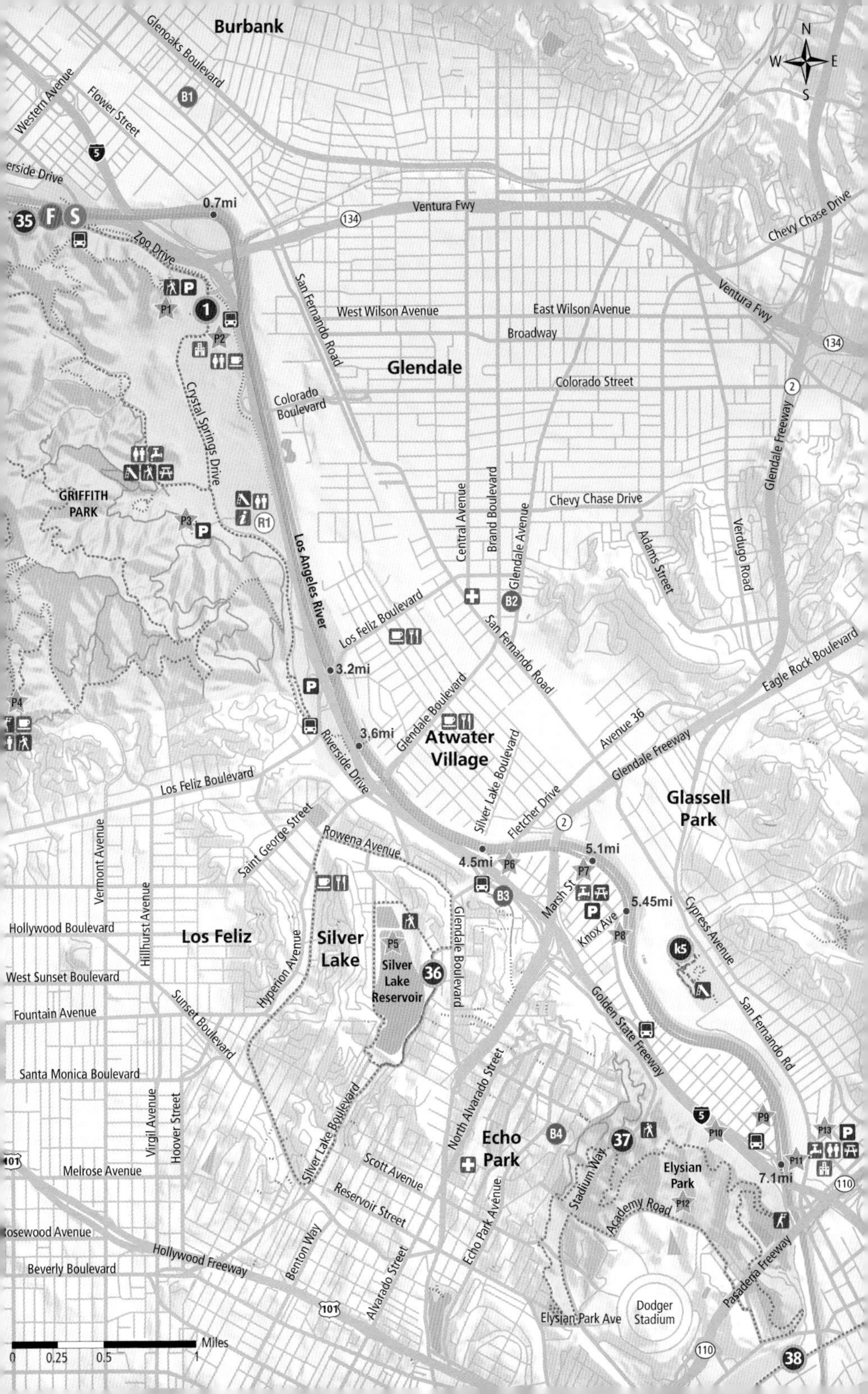

Burbank
Glendale
GRIFFITH PARK
Los Feliz
Silver Lake
Silver Lake Reservoir
Atwater Village
Glassell Park
Echo Park
Elysian Park
Dodger Stadium
Glenoaks Boulevard
Western Avenue
Flower Street
Riverside Drive
Ventura Fwy
Zoo Drive
Chevy Chase Drive
San Fernando Road
West Wilson Avenue
East Wilson Avenue
Broadway
Colorado Street
Colorado Boulevard
Crystal Springs Drive
Glendale Freeway
Central Avenue
Brand Boulevard
Glendale Avenue
Adams Street
Verdugo Road
Los Angeles River
Los Feliz Boulevard
Eagle Rock Boulevard
Glendale Boulevard
Avenue 36
Silver Lake Boulevard
Fletcher Drive
Saint George Street
Rowena Avenue
Vermont Avenue
Hillhurst Avenue
Hollywood Boulevard
West Sunset Boulevard
Fountain Avenue
Sunset Boulevard
Santa Monica Boulevard
Hyperion Avenue
Marsh St
Knox Ave
Cypress Avenue
Golden State Freeway
San Fernando Rd
North Alvarado Street
Virgil Avenue
Hoover Street
Melrose Avenue
Rosewood Avenue
Beverly Boulevard
Hollywood Freeway
Benton Way
Alvarado Street
Echo Park Avenue
Scott Avenue
Reservoir Street
Stadium Way
Academy Road
Elysian Park Ave
Pasadena Freeway
0.7mi
3.2mi
3.6mi
4.5mi
5.1mi
5.45mi
7.1mi
Miles
0
0.25
0.5
1

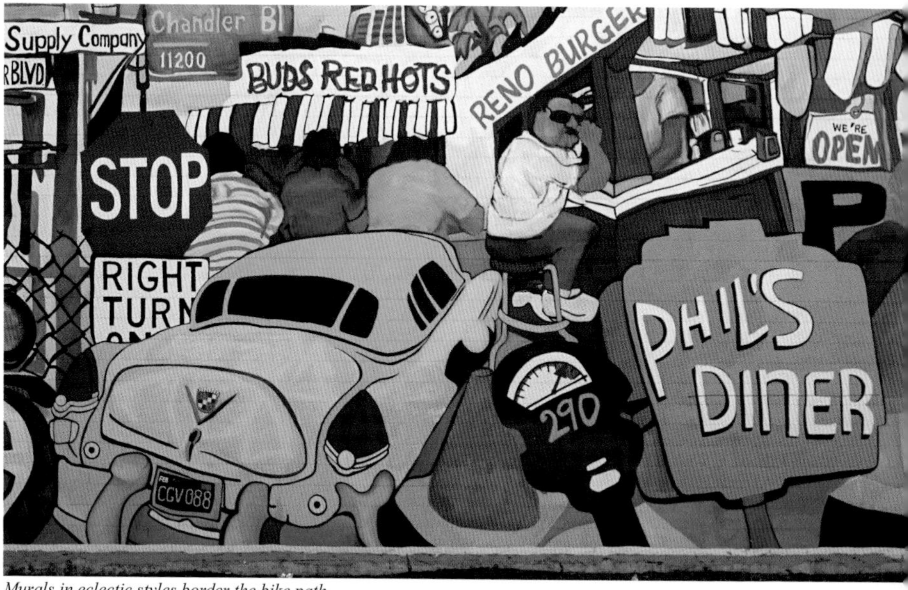


*Murals in eclectic styles border the bike path.*

## At a Glance

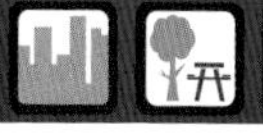

**Distance** 6.6 miles **Elevation Gain** 200 feet

### Terrain

From start to finish, this bikeway is flat and smoothly paved in concrete.

### Traffic

Though the path is free of vehicular traffic, it intersects several street crossings, where cyclists need to obey traffic lights and stop signs.

### How to Get There

The bikeway begins at the intersection of Chandler Boulevard and Vineland Avenue. Ample free parking is just to the west, at the North Hollywood Metro station. Exit the 170 Freeway at Magnolia Boulevard. Travel east and turn left (north) onto Lankershim Boulevard; continue about three bocks to parking. The North Hollywood Metro station is accessible via the Red Line subway from downtown or the Orange Line from points west.

### Food and Drink

You'll find snack options along Chandler Boulevard across from the Metro station.

### Side Trip

The bikeway links to the up-and-coming North Hollywood (NoHo) Arts District's theaters, music spots, recording studios, art galleries and restaurants, all within a few blocks of this ride's western end. The neighborhood centerpiece is the 1926 El Portal Theatre (Lankershim Boulevard at Weddington Street), a venue originally devoted to Vaudeville, later to silent pictures and now, with its three modern stages, to theatrical productions often featuring celebrities.

**Links to** 

**Where to Bike Rating** 

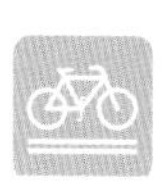   

# About...

The Chandler Bikeway is a Rails-to-Trails project that transformed part of Southern Pacific Railroad's defunct Burbank Branch into a wide median park with a bike path running its entire length. Six-plus miles round-trip, it's a pretty ride that will get even better as the landscaping matures. Beginning at a Metro train station, near the NoHo Arts District's epicenter, the bikeway also serves as an excellent connector to adjacent neighborhoods.

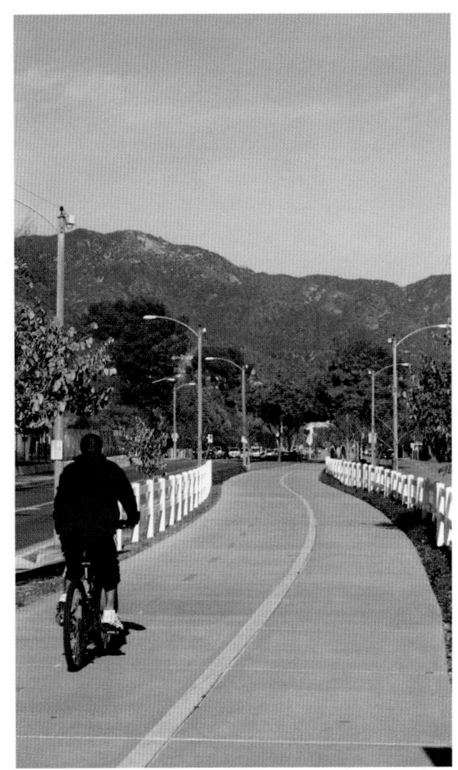

*Flat easy riding.*

The first half-mile of the ride passes through the Chandler Outdoor Gallery, or Murals, a 10-block corridor lined with 19 outdoor paintings on the walls of lumberyards, auto body shops, and other industrial structures. Larger-than-life depictions of peach orchards, steam locomotives, haciendas, pioneering aircraft, butterflies, movie sets, rock n' rollers and other icons of local history provide visual entertainment. While many of these paintings are *trompe l'oeil,* playfully evoking 3-D objects and spaces, other artworks along the bikeway are actually sculptural, such as Gary Lee Price's "*Family Outing,*" at the intersection of Hollywood Way: a hyper-literal depiction of a father and his kids out for a bike ride.

As it happens, the Chandler Bikeway is particularly well suited to just that: family outings. It's a great place to take young cyclists, even those still gaining their balance on wheels. One caveat, however: Since the bikeway crosses several busy streets, we recommend that parents supervise the crossings.

You might even want to take the kids on an early evening ride when the Sidewalk Astronomers set up telescopes at the intersection of Lima Street and the bikeway (once a month, beginning around 6:30 or 7:30 p.m., depending on the season. Call 818-238-5378 for exact times). With the right weather and celestial positions, the moon, Saturn, Venus and Jupiter may be visible.

Or you might be inspired to check out the thriving dining and entertainment scene in downtown Burbank, a short distance beyond this mini "cycling freeway." (At the end of the bikeway, turn right on Mariposa Street to Magnolia Boulevard, then left for several blocks to the town center.) On Thursday nights in July and August, ride into Burbank for its Come Out & Dance music festival. Or, for an ambitious daytime adventure, continue all the way to Griffith Park. (From Magnolia Boulevard, turn right onto Victory Boulevard, and a few blocks later, just past Verdugo Avenue, angle off to the right onto Main Street. Where Main joins Riverside Drive, turn left and follow the signs to Griffith Park.) The Bikeway also connects Burbank to points west in the San Fernando Valley.

# Ride Log

**0.0** From the North Hollywood Metro station's parking area, cross to the south side of Chandler Blvd (use the pedestrian crosswalk at Lankershim Blvd). Ride east, towards the mountains, in the bike lane on Chandler Blvd.

**0.4** Turn left on Vineland and join the Chandler Bikeway at the next signal.

**0.9** Cross Cahuenga Blvd.

**1.7** Cross North Hollywood Way.

**1.9** Pass Lima St.

**2.7** Pass Keystone St.

**3.3** Arrive at Mariposa St, make a U-turn and ride back along the bikeway.

**6.6** Back at parking area. End of ride.

*P1* El Portal Theatre
*P2* Chandler Outdoor Gallery
*P3* Family Outing sculpture
*P4* Sidewalk Astronomers (once a month)
*P5* The Wagon Pull sculpture
*P6* Trackwalker sculpture

*B1* Bicycle John's
1038 North Hollywood Way, Burbank
*B2* H&S Bicycles
509 North Victory Blvd, Burbank
*B3* Burbank Bike Shop
4400 West Victory Boulevard, Burbank
*B4* Metropolis Bikes
4660 Lankershim Blvd, North Hollywood

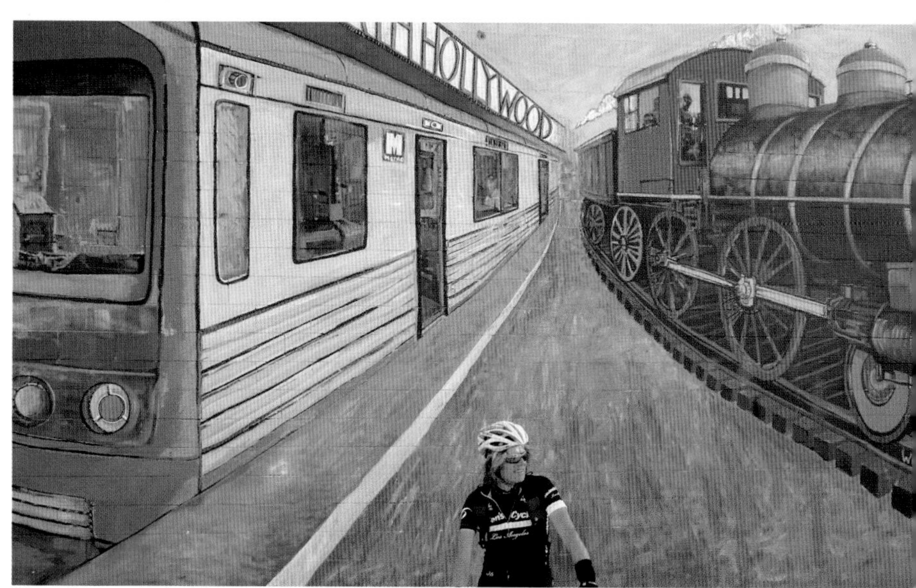


*Many of the murals playfully reinvent local scenes.*

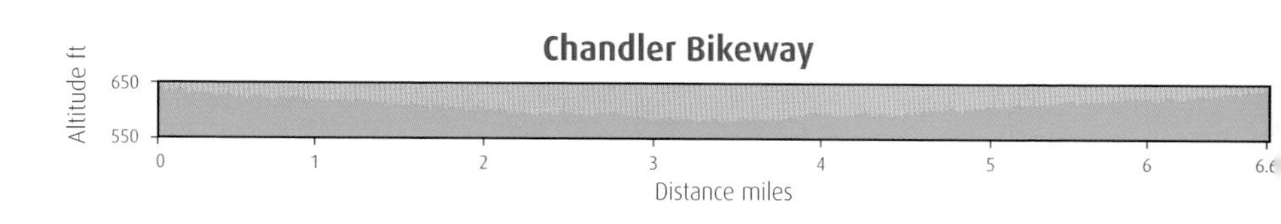

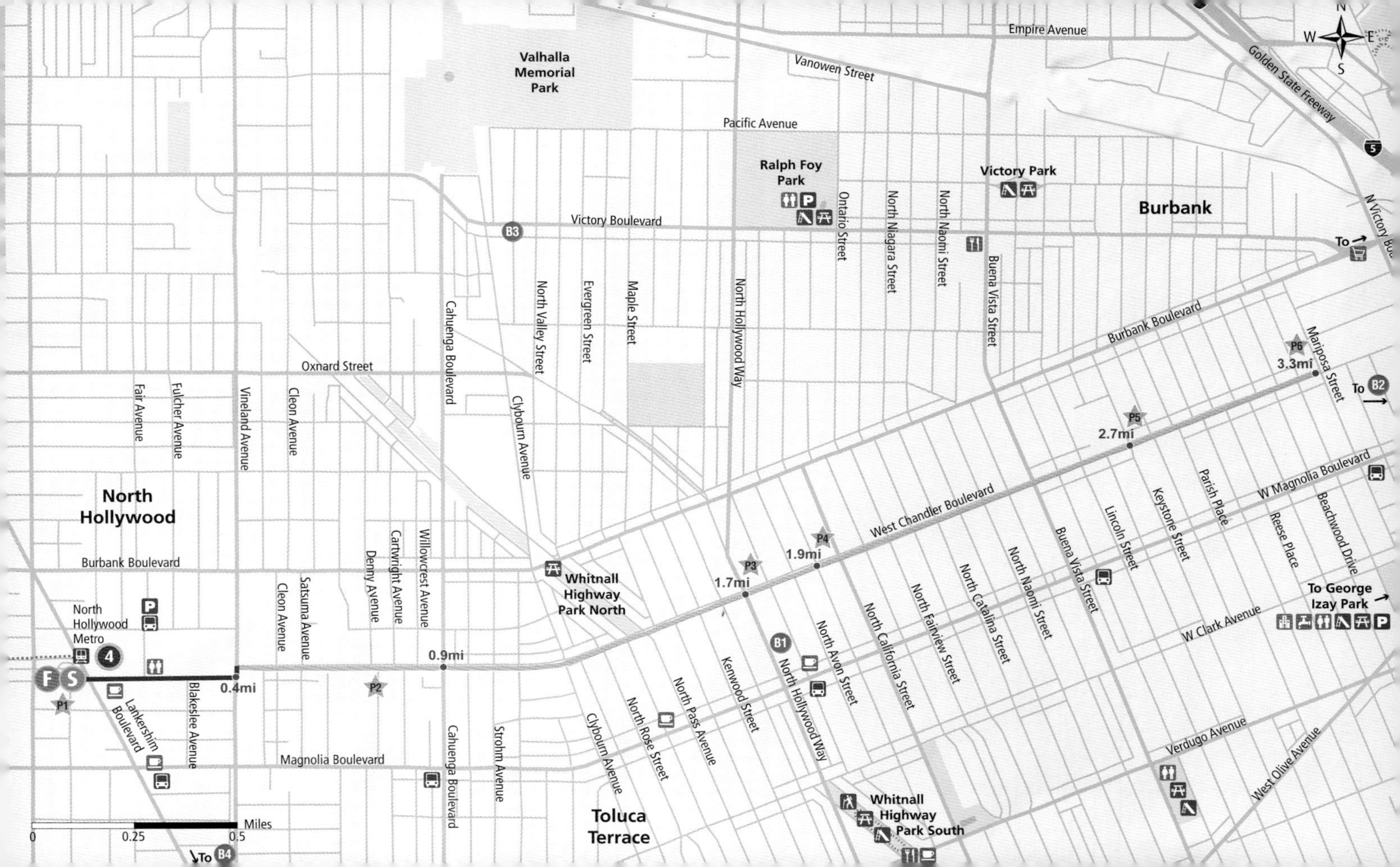

N
W
E
S
Empire Avenue
Valhalla Memorial Park
Vanowen Street
Golden State Freeway
5
Pacific Avenue
Ralph Foy Park
Victory Park
Burbank
N Victory Bou
Victory Boulevard
B3
Ontario Street
North Niagara Street
North Naomi Street
To
Buena Vista Street
Burbank Boulevard
North Valley Street
Evergreen Street
Maple Street
North Hollywood Way
Cahuenga Boulevard
Mariposa Street
P6
3.3mi
To B2
Oxnard Street
Fair Avenue
Fulcher Avenue
Vineland Avenue
Cleon Avenue
Clybourn Avenue
P5
2.7mi
W Magnolia Boulevard
Parish Place
Keystone Street
Beachwood Drive
North Hollywood
West Chandler Boulevard
Reese Place
Lincoln Street
P4
1.9mi
Burbank Boulevard
Whitnall Highway Park North
P3
1.7mi
North Naomi Street
Buena Vista Street
North Catalina Street
North Fairview Street
To George Izay Park
North Hollywood Metro
W Clark Avenue
Cleon Avenue
Satsuma Avenue
Denny Avenue
Cartwright Avenue
Willowcrest Avenue
0.9mi
B1
4
North Avon Street
North California Street
F
S
0.4mi
P2
P1
Lankershim Boulevard
Blakeslee Avenue
Kenwood Street
North Hollywood Way
North Pass Avenue
North Rose Street
Magnolia Boulevard
Cahuenga Boulevard
Strohm Avenue
Clybourn Avenue
Verdugo Avenue
West Olive Avenue
Whitnall Highway Park South
Toluca Terrace
Miles
0
0.25
0.5
To B4

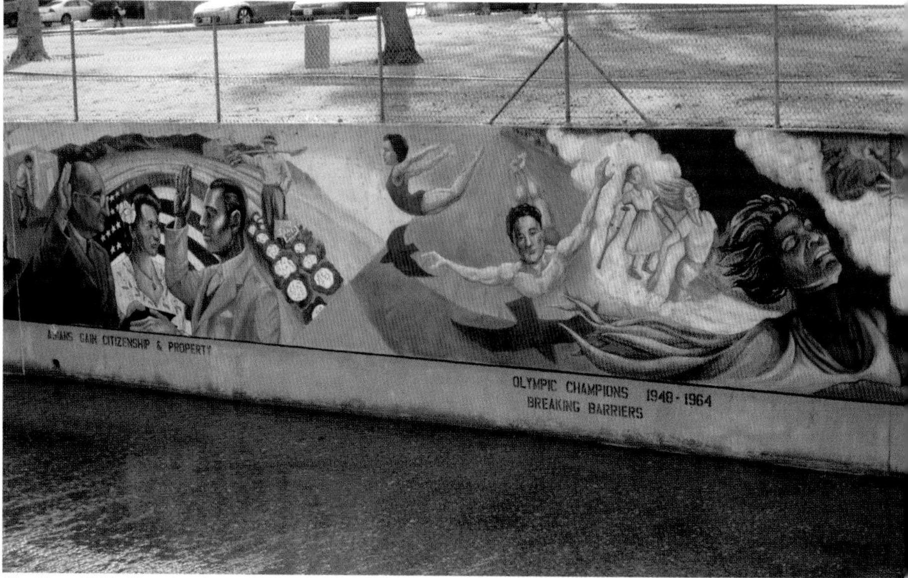


*The Great Wall of Los Angeles makes an excellent side trip from the Orange Line.*

## At a Glance

**Distance** 29.1 miles **Elevation Gain** 600 feet

### Terrain

This ride is virtually flat bike path and lanes with good pavement.

### Traffic

The route is car-free, except for bike lane at the beginning and end. The bike path intersects a series of cross streets where cyclists must respect traffic lights.

### How to Get There

Begin at the North Hollywood Metro station, at the intersection of Chandler and Lankershim boulevards. From the 170 Freeway, exit at Magnolia Boulevard and travel east to Lankershim. There's free parking two blocks north at the Metro lot. Alternatively, you can reach the North Hollywood Metro station via the Red Line subway from Downtown or the Orange Line bus from the west.

### Food and Drink

Along the entire route you'll find convenience stores on the streets surrounding the Orange Line. Near the North Hollywood Metro station, the many eateries include Panera Bread and Pitfire Pizza, both on Lankershim.

### Side Trip

A slight detour to the Pierce College farm stand will be worth your while, especially in strawberry season. At De Soto Avenue (mile 13.7), cross Victory Boulevard to the store, where you can buy fresh-picked produce and support the work of this agricultural college's budding young farmers.

**Links to** 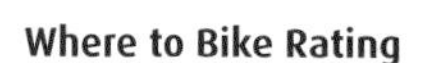

**Where to Bike Rating** 

# About...

This landscaped (though more practical than scenic) route provides for an easy, car-free journey across much of the San Fernando Valley. The bike path parallels the Orange Line busway, sharing its right-of-way while remaining well separated by a planted buffer zone. Many valley destinations are accessible by bike from this path or via intersecting bus routes (don't forget the buses have bike racks). And, of course, the Red Line subway from North Hollywood station links this entire network to Downtown L.A.

he Orange Line bike path is a cousin of rails to trails. ut instead of totally transforming a defunct rail route nto a bucolic trail, it's an agreeable urban compronise: the reincarnation of a long-dormant train and rolley right-of-way into a new rapid transit route with n integral bike path. Part of the beauty of this sleekly conomical solution is a quiet express bus that travls unobtrusively in its own "slot" without impinging n the bike trail or surrounding neighborhoods. At the ame time, the transit right-of-way enables cyclists o traverse the San Fernando Valley without vehicuar traffic nipping at their heels. (Intersecting routes cross the valley, plus a swift connection to Downtown .A. via the Red Line subway from North Hollywood tation further expand your reach.) And if you need a reak from pedaling, there's the option of hopping an )range Line bus, with your bike on its rack.

The 14-mile bike path will add four more miles vhen the Canoga Station-to-Chatsworth section reachs completion, expected in 2012. But already, the exensive and highly functional trail is smooth-surfaced, vell lit, regularly maintained and edged in seasonally lowering trees, plants and vine-covered walls. Beause the bikeway is at grade, however, cross-streets intersect it, punctuating (or breaking) your rhythm with obligatory stops at red lights.

Midway through the ride, the path jogs across and partially around the Sepulveda Basin Recreation Area, making it easy to combine your journey with the parkland's many offerings.

For a completely different experience, we recommend a detour to "The Great Wall of Los Angeles." A brainchild of artist Judith Baca, this half-mile-long mural was painted by local youth through the Social and Public Art Resource Center (SPARC) beginning in the 1970s. Lining a vertical wall of the Tujunga Wash, the painting traces California history, focusing on people disenfranchised or "left out of the history books," says Baca, who envisioned the mural as a "tattoo over the scar where the river once ran" (before becoming a concrete-lined channel). From the Orange Line, turn north at Coldwater Canyon (about 2.1 miles west of the North Hollywood Metro station) and pick up the path through the greenway along Coldwater's east side. Cross Burbank Boulevard at the crosswalks and continue through the Tujunga Wash Greenway until you see murals below you at left.

# Ride Log

**0.0** From the Metro parking lot, cross Lankershim Blvd at Chandler Blvd. Commence riding west along Chandler using the bike lane.

**1.1** Cross Laurel Canyon Blvd (Orange Line station).

**2.3** Angle slightly to the right where Chandler crosses the busway to begin the Orange Line Bikeway.

**2.7** Cross Burbank Blvd and Fulton Ave using the crosswalks.

**4.5** Cross Van Nuys Blvd (Orange Line station).

**5.5** Cross Sepulveda Blvd (Orange Line station).

**5.7** Cross Haskell Ave and ride along the sidewalk/bike path.

**6.3** Cross Haskell Ave again and enter the Sepulveda Dam Recreation Area.

**6.7** Cross Woodley (Orange Line station).

**7.7** Turn left at Balboa Blvd and then, cross the bus-

## Ride Log continued...

way. Ride straight along Balboa using the bike path.

**8.2** Cross the Los Angeles River.

**8.3** Turn left and then cross under Balboa Blvd.

**8.5** Turn right at the parking lot.

**8.7** Follow the bike path out of the Sepulveda Dam Recreation Area.

**9.5** Cross White Oak Ave and re-enter the bikeway.

**11.5** Cross Tampa Ave (Orange Line station).

**12.6** Cross Winnetka (Orange Line station).

**13.7** Cross De Soto Ave.

**13.9** Stay to the right at the Y in the bikeway.

**14.2** Canoga Ave (Orange Line station). Return by bike or by bus along the same route.

**14.8** Cross De Soto Ave.

**19.1** Cross White Oak Ave.

**19.6** Continue straight on the bike path, passing the Encino Velodrome.

**19.9** Enter the Sepulveda Dam Recreation Area.

**20.1** Turn left at the parking lot and cross under Balboa Blvd.

**20.3** Continue north along Balboa Blvd a short distance.

**20.4** Turn right at the Y and ride parallel to the Los Angeles River.

**20.7** Turn right on North Balboa Blvd.

**20.9** Ride around Lake Balboa.

**22.2** Turn left on Woodley Ave.

**22.3** Cross the busway, then cross Woodley at Victory Blvd.

**22.8** Leave the Sepulveda Dam Recreation Area, cross Haskell Ave.

P *P1* Universal Studios Hollywood / Universal CityWalk
*P2* The Great Wall of Los Angeles
*P3* Castle Park Entertainment Center
*P4* Japanese Tea Garden
*P5* Sepulveda Basin Wildlife Reserve
*P6* Lake Balboa Park
*P7* Encino Velodrome (Ride 6)
*P8* Los Encinos State Historic Park
*P9* Pierce College Farm Center

B *B1* Pedalers West Bike Shop
5616 Van Nuys Blvd, Van Nuys
*B2* Europa Bicycles
14764 Ventura Blvd, Sherman Oaks
*B3* The Bike Connection
13711 Ventura Blvd, Sherman Oaks
*B4* Custom Bicycle Sales
18424 Ventura Blvd, Tarzana
*B5* Bike Warrior
19449 Ventura Blvd, Tarzana
*B6* Performance Bicycle Shop
6400 Owensmouth Ave, Woodland Hills
*B7* Valley Bikery
14416 Victory Blvd, Van Nuys
*B8* Reseda Bicycles
7056 Reseda Blvd, Reseda

R *R1* Wheel Fun Rentals, Lake Balboa Park

**23.3** Cross Haskell Ave.

**23.5** Cross Sepulveda Blvd.

**26.3** Cross Burbank Blvd and Fulton Ave using the crosswalks.

**26.7** The bike path ends as it crosses the Orange Line Continue east along Chandler Blvd using the bike lane

**27.9** Cross Laurel Canyon Blvd.

**29.1** Turn Left on Lankershim Blvd and enter the Metro parking lot.

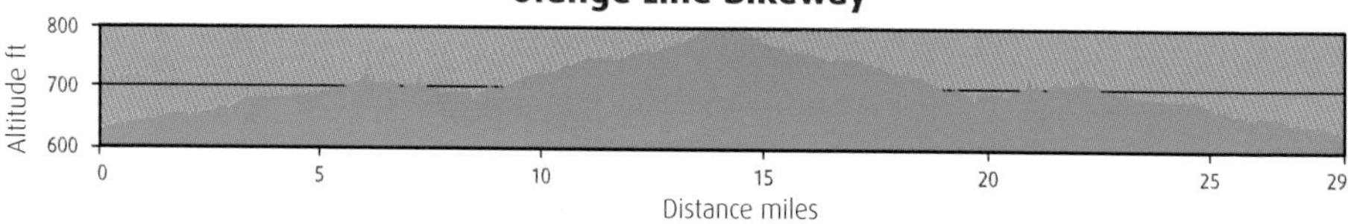

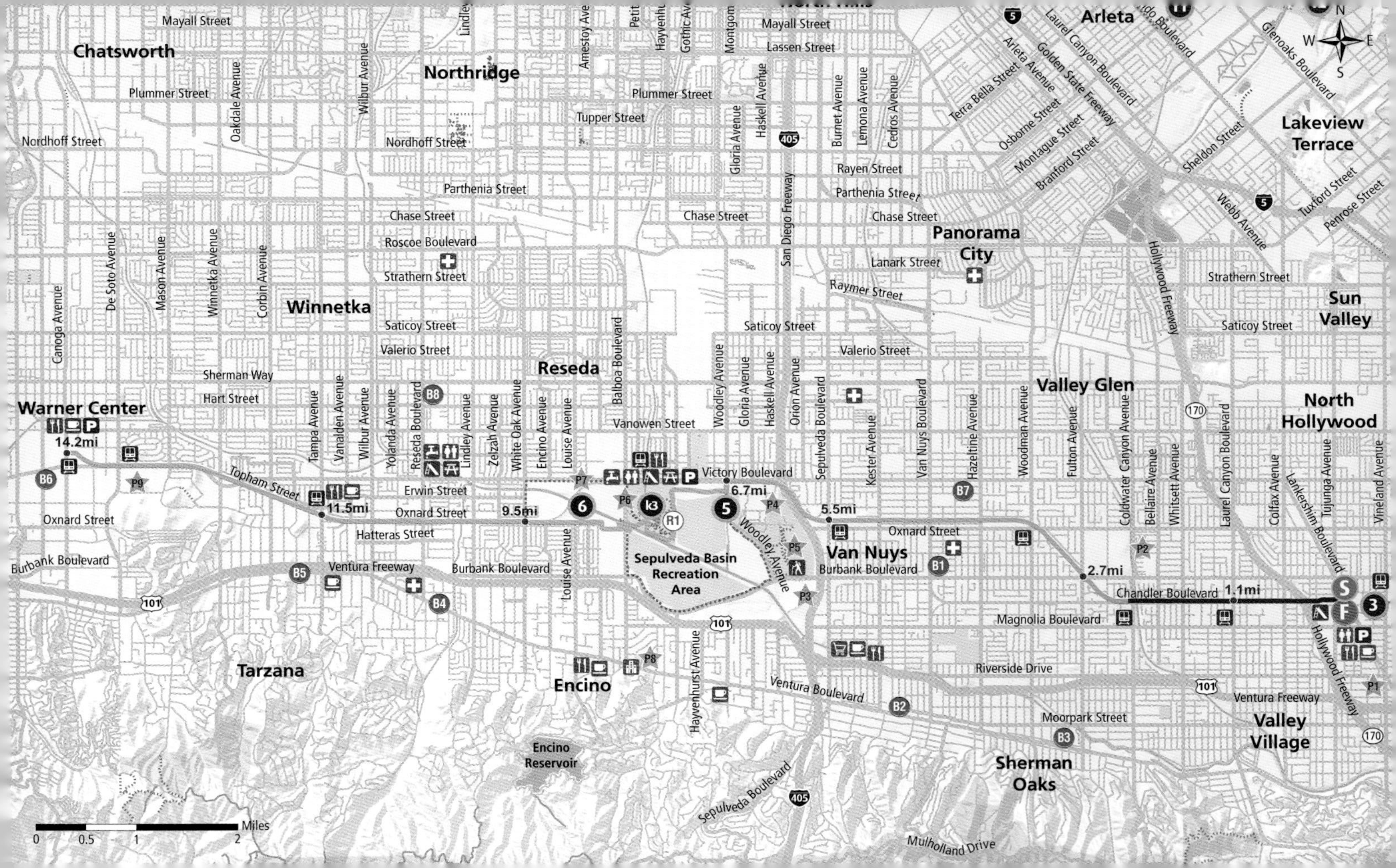

Chatsworth
Northridge
Winnetka
Warner Center
Reseda
Tarzana
Encino
Encino Reservoir
Van Nuys
Sepulveda Basin Recreation Area
Panorama City
Valley Glen
Sherman Oaks
Valley Village
North Hollywood
Sun Valley
Lakeview Terrace
Arleta
14.2mi
11.5mi
9.5mi
6.7mi
5.5mi
2.7mi
1.1mi
Hollywood Freeway
San Diego Freeway
Ventura Freeway
Golden State Freeway
Ventura Boulevard
Victory Boulevard
Chandler Boulevard
Burbank Boulevard
Oxnard Street
Topham Street
Woodley Avenue
Sepulveda Boulevard
Mulholland Drive
Riverside Drive
Magnolia Boulevard
Moorpark Street
Lankershim Boulevard
Laurel Canyon Boulevard
Canoga Avenue
De Soto Avenue
Mason Avenue
Winnetka Avenue
Corbin Avenue
Tampa Avenue
Reseda Boulevard
Balboa Boulevard
Van Nuys Boulevard
Woodman Avenue
Coldwater Canyon Avenue
Vineland Avenue
Nordhoff Street
Plummer Street
Saticoy Street
Strathern Street
Roscoe Boulevard
Sherman Way
Vanowen Street
Miles
0
0.5
1
2

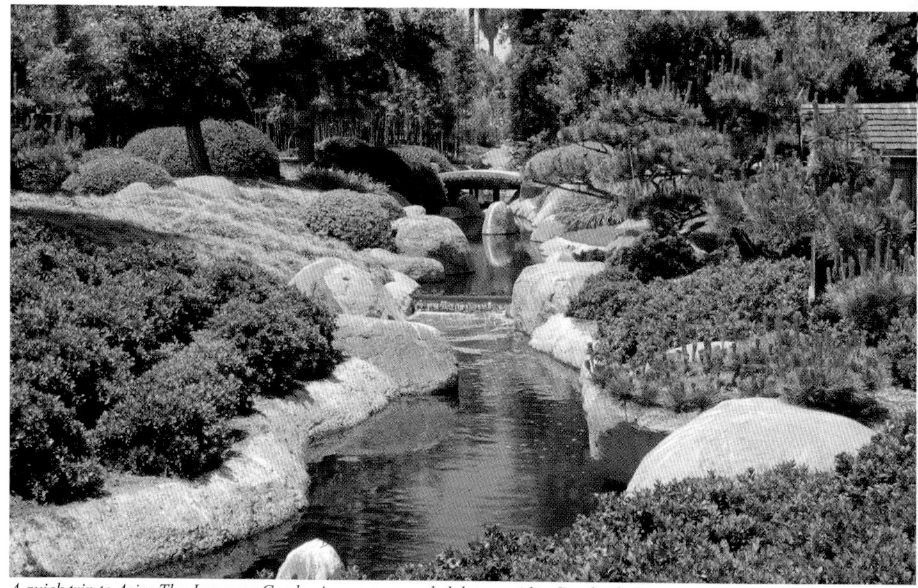

*A quick trip to Asia: The Japanese Garden is a recommended detour within Sepulveda Basin.*

## At a Glance

**Distance** 7.9 miles **Elevation Gain** 300 feet

### Terrain

The path is paved and the parkland virtually flat.

### Traffic

Except for few of blocks of bike lane along White Oak Avenue, this loop follows dedicated bicycle paths within the extensive Sepulveda Basin network.

### How to Get There

Sepulveda Basin Recreation Area (SBRA) lies at the intersection of the 101 and 405 freeways, easily accessible from most of L.A. Exit the 101 onto Balboa Boulevard and go north to Anthony C. Beilenson Park. Or, from the 405, exit at Burbank Boulevard, head west, then north on Balboa to the park. Parking is free in lots throughout SBRA or along Lake Balboa's access road. The Orange Line bus also stops nearby, at its Balboa and Woodley stations.

### Food and Drink

Victory Boulevard, on SBRA's north side, offers fast food and convenience stores. Hotdog or ice cream vendors sometimes roam the park and periphery.

### Side Trip

Sepulveda Basin has its own 225-acre wildlife reserve, with native willows and migratory waterfowl, and a 6.5-acre Japanese Garden (on the grounds of the Tillman water reclamation plant), evoking 18th and 19th century "wet gardens," while showcasing water reclamation benefits. (Sunday through Thursday, 10 a.m. to 4 p.m. **www.thejapanesgarden.com**. Entry fee: $3)

**Links to**   

**Where to Bike Rating** 

# About...

This paved loop allows you to explore the Sepulveda Basin Recreation Area, with its vast array of leisure activities. Amid lawns and shade trees, you'll bike by Lake Balboa and athletic fields, golf courses, an outdoor velodrome and more. The bike path also provides easy access to such venues as the Sepulveda Basin wildlife reserve, Japanese Garden and model aircraft field. During L.A.'s exceedingly rare instances of heavy flooding—when you'd want to retreat indoors anyway—this entire area performs as a flood-control reservoir, closed to the public.

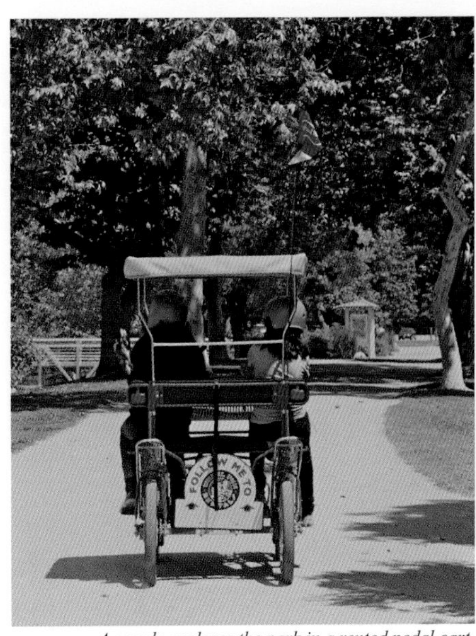

*A couple explores the park in a rented pedal cart.*

The Sepulveda Basin—2,100 acres of lowlands—is a vast flood-control catchment for the Los Angeles River and entire San Fernando Valley watershed. To protect the surrounding communities from torrential floods in rare episodes of dramatic rainfall, the Army Corps of Engineers has restricted building in the basin to a minimum and erected the Sepulveda Dam, completed in 1941, on its southeastern edge. Since this great "reservoir" remains dry most the time, the Army Corps has leased it long-term to the City of Los Angeles Department of Recreation & Parks. With the most extensive parkland in the San Fernando Valley, the basin includes athletic fields, three golf courses, an 11-acre fishing lake, tennis courts, a skate park, community garden plots, an outdoor velodrome (see Ride 6), an evolving wildlife reserve, a model-aircraft field, several miles of easy cycling (and jogging) path.

The ride begins near the bike-and-pedal-car rental kiosk at Lake Balboa, in Anthony C. Beilenson Park. You may want to focus purely on this leisurely cycling loop—or take advantage en route of the many activity and detour options. After the first couple of turns, you'll reach the access road, on your right, to the Apollo 11 model aircraft field, where you can watch radio-controlled planes overhead, on the runway and in the benching area (where aficionados tinker with mini engines and wing flaps). But if you continue along the bike path, you'll soon have the option, via a turn-off on your left, to visit the Japanese Garden on foot or hike into the Sepulveda Basin wildlife reserve, which features native flora and a pond with a migratory bird refuge island. (Binoculars are recommended for a good look at snowy egrets, great blue herons, red-tailed hawks and other winged creatures). Back on the bike path, you'll cross over a stream, which is actually one of the rare soft-bottomed stretches of the L.A. River. Soon the route passes the Encino and Balboa golf courses and then skirts by the Encino Velodrome where you can watch racing cyclists for free. The path ultimately loops back to the lake, where you might want to wrap up the outing in a rented paddleboat. Or you can save all the detours for later—and just enjoy meandering through the parkland, with its shady trees and lawns.

*While Ride 5 has not been deemed kid-friendly in its entirety, it does include substantial sections which are entirely safe for family use.*

# Ride Log

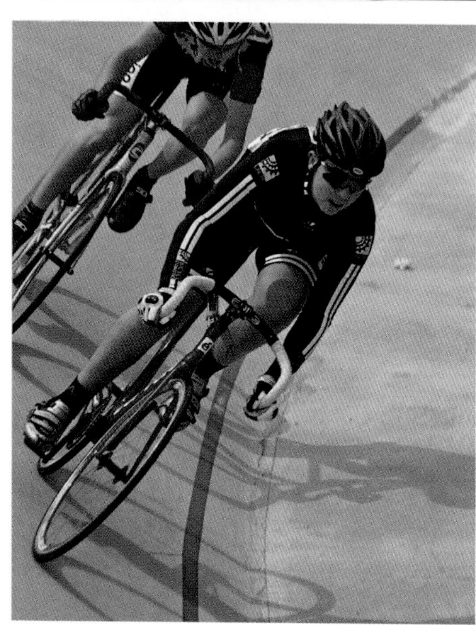

*Right en route, at the Encino Velodrome, you can watch racing cyclists (for free).*

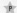

*P1* Apollo XI Model Airplane Field
*P2* Japanese Garden
*P3* Sepulveda Basin Wildlife Reserve
*P4* Castle Park Entertainment Center
*P5* Los Encinos State Historic Park
*P6* Encino Velodrome

*B1* Custom Bicycle Sales
18424 Ventura Blvd, Tarzana
*B2* Europa Bicyles
14764 Ventura Blvd, Sherman Oaks
*B3* The Bike Connection
13711 Ventura Blvd, Sherman Oaks
*R1* Wheel Fun Rentals, Lake Balboa Park

**0.0** From the Anthony C. Beilenson Park/Lake Balboa parking area nearest to the pedal car/bicycle rental facility, turn left onto the bike path and follow it over the small hill.

**0.2** Follow the bike path as it continues along North Balboa Blvd.

**0.8** Turn right on the path running along the west side of Woodley Ave.

**1.1** Pass the access road to the model airplane runways.

**1.8** Follow the bike path as in bears to the right just before Burbank Blvd.

**2.0** Cross the Los Angeles River.

**3.0** Follow the bike path to the right around the Balboa Golf Course parking lot and past the golf course clubhouse.

**3.6** Turn right just before Balboa Blvd.

**4.0** Take the right side of the Y just before the Los Angeles River.

**4.1** Cross under Balboa Blvd.

**4.2** Turn right where the bike path meets the parking lot.

**4.5** Make a right turn, then a left, and exit Sepulveda Dam Recreation Area, continuing west on Oxnard St.

**4.7** Pass Encino Velodrome.

**5.2** Turn right on White Oak Ave.

**5.6** Cross the Los Angeles River and transition back to the bike path.

**5.7** Turn right just before Victory Blvd.

**6.7** Cross Balboa Blvd at the signal, then turn right on the bike path running along the east side of Balboa Blvd.

**6.8** Take the left side of the Y in the bike path (don't continue along Balboa).

**7.1** Cross the access road to Anthony C. Beilenson Park.

**7.3** Arrive back at Lake Balboa.

**7.9** End the loop at the parking lot.

**Sepulveda Basin**

Altitude ft: 750, 650
Distance miles: 0, 2, 4, 6, 8, 7.9

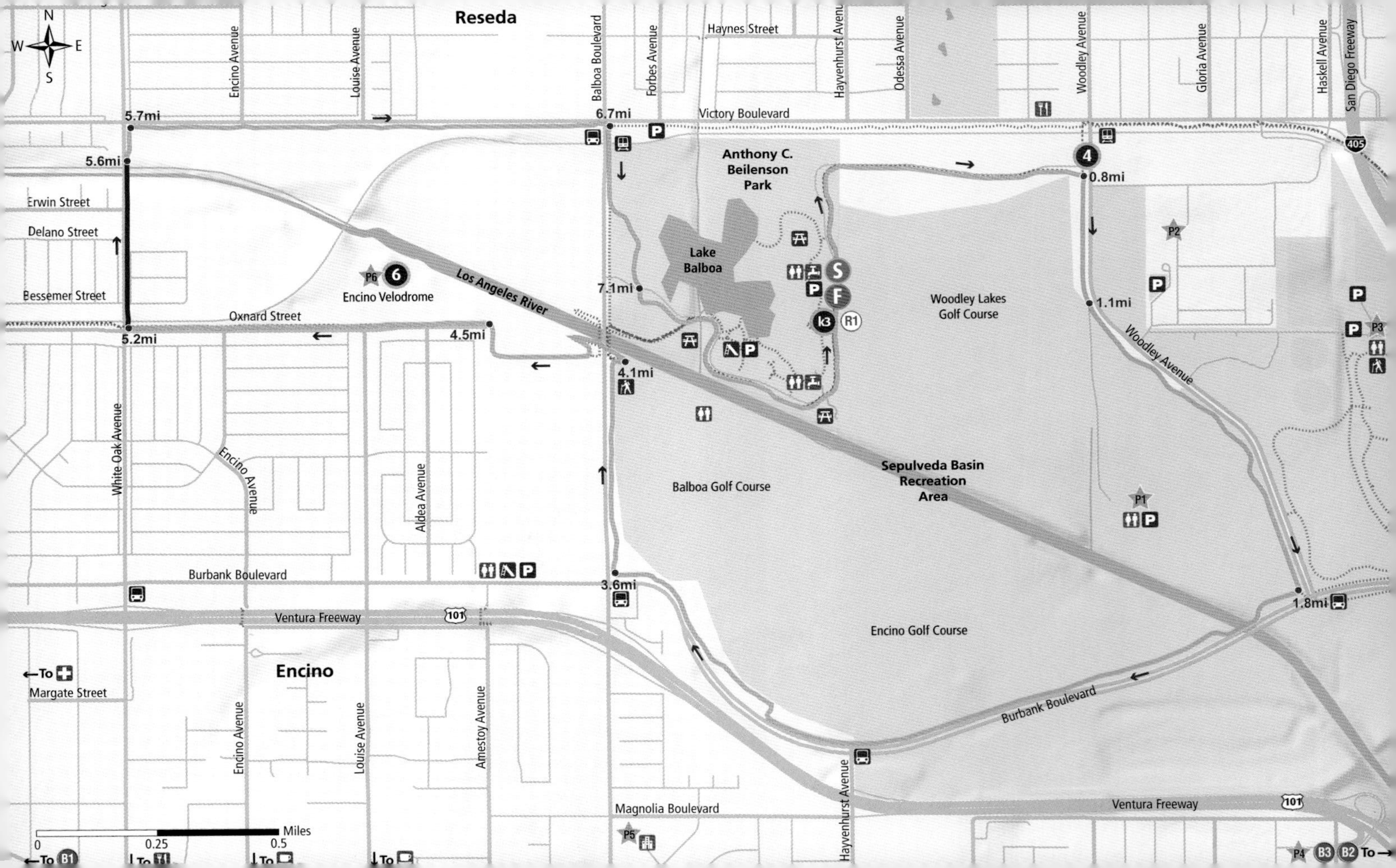

Reseda
Encino
N
E
S
W
Encino Avenue
Louise Avenue
Balboa Boulevard
Forbes Avenue
Haynes Street
Hayvenhurst Avenue
Odessa Avenue
Woodley Avenue
Gloria Avenue
Haskell Avenue
San Diego Freeway
405
Victory Boulevard
5.7mi
6.7mi
5.6mi
Erwin Street
Delano Street
Bessemer Street
Anthony C. Beilenson Park
Lake Balboa
P6
6
Encino Velodrome
Los Angeles River
7.1mi
Oxnard Street
5.2mi
4.5mi
4.1mi
4
0.8mi
1.1mi
P2
P3
Woodley Lakes Golf Course
Woodley Avenue
S
F
k3
R1
White Oak Avenue
Encino Avenue
Aldea Avenue
Balboa Golf Course
Sepulveda Basin Recreation Area
P1
Burbank Boulevard
3.6mi
1.8mi
Ventura Freeway
101
Encino Golf Course
To
Margate Street
Encino Avenue
Louise Avenue
Amestoy Avenue
Burbank Boulevard
Hayvenhurst Avenue
Magnolia Boulevard
P5
Ventura Freeway
101
Miles
0
0.25
0.5
To B1
To
To
To
P4
B3
B2
To

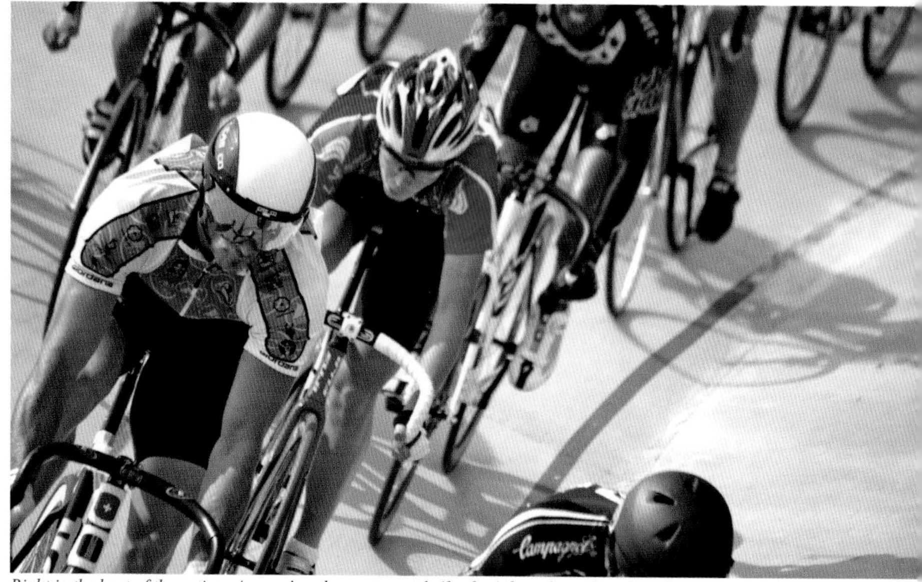

*Right in the heat of the action: Anyone's welcome to watch (for free) from the rails or bleachers.*

## At a Glance

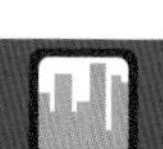

**Distance** 0.2 miles **Elevation Gain** 00.0

### Terrain

This outdoor, oval-shaped track has super-smooth concrete riding surfaces, highlighted by steeply banked turns and straights.

### Traffic

This is a 100% car-free ride.

### How to Get There

Exit the 101 Freeway at White Oak Avenue, head north and turn right onto Oxnard Street. Within half a block, enter just past the "Encino Velodrome" sign on the left. Follow the driveway into the rear parking area. Alternatively, take the Orange Line bus to the Balboa stop, then ride your bike or walk to the track.

### Food and Drink

Concession stands at the nearby baseball fields may be open, but you'll find better eats along Ventura Boulevard, particularly around White Oak Avenue.

### Side Trip

Watching one of the many racing events here is an exciting alternative to riding the track yourself—and it's admission free. The arena's annual highlights include the Hansing Memorial Cup in the spring and the Far West Encino Velodrome Championships in the fall. To combine a spectator experience with your own pre-event workout, pick a departure point, say the North Hollywood Metro station and pedal to the velodrome (for directions, see Ride 4).

**Links to**  

**Where to Bike Rating** 

 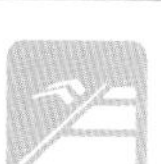 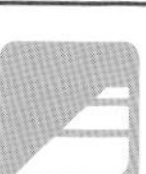 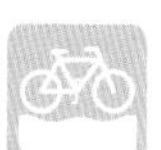

## About...

A velodrome is an arena for track cycling. And the Encino Velodrome is no exception, offering a change of pace, literally and figuratively. The 250-meter circuit combines a pair of short straights with two 180-degree turns. You'll go round and round, sped along by banked surfaces. If you want to try this brand of cycling just for fun, or test your mettle as a track racer, Encino is the perfect place. Start with an introductory lesson. We've found the riders, coaches and instructors here unassuming, friendly and encouraging.

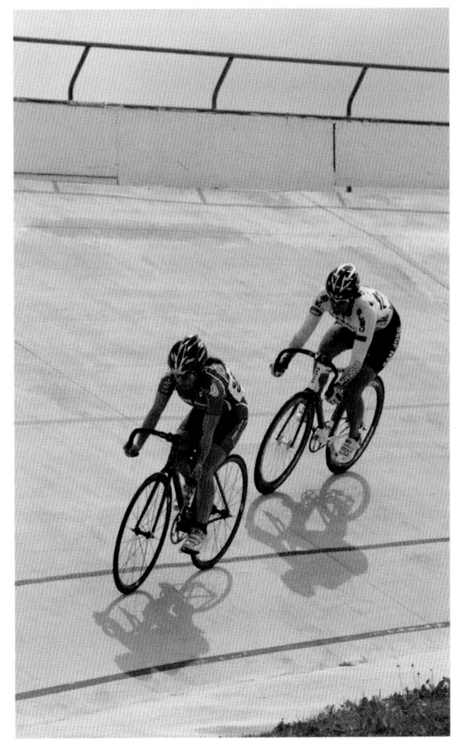

*Women and girls rank among the contenders here.*

The Encino Velodrome was inspired by a conversation among four cycling buddies out on a ride, back in 1953. Over the next few years, George Garner, Bob Hansing, Jack Kemp and Charlie Morton gained the support of friends, the bicycling community, local businesses and the Army Corps of Engineers, and after investing some of their own funds, brought the velodrome to life in 1961. The place became such a hit for riding, training and racing that, only two years later, the original asphalt track got a concrete facelift, yielding an even smoother ride. For more than 50 years, these banked surfaces (28 to 32 degrees in the turns, 15 degrees on the straights) have been legendary in Southern California.

You might ask, can an ordinary rider use the velodrome? The answer is absolutely yes. Encino, like most velodromes, offers a beginners' class for cyclists curious to give track riding a whirl. This course is a 2.5 hour session that costs $40, including the use of a track bike, and is usually taught by Ken Avchen, the velodrome's president. The instructor will teach you to ride track bikes, those fixed gear two-wheelers that don't free wheel, or coast, when you stop pedaling and have no hand brakes. You might gasp—what no brakes! Not to worry, the steeply banked track helps with that: You slow down by riding "up" the track and accelerate by aiming "down" it. You'll also learn track etiquette, safe riding practices and basic racing skills. As the session wraps up, you may get to compete in your first track racing events, such as a "Flying 200," a time trial that pits riders against the clock over the last 200 meters of the course. Another event you might get to try is the Pursuit Race, in which two riders try to overtake one another, beginning from stationary positions on opposite sides of the track.

Completion of the class qualifies you to use the velodrome during the training sessions Monday to Thursday evenings (starting about 5:30 p.m.—the track is lit) and on some weekends. The cost is incredibly modest: $5.00 per session. Bike rentals are correspondingly cheap, at $5.00 per session. For more information, including class and training schedules, visit **www.encinovelodrome.org**.

## Ride Log

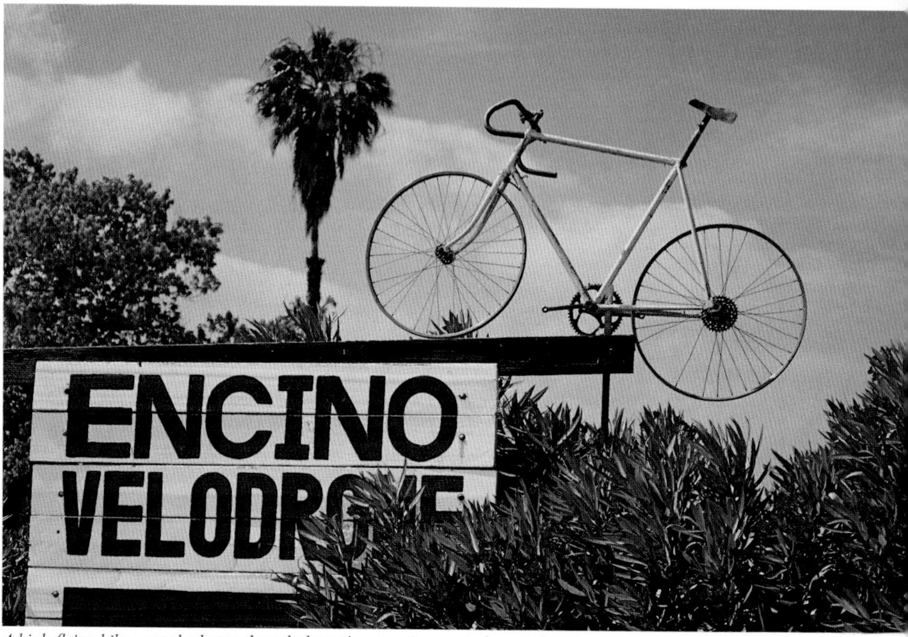


*A high-flying bike—perched atop the velodrome's entry sign—sets the mood.*

**This isn't your regular ride log:** From the office, grandstand and announcer's booth area, open the low gate and, with your bike, cross the track at the start/finish line. Be sure to look to the left for other riders already in motion. From this point, always start with a few laps on the circular warm-up track, riding counter-clockwise. Then, briskly ride onto the main track by crossing the narrow, flat apron (also called the *Côte d'Azur*), entering only on the "home-stretch" side. Watch for other riders from the right. Ride as many laps as you like. When finished, slow and exit onto the warm-up track, but only from the backstretch. Be respectful of other riders by hand signaling before you exit.

 *P1* Sepulveda Basin Recreation Area

 *R1* Encino Velodrome

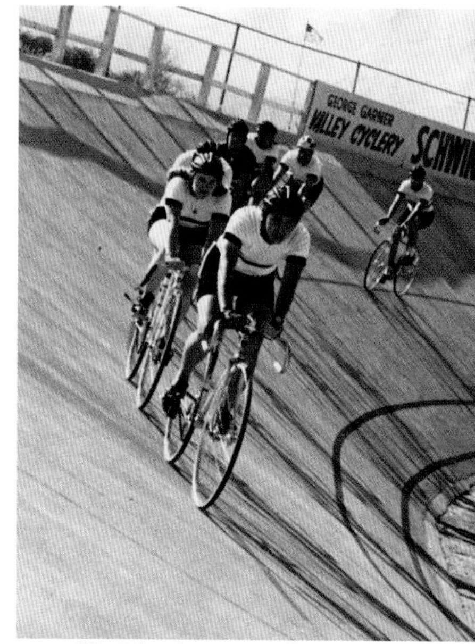


*Wheels have been spinning here since the early '60s.*

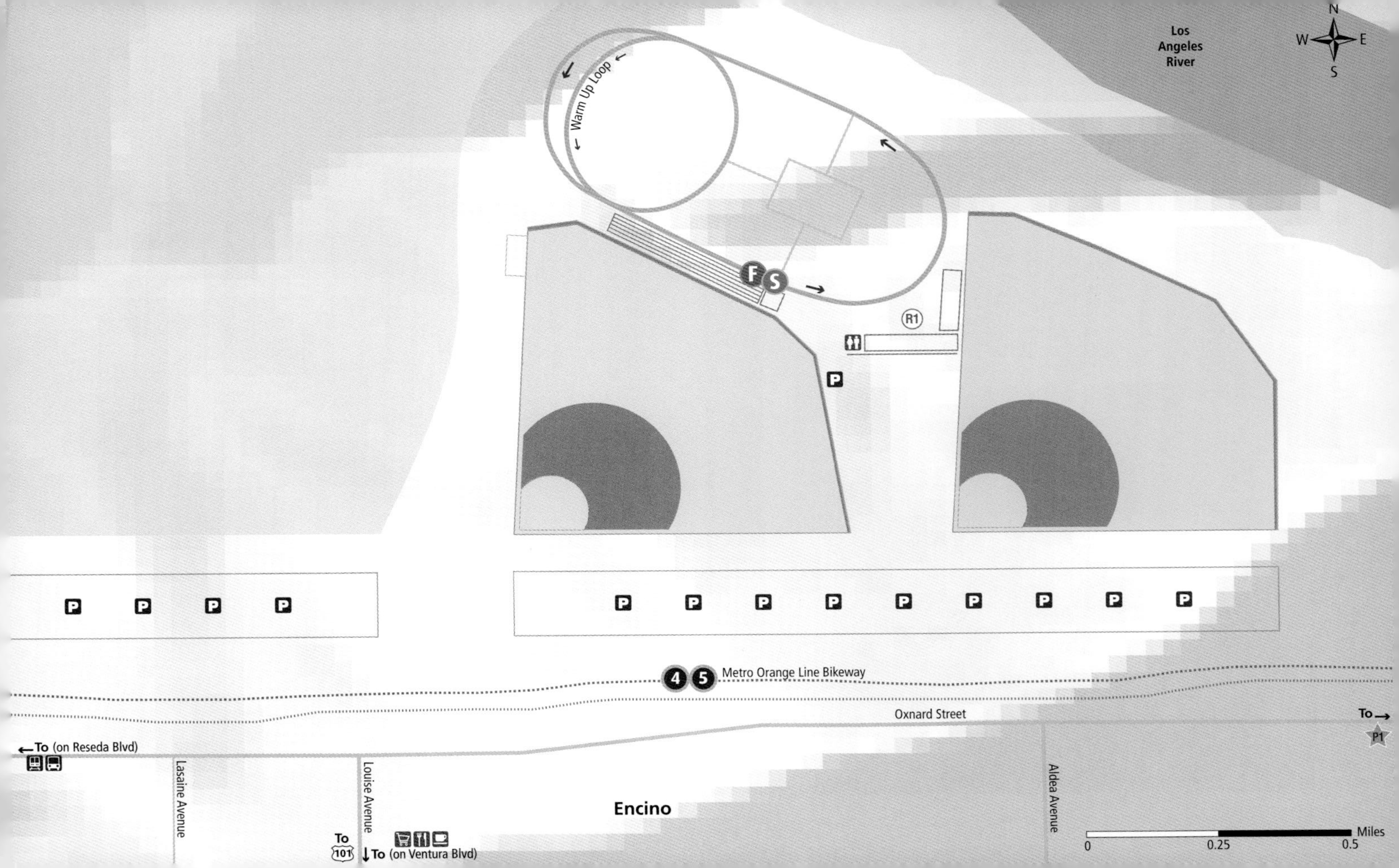
Los Angeles River
N
W
E
S
Warm Up Loop
F
S
R1
P
P
P
P
P
P
P
P
P
P
P
P
P
P
4
5
Metro Orange Line Bikeway
Oxnard Street
To
P1
To (on Reseda Blvd)
Lasaine Avenue
Louise Avenue
Encino
Aldea Avenue
To 101
To (on Ventura Blvd)
0
0.25
0.5
Miles

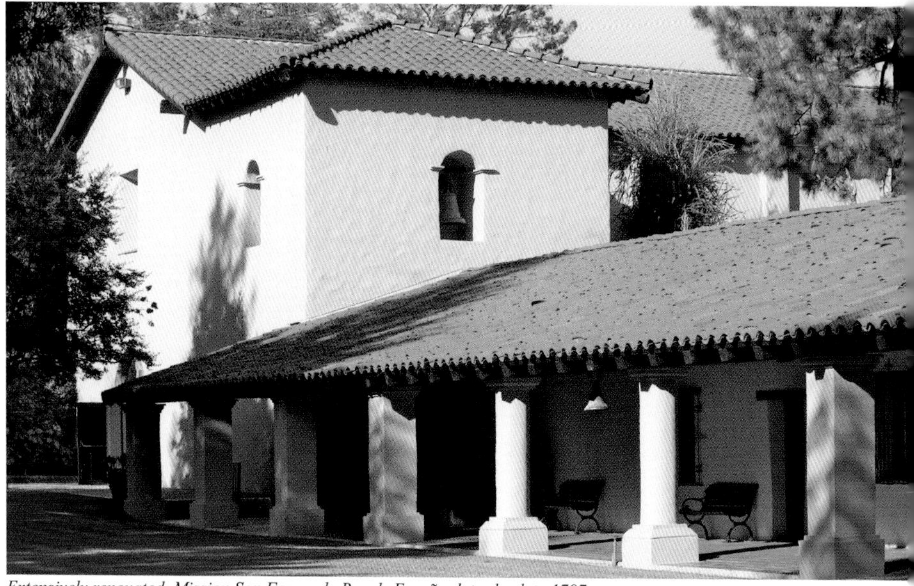

*Extensively renovated, Mission San Fernando Rey de España dates back to 1797.*

## At a Glance

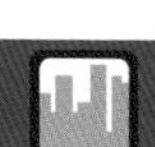

**Distance** 27.0 miles **Elevation Gain** 1,700 feet

### Terrain

The eight-mile stretch on Rinaldi Street undulates over rolling foothills. The rest tends to be flat. The optional climb up Reseda Boulevard to Palisades Park rises about 400 feet over a mile.

### Traffic

Expect typical city traffic on Rinaldi, heavier near access points to the 405 and 5 freeways. The areas near the parks get little traffic.

### How to Get There

Exit the 5 or 405 freeways onto San Fernando Mission Boulevard. Continue northeast to the T, turn left onto Truman Street, right onto Hubbard Avenue and then, an immediate left into Metrolink parking.

### Food and Drink

The Munch Box—an authentic 1950s-era burger stand and cultural heritage site—serves famous hickory burgers, chili-burgers, fries and drinks from a yellow-and-red stand on Devonshire Street in Chatsworth. Its food, service and "vintage" low prices get raves. Elsewhere along the route, you'll find convenience stores, selling 21st century fare.

### Side Trip

Palisades Park in Porter Ranch, a sliver of open space between Reseda Boulevard, Tampa Avenue and Braemore Road, offers panoramic views of the whole San Fernando Valley. Just below the ridgeline, a hiking-equestrian trail runs the length of the park.

**Links to** 

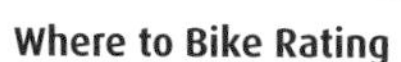

**Where to Bike Rating** 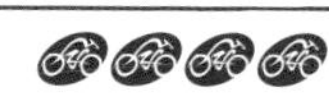

# About...

Rinaldi Street spans nearly the entire San Fernando Valley, extending across its northern edge from the city of San Fernando to the Santa Susana Pass in Chatsworth. At times a mundane residential and commercial artery, its triumph is connecting the historic Mission San Fernando, a nexus of Latino culture at the ride's eastern end, with the Simi Hills' rugged rock formations, chaparral-covered slopes, oak groves, hiking trails and grasslands at this route's western terminus.

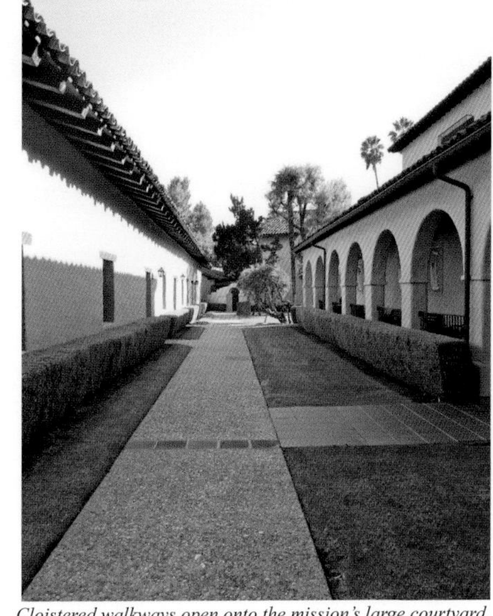

*Cloistered walkways open onto the mission's large courtyard.*

Although the San Fernando Valley, as it's now called, thrived under the Tongva and other indigenous peoples, the region's Spanish "discoverers" overrode the native culture beginning in 1797. That year, Father Fermín Francisco de Lausén founded the Mission San Fernando Rey De España here—a landmark you'll encounter early in this ride.

Between 1769 and 1823, Spain's mission system established itself throughout California to convert native tribes to Catholicism and secure a colonial foothold here. But, after Mexico's successful revolt against Spain, in 1821, a breakdown of the mission system ensued, bringing an avalanche of change: Mission San Fernando, already damaged by the 1812 earthquake (and gold-diggers hacking into the church floor) successively served as Governor Pio Pico's headquarters, a stagecoach station, a water warehouse and even a hog farm. In the 1920s, the sanctuary was finally reclaimed as a church, and later, the Hearst Foundation funded its restoration. The Sylmar earthquake of 1971 prompted yet another round of reconstruction.

Now well tended, the mission is focal to the Latino community, drawing an amazing profusion of weekend wedding and *quinceañera* ("sweet 15") gatherings—here and at Brand Park Memory Garden, directly across the street—amid rose bushes, fountains and pergolas.

From here, the ride proceeds for six miles on Rinaldi Street, an artery with wide bike lanes and occasional glimpses of undeveloped hillsides. At Reseda Boulevard, an optional loop ascends along Palisades Park, through Porter Ranch (once vast pastures, now a planned community) with a panoramic overlook at mile 8.4. After winding through residential Chatsworth, you'll reach Chatsworth Park North—nestled with Chatsworth Park South, Stoney Point Park, Santa Susana Pass State Historic Park and Garden of the Gods at the foot of the Simi Hills.

These rustic parks share scenic traits: massive sandstone outcroppings against native chaparral and oak. The Santa Susana Pass, between the Simi Hills and Santa Susana Mountains, is a vital wildlife corridor for birds, mammals, and reptiles. It was also an essential tribal route for an estimated 8,000 years.

The pass became a 19th century stagecoach road infamous for its "Devil's Slide"—a stretch so precipitous that horses had to be blindfolded to descend and chains used to augment brakes. In the 20th century, the pass was a Western film location. Why not tie up your "steed" and hike an easy piece of this striking terrain?

# Ride Log

**0.0** Start by turning right out of the Metrolink station parking lot, and then right onto Hubbard Ave, cross Truman St and then, make a left onto San Fernando Rd.
**0.5** Turn right onto Workman St.
**1.3** Pass under the 5 Freeway where Workman becomes Rinaldi St. Join the bike lane.
**2.1** Cross Sepulveda Blvd. To reach the San Fernando Mission, turn left onto Sepulveda, then left onto San Fernando Mission Rd. The mission is 0.3 miles down on the left. After visiting it, retrace this route back to Rinaldi.
**6.0** Turn right on Reseda Blvd, joining the bike lane. (But if you prefer a "lowlands" route, avoiding a mile-long climb up Reseda, continue straight on Rinaldi St to Mason Ave, then turn left. If traffic conditions warrant, use the crosswalk at Rinaldi and Mason.)
**7.1** Turn left onto Braemore Rd.
**8.0** Turn right onto Tampa Ave.
**8.3** Turn left onto Sesnon Blvd.
**10.2** Turn left onto Mason Ave.
**11.6** Cross Rinaldi St and continue on Mason Ave.
**12.4** Turn right onto Chatsworth St.
**13.1** Turn left onto Variel Ave.
**13.6** Turn right onto Devonshire St.
**14.7** Turn right onto Valley Circle Blvd.
**15.1** Turn left onto Germain St, then right into Chatsworth Park North. When your are ready to return, exit Chatsworth Park North, make a left onto Germain St, then right onto Valley Circle Blvd.
**15.5** Turn left onto Devonshire St.
**16.6** Turn left onto Variel Ave.

*P1* Forneris Farm Market and Corn Maze
*P2* Aliso Canyon Park
*P3* Palisades Park
*P4* Limekiln Canyon
*P5* The Old Mission Trail
*P6* Homestead Acre/Hill Palmer House
*P7* Chatsworth Park South
*P8* Chatsworth Park North
*P9* Stony Point Park
*P10* Garden of the Gods
*P11* Santa Susana Pass State Historic Park
*P12* The Munch Box
*P13* California State University Northridge
*P14* Mission San Fernando Rey de Espana
*P15* Brand Park Memory Gardens (rose gardens)
*P16* Andres Pico Adobe Park

**17.1** Turn right onto Chatsworth St.
**17.9** Turn left onto Mason Ave at the stoplight.
**18.6** Turn right onto Rinaldi St.
**24.9** Pass under the 405 Freeway.
**25.7** Pass under the 5 Freeway. Bike path ends and Rinaldi St becomes Workman St.
**26.5** Workman St ends. Turn left onto Truman St.
**27.0** Turn right onto Hubbard St, left onto Frank Modugno Dr and then, left into the Metrolink station parking lot. End of ride.

**Note:** *You can combine a one-way trip with a Metrolink leg. But here's the catch: The Chatsworth and Sylmar/San Fernando stations are on different lines, so trip requires a transfer at the Downtown Burbank station (45 minutes on the trains, plus transfer time).*

## San Fernando to Santa Susana Pass

*Please note: the profile for Ride 7 is depicted in 200ft vertical increments due to unusually high elevation.*

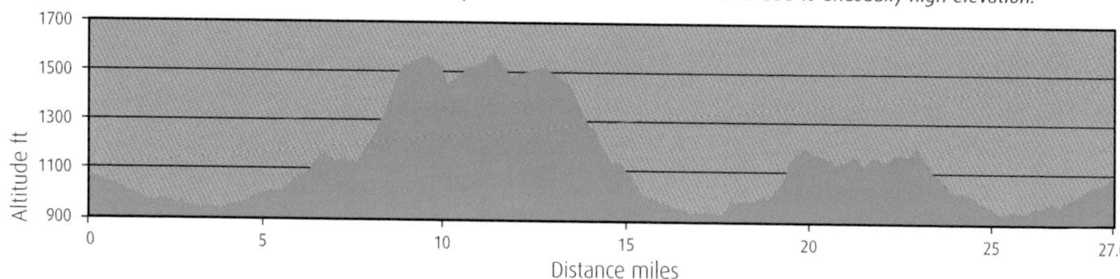

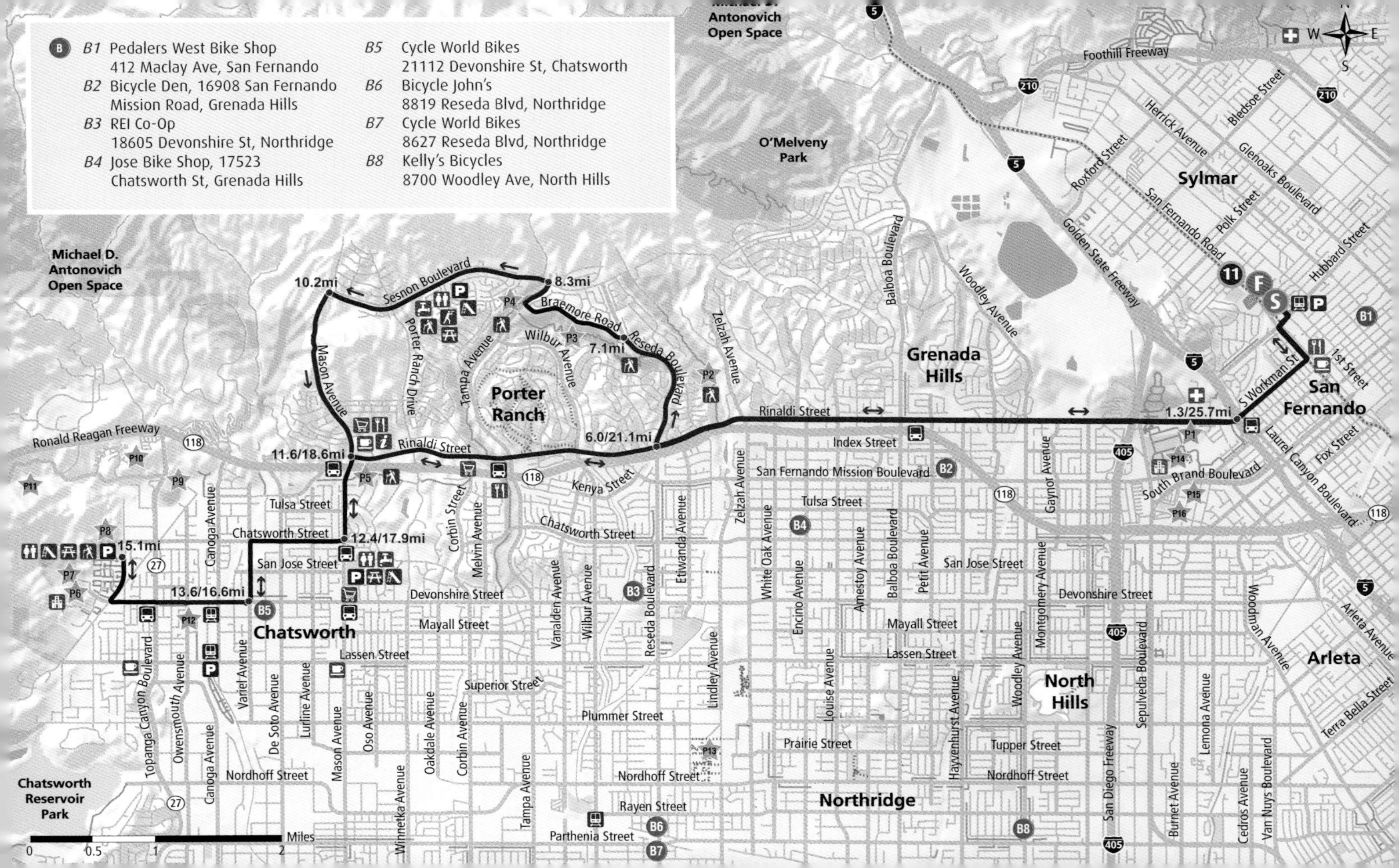

B1 Pedalers West Bike Shop
412 Maclay Ave, San Fernando
B2 Bicycle Den, 16908 San Fernando Mission Road, Grenada Hills
B3 REI Co-Op
18605 Devonshire St, Northridge
B4 Jose Bike Shop, 17523 Chatsworth St, Grenada Hills
B5 Cycle World Bikes
21112 Devonshire St, Chatsworth
B6 Bicycle John's
8819 Reseda Blvd, Northridge
B7 Cycle World Bikes
8627 Reseda Blvd, Northridge
B8 Kelly's Bicycles
8700 Woodley Ave, North Hills
Michael D. Antonovich Open Space
O'Melveny Park
Sylmar
San Fernando
Grenada Hills
Porter Ranch
Chatsworth
North Hills
Northridge
Arleta
Chatsworth Reservoir Park
Foothill Freeway
Golden State Freeway
Ronald Reagan Freeway
San Diego Freeway
Sesnon Boulevard
Mason Avenue
Braemore Road
Reseda Boulevard
Rinaldi Street
Wilbur Avenue
Tampa Avenue
Porter Ranch Drive
Zelzah Avenue
Balboa Boulevard
Woodley Avenue
San Fernando Road
Roxford Street
Herrick Avenue
Bledsoe Street
Glenoaks Boulevard
Polk Street
Hubbard Street
1st Street
S Workman St
Laurel Canyon Boulevard
Fox Street
South Brand Boulevard
Index Street
San Fernando Mission Boulevard
Tulsa Street
Chatsworth Street
San Jose Street
Devonshire Street
Mayall Street
Lassen Street
Superior Street
Plummer Street
Prairie Street
Tupper Street
Nordhoff Street
Rayen Street
Parthenia Street
Kenya Street
Corbin Street
Melvin Avenue
Topanga Canyon Boulevard
Owensmouth Avenue
Canoga Avenue
Variel Avenue
De Soto Avenue
Lurline Avenue
Oso Avenue
Winnetka Avenue
Oakdale Avenue
Corbin Avenue
Vanalden Avenue
Etiwanda Avenue
Lindley Avenue
White Oak Avenue
Encino Avenue
Louise Avenue
Amestoy Avenue
Petit Avenue
Hayvenhurst Avenue
Gaynor Avenue
Montgomery Avenue
Sepulveda Boulevard
Woodman Avenue
Burnet Avenue
Lemona Avenue
Cedros Avenue
Van Nuys Boulevard
Arleta Avenue
Terra Bella Street
1.3/25.7mi
6.0/21.1mi
7.1mi
8.3mi
10.2mi
11.6/18.6mi
12.4/17.9mi
13.6/16.6mi
15.1mi
Miles
0
0.5
1
2

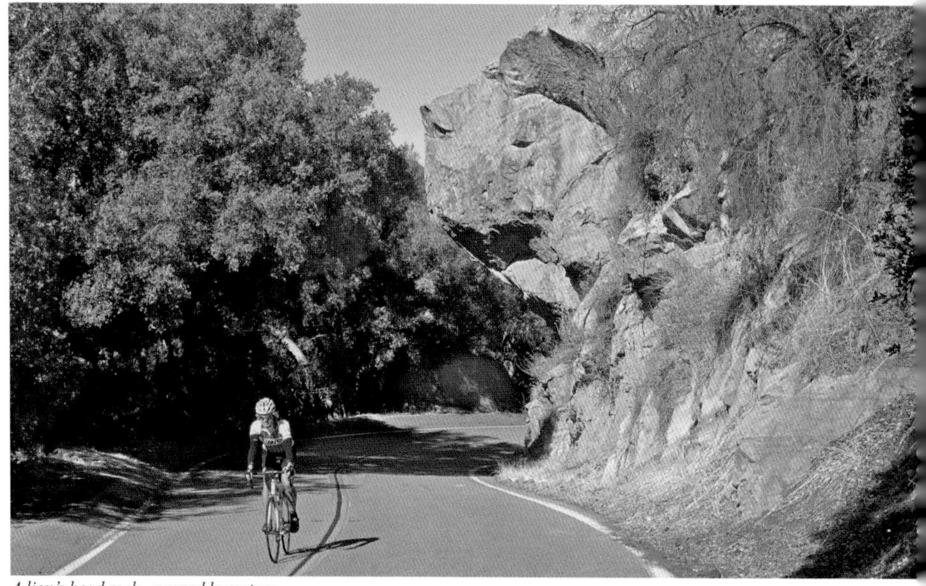

*A lion's head rock—carved by nature.*

## At a Glance

**Distance** 27.2 miles **Elevation Gain** 3,300 feet

### Terrain

With good road surfaces throughout, this ride has three ascents and one long, sweeping downhill—combining rolling coastline with canyon riding.

### Traffic

Expect moderate traffic. The roadway shoulders are usually as wide as bike lanes. Use extra caution through the Malibu Canyon Road tunnel, near the ride's end. The route is best on weekend mornings.

### How to Get There

The start is near Malibu Creek State Park. From the 101 Freeway, exit at Las Virgenes Road and drive about four miles south. Or from Pacific Coast Highway, take Malibu Canyon Road north roughly six miles. Park along Mulholland Highway's shoulder or in the park's paid lot.

### Food and Drink

The Rock Store offers food and drink, but the fare's better at Rustic Canyon General Store & Grill, at the intersection of Sierra Creek and Kanan roads, about three-tenths of a mile north of Mulholland Highway. Rustic has tasty BBQ, burgers and snacks.

### Side Trip

To glimpse at Malibou Lake, its lodge and weekend retreat cabins, once a hunting and fishing club (founded in 1922), turn left onto Lake Vista Drive for about a mile. (This stunning setting has appeared in many movies, including *The Postman Always Rings Twice*, in 1946.)

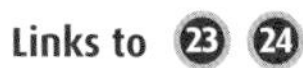

**Where to Bike Rating** 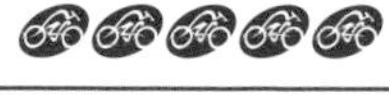

 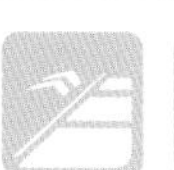  

# About...

Named for the famous Rock Store Café, where motorcyclists and sports car drivers congregate, this ride along the San Gabriel Valley's southwest edge explores the rural countryside at the western end of the Santa Monica Mountains. Cyclists frequent these roads daily. The centerpiece of this bicycling adventure is the legendary, serpentine Rock Store Climb, out of the valley towards the ocean—but the refreshing six-mile cruise that follows, along the ocean to Malibu and Malibu Canyon Road, is also great in its own right.

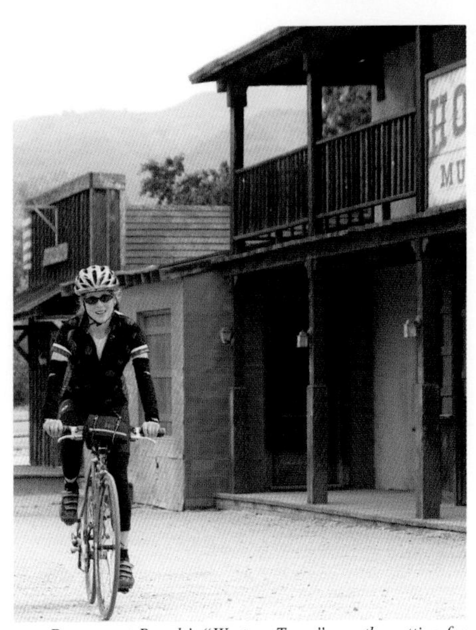

*Paramount Ranch's "Western Town" was the setting for many Hollywood movies.*

As you ride north on Mulholland Highway from the start at Malibu Creek, you might recognize the jagged peaks to your left. Think Korean War, tents and the whoop-whoop of helicopters….Yes, this was the film location for the popular TV show M*A*S*H during its 11-season run. You can actually hike to the rusting remains of the set, in Malibu Creek State Park, formerly the 20th Century Fox movie ranch. And this isn't the only bit of Hollywood history you'll pass along Mulholland Highway. Also out here is Paramount Ranch, Paramount Pictures' Western-town backlot, now in the Santa Monica Mountains National Recreation Area.

Further along Triunfo Valley, past Malibou Lake, once a hunting and fishing club, and Peter Strauss Ranch, an oak woodlands park, you'll arrive at the Rock Store, a famous watering hole. Originally a stagecoach stop, hewn from volcanic stone, this hangout is crowded every weekend with leather-clad and leather-skinned bikers (as in motorcyclists) riding the mountain and canyon roads to see and be seen. Bicyclists also come here on weekends, but typically for the fabled 2.5-mile Rock Store Climb that starts a few hundred yards west of the café.

This famous ascent was part of the Tour of California. And it is the course for the home grown Rock Store Time Trial (see: **rockstoretimetrial.com**), challenging riders *contre la montre* (against the clock) in early evening two or three times each summer. Though you may feel tempted to test yourself against the best times (typically in the 11 to 12-minute range), we encourage a more leisurely pace because the eight switchbacks beneath oak-tree canopies are downright enjoyable and the valley panoramas not to be missed.

After the climb, the course turns south on Kanan Dume Road, where a hiccup of an uphill leads to a six-mile downhill to the ocean. Mind your speed, of course. At Pacific Coast Highway, the route turns west for a leisurely, undulating spin along the ocean. A left-hand turn at Pepperdine University takes you onto Malibu Canyon Road for more than five miles of majestic canyon riding. Several turnouts along this stretch overlook red rock formations, the canyon and Malibu Creek: all amazing landscapes that register seasonal change, most strikingly with bright green hillsides, wildflowers and flowing streams in spring; bright red, orange and yellow leaves in the fall.

# Ride Log

P1 Malibu Creek State Park
P2 The TV show M*A*S*H*'s filming location
P3 King Gillette Ranch Park
P4 Paramount Ranch
P5 Malibou Lake
P6 Peter Strauss Ranch
P7 Rustic Canyon General Store & Grill
P8 The Rock Store
P9 Rocky Oaks Park
P10 Zuma Beach
P11 Paradise Cove
P12 Malibu Bluffs Park
P13 Tapia County Park
P14 Escondido Canyon Park

B1 Sundance Cycles
5019 Kanan Road, Agoura Hills
B2 Bicycle John's
29041 Thousand Oaks Blvd, Agoura Hills
B3 Win's Wheels
30941 Agoura Rd, Westlake Village
B4 Cycle Design at Malibu
29575 Pacific Coast Highway, Malib

**0.0** From Las Virgenes Rd, ride across the low bridge over Malibu Creek west on Mulholland Hwy.

**1.8** Summit.

**3.2** Pass Lake Vista Dr/Cornell Rd (turn right to Paramount Ranch, left to Malibou Lake).

**5.1** Pass Peter Strauss Ranch.

**5.4** Pass Sierra Creek Rd.

**5.8** Pass the Rock Store. Begin the Rock Store climb.

**8.5** Summit.

**8.8** Turn left on Kanan Dume Rd. Cross traffic does not stop, so exercise extreme caution at this intersection.

**15.0** Turn left on Pacific Coast Hwy.

**16.0** Pass the entrance to Paradise Cove beach.

**20.9** Turn left on Malibu Canyon Rd.

**23.7** Summit (no more climbing!).

**24.4** Pass through the tunnel. There's a single traffic lane in each direction through the tunnel, so exercise extreme caution.

**27.2** Turn left on Mulholland Hwy. End of the ride.

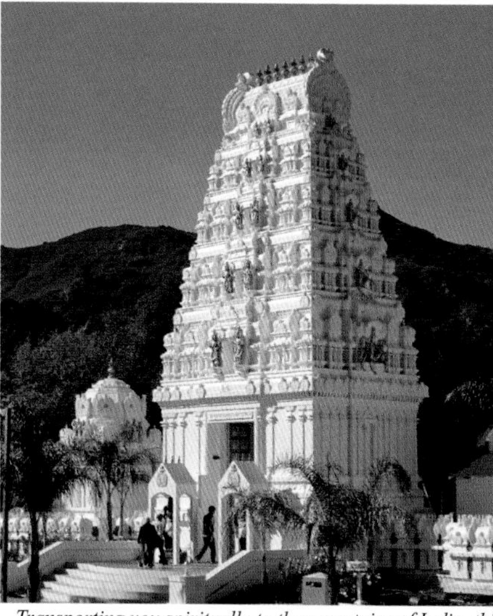

*Transporting you spiritually to the mountains of India, this Hindu temple complex (ca. 1981) is near Calabasas.*

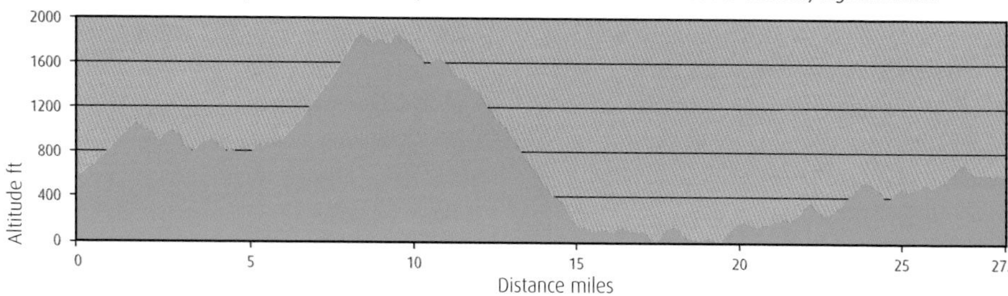

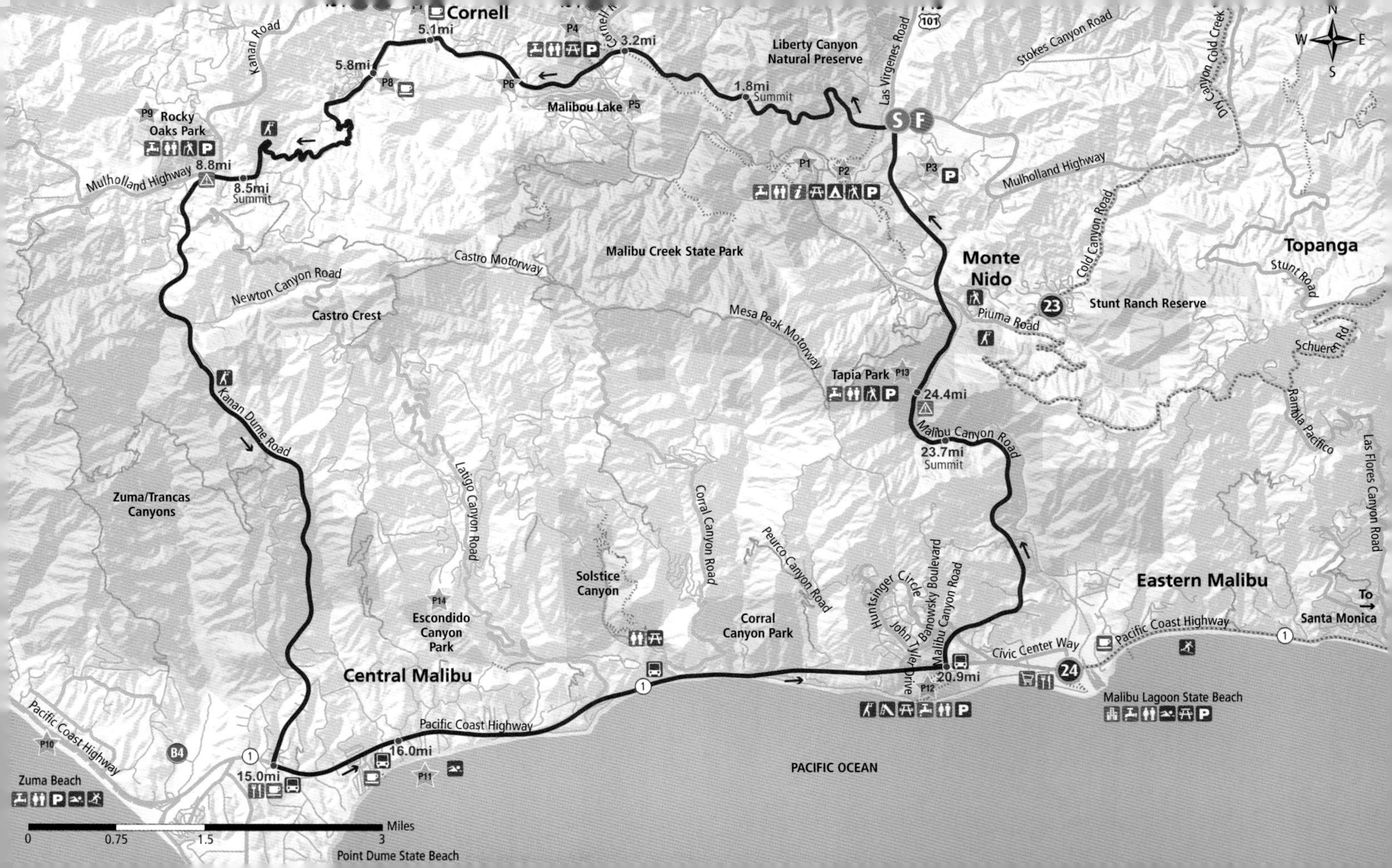
Cornell
5.1mi
5.8mi
P8
P4
3.2mi
P6
Liberty Canyon
Natural Preserve
Las Virgenes Road
101
Stokes Canyon Road
Dry Canyon Cold Creek
1.8mi
Summit
Malibou Lake
P5
Kanan Road
P9
Rocky
Oaks Park
Mulholland Highway
8.8mi
8.5mi
Summit
P1
P2
P3
Mulholland Highway
Cold Canyon Road
Topanga
Stunt Road
Malibu Creek State Park
Castro Motorway
Newton Canyon Road
Castro Crest
Monte
Nido
Piuma Road
23
Stunt Ranch Reserve
Schueren Rd
Mesa Peak Motorway
Tapia Park
P13
24.4mi
Rambla Pacifico
Kanan Dume Road
Malibu Canyon Road
23.7mi
Summit
Las Flores Canyon Road
Zuma/Trancas
Canyons
Latigo Canyon Road
Corral Canyon Road
Peurco Canyon Road
Solstice
Canyon
Huntsinger Circle
Banowsky Boulevard
Malibu Canyon Road
John Tyler Drive
Eastern Malibu
To
Santa Monica
P14
Escondido
Canyon
Park
Corral
Canyon Park
Pacific Coast Highway
Civic Center Way
24
20.9mi
P12
Malibu Lagoon State Beach
Central Malibu
1
Pacific Coast Highway
Pacific Coast Highway
P10
B4
16.0mi
15.0mi
P11
PACIFIC OCEAN
Zuma Beach
Miles
0
0.75
1.5
3
Point Dume State Beach

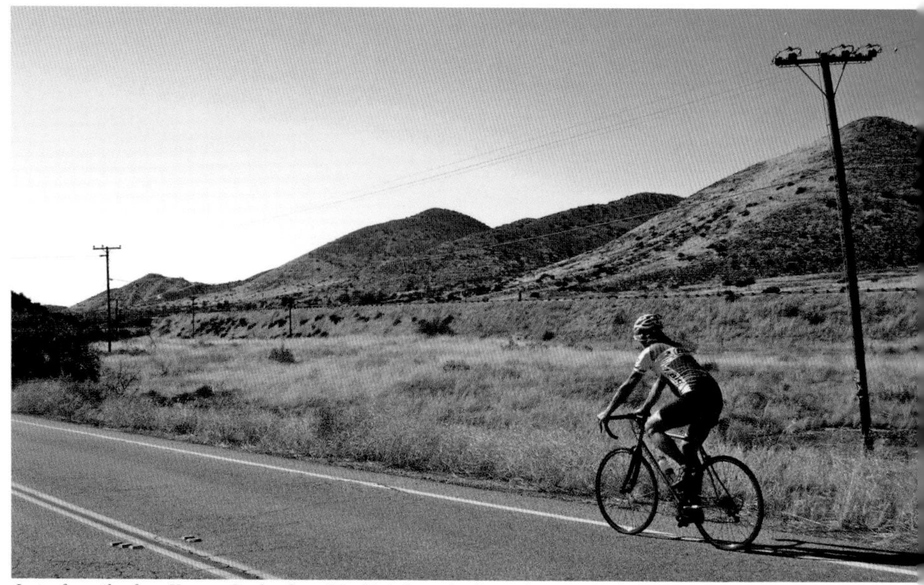

*Just a few miles from Vasquez Rocks, the golden high desert landscape has an entirely different character.*

## At a Glance

**Distance** 23.3 miles **Elevation Gain** 1,800 feet

### Terrain

These undulating, high desert country roads are in good condition. The only sustained climb is just beyond Acton. Occasionally, stiff afternoon winds can turn "flats into hills" or "downhills into flats."

### Traffic

Maybe cars outnumber tumbleweeds in these parts, but just barely. These back roads have very little traffic, even on weekends.

### How to Get There

Vasquez Rocks Natural Area Park is outside the small town of Agua Dulce. Exit the 14 Freeway north onto Agua Dulce Canyon Road. Continue north approximately one and one-half miles, then turn right onto Morgan Road to the park.

### Food and Drink

The old Western town of Agua Dulce (meaning "sweet water," in Spanish) naturally has a Sweetwater Café, a laid-back place with a 13-page menu (listing items from coffee and nibbles to full entrees). Drinks are served in mason jars. The town also has a general store where you can buy cold drinks and snacks.

### Side Trip

Consider scheduling a mid-ride break at Shambala Preserve, founded in 1983 by actress Tippi Hedren. This sanctuary for more than 60 big cats—including lions, tigers, leopards and cougars—rescues exotic felines from harsh conditions and gives them a natural habitat. The preserve is open once a month for safari-like tours (**www.shambala.org**).

**Where to Bike Rating** 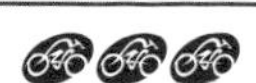

 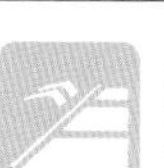  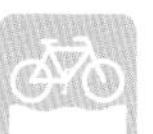

# About...

Set in the eastern Santa Clarita Valley, this ride winds through scenic desert landscapes: dry river washes, hillsides thick with sagebrush and, most famously, tawny gray and red sandstone formations, dramatically tilted up by millions of years of earthquake activity. Encircling Parker Mountain, this journey first heads eastward, through a canyon cut by the Santa Clara River en route from its headwaters, in the San Gabriel Mountains. In the old gold-mining town of Acton, the ride turns west, heading to another vintage town, Agua Dulce.

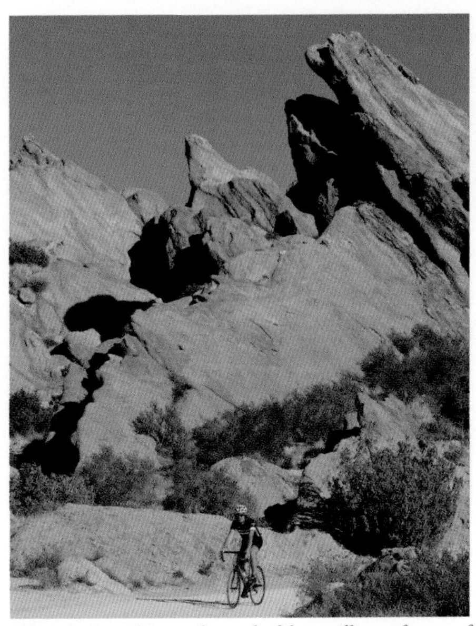

*Great jutting, tilting rocks resulted from millions of years of earthquake activity.*

As you unload the bikes and gear up, it's hard not to be mesmerized by this landscape. Huge tilted rocks in grays and reds jut up from the ground. The steeply canted sandstone formations look like scenery straight out of a Western saga. And, as a matter of fact, they are. Vasquez Rocks provided the backdrop for the real-life drama of the notorious bandito Tiburcio Vasquez, who holed up here during the 1870s. And then, beginning in the1930s, this same area became a filming location for dozens of Westerns and, later, other films and even TV shows, from *The Flintstones* and *Planet of the Apes* movies to *Star Trek* episodes. But the story of Mr. Vasquez, for whom this place was named, remains as dramatic as any fiction. While this handsome, guitar-playing outlaw was busy building a reputation with the *señoras* and *señoritas* for his dance moves and charms as a buckaroo, he was robbing, pillaging, kidnapping and killing his way through California. In 1874, after 20 years of this wild living, he was captured near Hollywood, charged with multiple murders, convicted and hanged the following year in San Jose. He remains a folk hero for his dashing exploits and because he championed Hispanic and Mexican-American rights.

Rolling out from Tiburcio's former hang-out, you'll descend to Soledad Canyon Road, aptly named because it traverses some pretty remote territory. The road cuts a line between radically different geologies: sandstone formations to the north and granite-strewn San Gabriel foothills to the south. The Santa Clara River occasionally flows through this canyon, too, but only after severe summer thunderstorms or long winters of rain and mountain snowfall.

For the next 10 miles, the road through Soledad Canyon climbs gradually. Soon after the 14-mile marker, you'll blow into the small town of Acton, a gold- and copper-mining hub, once promoted to become the new state capital. Nowadays it makes a good waypoint. The 49er Bar and Grill, on Crown Valley Road just north of Soledad Canyon Road, has been in business since 1889, offering saloon fare (burgers, cold drinks and rye whiskey). You'll still find a hitching post (aka: bike rack) out front. From here, the climb continues about four more miles before you descend into the Sierra Pelona Valley, a rift created by the same seismic forces that formed Vasquez Rocks.

# Ride Log

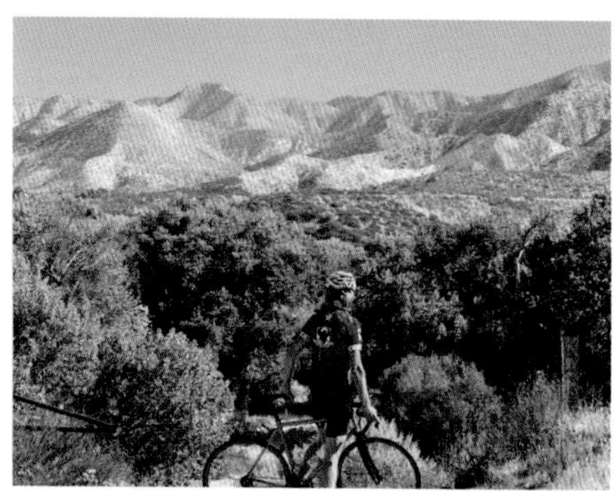

*A few miles from Vasquez Rocks, cottonwoods give way to the San Gabriel Mountains' bald peaks.*

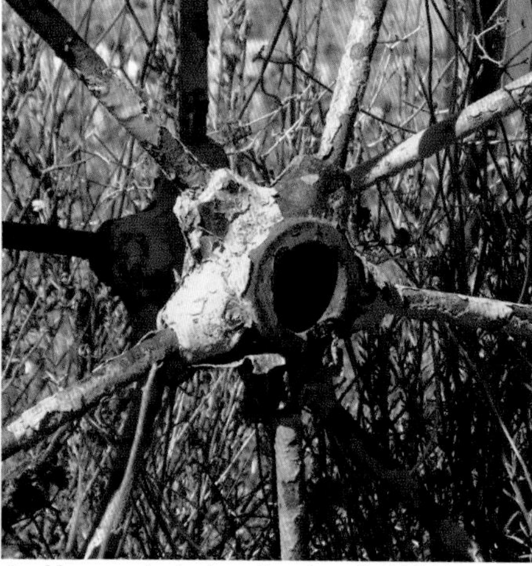

*An old wagon wheel echoes the colors of wild field grasses.*

**0.0** From the entrance of Vasquez Rocks Natural Area Park, turn left and start pedaling west along Escondido Canyon Rd.

**0.6** Turn left after the stop sign, continuing on Agua Dulce Canyon Rd.

**2.2** Cross under the 14 Freeway.

**4.5** Turn left onto Soledad Canyon Rd.

**10.0** Shambala Preserve.

**12.2** Angle to the right onto Crown Valley Rd, running parallel to Soledad Canyon Rd.

**14.4** Cross Soledad Canyon Rd.

**14.8** Turn left onto Syracuse Ave, which becomes Escondido Canyon Rd at Acton Park (where you'll find shade, restrooms and drinking water).

**17.6** Pass Ward Rd.

**21.0** Cross over the 14 Freeway.

**23.3** Arrive at Vasquez Rocks Park. End of ride.

P *P1* Vasquez Rocks Park
*P2* Agua Dulce
*P3* Rio Cafe and Grocery
*P4* Shambala Preserve
*P5* Acton Wash Wildlife Sanctuary
*P6* Acton
*P7* Agua Dulce Winery

B *B1* Bicycle John's
26635 Valley Circle Dr, Santa Clarita.

## Vasquez Rocks

*Please note: the profile for Ride 9 is depicted in 300ft vertical increments due to unusually high elevation.*

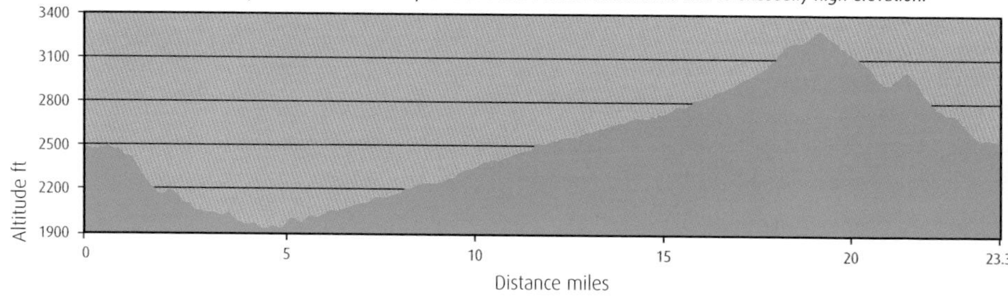

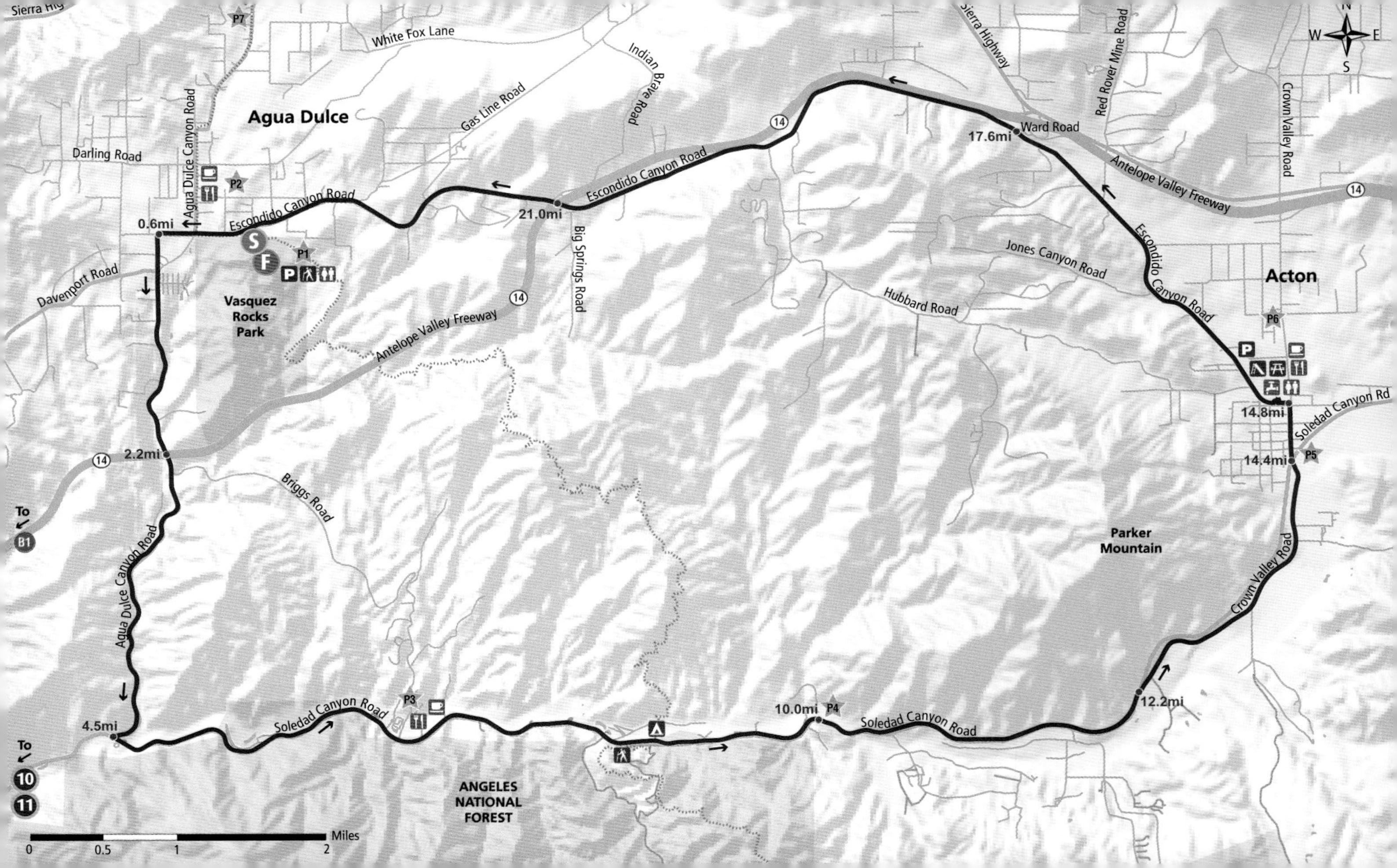

Agua Dulce
Acton
Parker Mountain
Vasquez Rocks Park
ANGELES NATIONAL FOREST
White Fox Lane
Indian Brave Road
Gas Line Road
Darling Road
Agua Dulce Canyon Road
Escondido Canyon Road
Davenport Road
Antelope Valley Freeway
Big Springs Road
Sierra Highway
Red Rover Mine Road
Ward Road
Crown Valley Road
Jones Canyon Road
Hubbard Road
Soledad Canyon Rd
Soledad Canyon Road
Briggs Road
14
0.6mi
2.2mi
4.5mi
10.0mi
12.2mi
14.4mi
14.8mi
17.6mi
21.0mi
P1
P2
P3
P4
P5
P6
P7
S
F
P
To B1
To 10 11
Miles
0
0.5
1
2
N
E
S
W

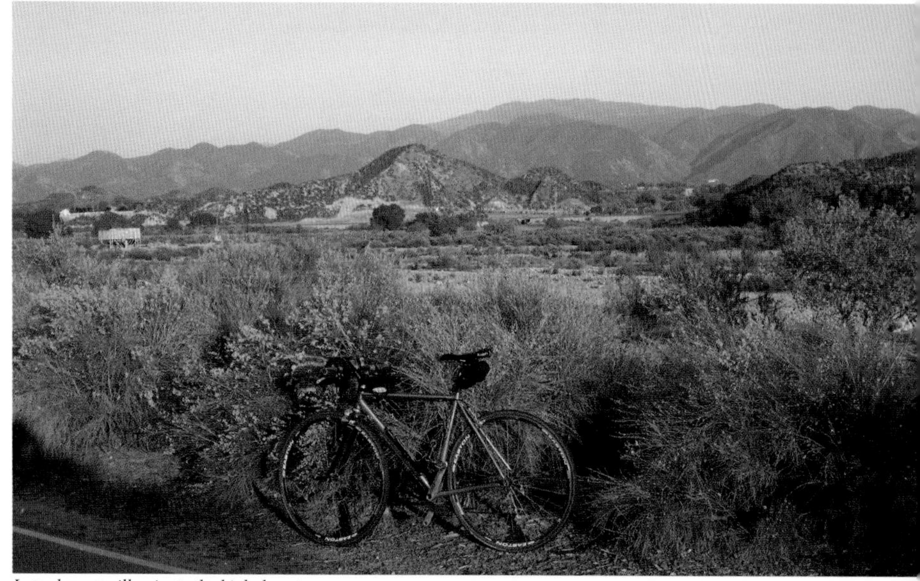

*Late-day rays illuminate the high desert.*

## At a Glance

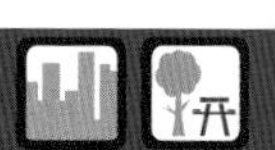

**Distance** 24.9 miles **Elevation Gain** 1,300 feet

### Terrain

Throughout Santa Clarita, the bike paths are smooth asphalt or concrete. There's one moderate hill, up Golden Valley Road, and small grade changes where the paths cross under boulevards.

### Traffic

Except for two short sections, this ride follows a network of bike paths lacing through the valley.

### How to Get There

Exit the 5 Freeway onto Magic Mountain Parkway eastbound. Turn left onto McBean Parkway and then, left into the shopping center at the next traffic light. Park just north of McDonald's in the lot by the river. Or, take Metrolink's Antelope Valley line to Santa Clarita's station, cross Soledad Canyon Road and begin the Cloverleaf there.

### Food and Drink

Wolf Creek Restaurant and Brewing Company, at Decoro Drive and McBean Parkway, is a local microbrewery with pleasant food, drinks and outdoor seating—a good après-ride stop.

### Side Trip

Visit La Loma de los Vientos, the former ranch of William S. Hart, who starred in 65 silent movies, mostly Westerns, filmed nearby. The property is now a park with picnic grounds, hiking trails, a barnyard and a museum of period artifacts and Western art. The herd of bison descended from a gift by Walt Disney.

**Links to** 11 k1 k2

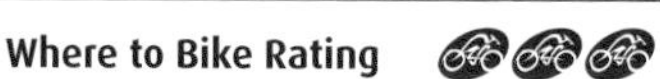

**Where to Bike Rating**

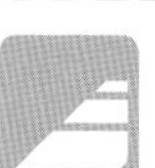

# About...

Our Dali-esque four-leaf clover traces the banks of the Santa Clara River and two of its tributaries through the Santa Clarita Valley. Unlike the rivers in the L.A. Basin, this one, also often a dry riverbed, remains largely in its natural state (i.e. not "channelized" in concrete). Sure, it has some strategically placed boulders and spillways, but otherwise the Santa Clara—a sandy, gravelly desert arroyo amid cottonwoods and rolling hills—probably appears much as it did to the first settlers who arrived here in the mid-1800s.

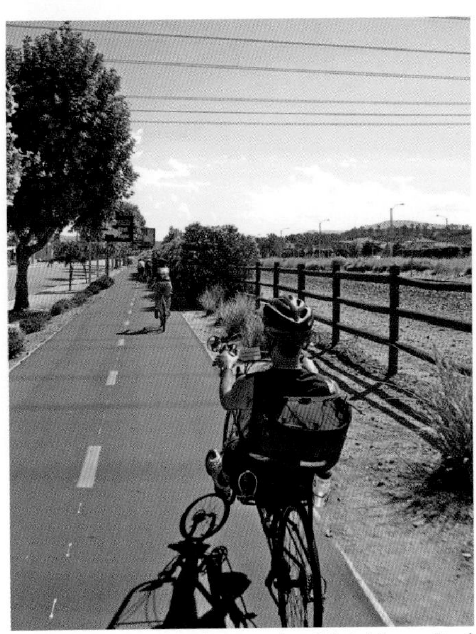

*Recumbent and upright, riders coast along Soledad Canyon Road.*

The Santa Clarita bike paths often form dividing lines between the tame and the seemingly wild: On one side are intermittent spurts of development (low-rise housing and shopping) and on the other, wide open terrain with hilly ranchland rolling out to the horizon.

As cities go, Santa Clarita is young, formed in 1987 through the union of the communities of Saugus, Newhall, Valencia and Canyon Country. But this valley's modern history actually began in 1875 when railroad baron Henry Newhall purchased the 46,460-acre Rancho San Francisco for two dollars an acre. Over subsequent decades, farming, ranching, oil-drilling, moviemaking and, ultimately, subdivision happened here.

As you pedal along, you'll encounter past and present. An 1898 rail bridge near the start now carries only cyclists and hikers. Fences reminiscent of the old San Francisquito Creek corrals edge the bike path. Tesoro Adobe, once home to silent Western superstar Harry Carey, and La Loma de los Vientos, the ranch of his silver-screen colleague William S. Hart, are now both memento-filled museums with grounds turned into county parks.

The beauty of this ride is the experience of the spare high-desert landscape. Late fall is an especially good time, when the leaves on the arroyos' ubiquitous cottonwoods turn bright yellow: brilliant flashes of color against the pale tawny terrain.

The Cloverleaf—an ultra-loosely formed four-leaf clover—offers the possibility of longer or shorter rides and multiple reconfigurations (for example, you can essentially clip it into a three-, two- or one-leaf clover, as desired). One option is a simple loop on the San Francisquito Trail. Another short loop combines the Santa Clara River Trail and Golden Valley Road from McBean Parkway. Or the South Fork and Santa Clara River trails can each become an enjoyable "out-and-back" spin with the turnaround near Orchard Village Road or Whites Canyon Road, respectively.

Of course, if one four-leaf clover isn't quite enough, you can extend the "stem" into a longer ride, popular with local cyclists, by continuing east from Whites Canyon Road along Soledad Canyon Road. The trail follows the river for several miles, entering less and less populated high-desert terrain. A good destination for this elongated route is Acton, with a rest stop at Acton Park and refreshments at the 49er Bar & Grill.

*While Ride 10 has not been deemed kid-friendly in its entirety, it does include substantial sections which are entirely safe for family use.*

# Ride Log

**0.0** Leave the parking lot, enter the South Fork Trail and ride west toward Six Flags Magic Mountain.
**0.5** Turn left just before the pocket park and follow the drive out to Magic Mountain Pkwy. You may have to walk around the low access gate.
**0.6** Turn right onto Magic Mountain Pkwy.
**0.9** Angle to the right, down a small ramp, then ride along a short dirt path to the old railroad bridge. By the time you read this, the city may have paved a path to the bridge.
**1.1** Turn right onto the San Francisquito Creek Trail.
**2.4** The trail stops. Ride up the ramp. At the top, turn left and ride north to Ave Tibbets/Dickason Dr. Cross Newhall Ranch Rd using the crosswalk. Turn right and ride along the sidewalk to re-enter the San Francisquito Creek Trail.
**3.5** Cross under Decoro Dr.
**5.0** Exit the bike trail where it stops. Cross the creek on Copper Hill Rd and turn right where the San Francisquito Creek Trail resumes.
**6.3** Cross under Decoro Dr.
**8.1** Bike trail stops. Turn left onto the short concrete walk then left onto the sidewalk running along McBean Pkwy. Cross at Ave Scott/Bridgeport Ln using the crosswalk. Make a right and ride along the sidewalk to the Santa Clara River Trail.
**9.6** Turn right onto bike path parallel to Newhall Ranch Rd and then right onto the Santa Clara River Trail.
**10.2** Cross under Bouquet Canyon Rd. Continue on the bike trail as it turns to the left and then parallels Newhall Ranch Rd.
**10.6** Stay to the left at the Y in the path, begin ride up the hill.
**12.3** Make a right onto Valley Center Dr.
**12.7** Cross Soledad Canyon Rd at the signal. Turn left onto the Chuck Pontius Commuter Rail Trail, parallel to Soledad Canyon Rd.
**14.5** Angle to the right for a short distance, then make a U-turn and return along the Chuck Pontius Commuter Rail Trail.
**16.9** Cross Soledad Canyon Rd via the crosswalk where the trail stops, opposite Santa Clarita Bowling Lanes. The bike path resumes parallel to the sidewalk.
**18.7** The path curves behind some local businesses, then crosses under Bouquet Canyon Rd.
**19.1** Angle to the right at the Y, just before the Mercedes Benz dealership.
**19.4** Pass the William S. Hart baseball fields.
**19.6** Turn right at Valencia Blvd and continue on the bike path across South Fork.
**19.7** Turn right down a short ramp, then right onto the South Fork Trail and then, pass under Valencia Blvd.
**21.9** Arrive at a pathway intersection (there's a wooden bike bridge on the left). This is the turnaround point. Return by the same route on the South Fork of the Santa Clara River.
**23.9** Cross under Valencia Blvd and then, continue straight on the South Fork Trail.
**24.9** Cross under McBean Pkwy and then, turn left into the parking area. End of ride.

**Santa Clarita: The Cloverleaf**

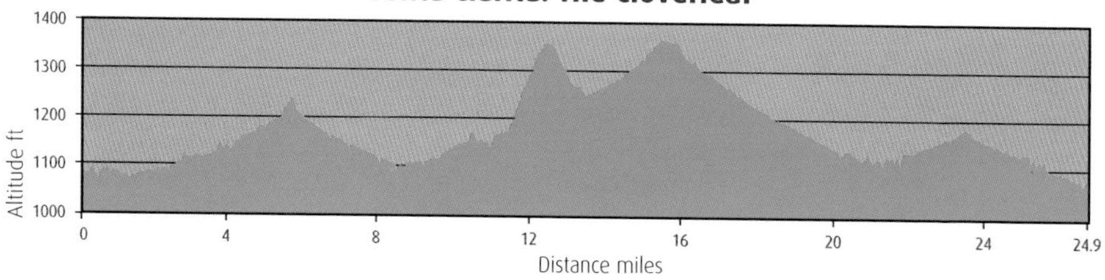

Altitude ft: 1000, 1100, 1200, 1300, 1400
Distance miles: 0, 4, 8, 12, 16, 20, 24, 24.9

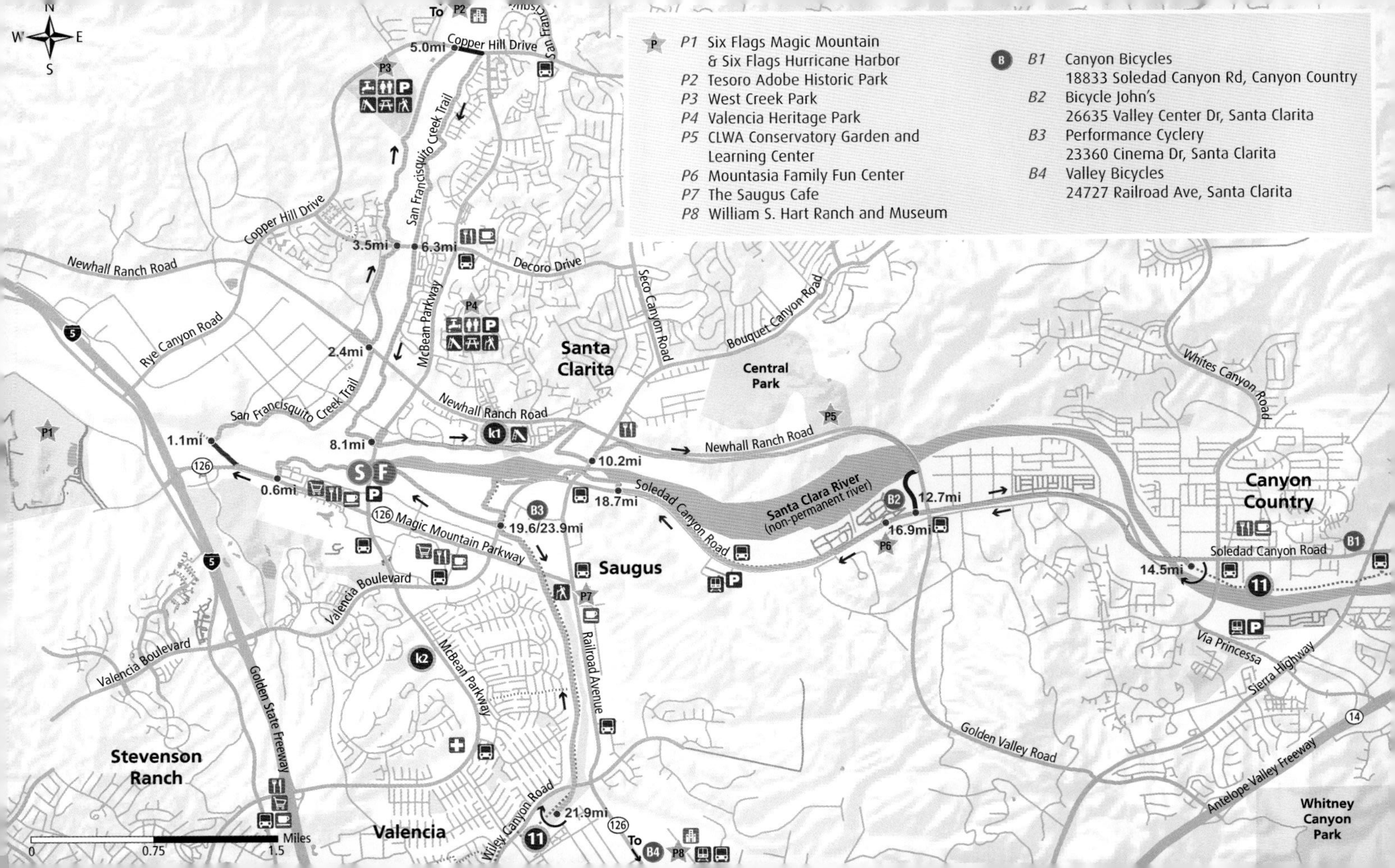
P1 Six Flags Magic Mountain & Six Flags Hurricane Harbor
P2 Tesoro Adobe Historic Park
P3 West Creek Park
P4 Valencia Heritage Park
P5 CLWA Conservatory Garden and Learning Center
P6 Mountasia Family Fun Center
P7 The Saugus Cafe
P8 William S. Hart Ranch and Museum
B1 Canyon Bicycles
18833 Soledad Canyon Rd, Canyon Country
B2 Bicycle John's
26635 Valley Center Dr, Santa Clarita
B3 Performance Cyclery
23360 Cinema Dr, Santa Clarita
B4 Valley Bicycles
24727 Railroad Ave, Santa Clarita
To P2
Copper Hill Drive
5.0mi
San Francisquito Creek Trail
3.5mi
6.3mi
Newhall Ranch Road
Decoro Drive
McBean Parkway
Rye Canyon Road
2.4mi
Santa Clarita
Seco Canyon Road
Bouquet Canyon Road
Central Park
Whites Canyon Road
1.1mi
8.1mi
10.2mi
0.6mi
18.7mi
Soledad Canyon Road
Santa Clara River
(non-permanent river)
12.7mi
16.9mi
Canyon Country
Magic Mountain Parkway
19.6/23.9mi
Saugus
Valencia Boulevard
Railroad Avenue
14.5mi
Via Princessa
Sierra Highway
Golden State Freeway
Golden Valley Road
Stevenson Ranch
Antelope Valley Freeway
Whitney Canyon Park
Wiley Canyon Road
21.9mi
Valencia
To B4
Miles
0
0.75
1.5

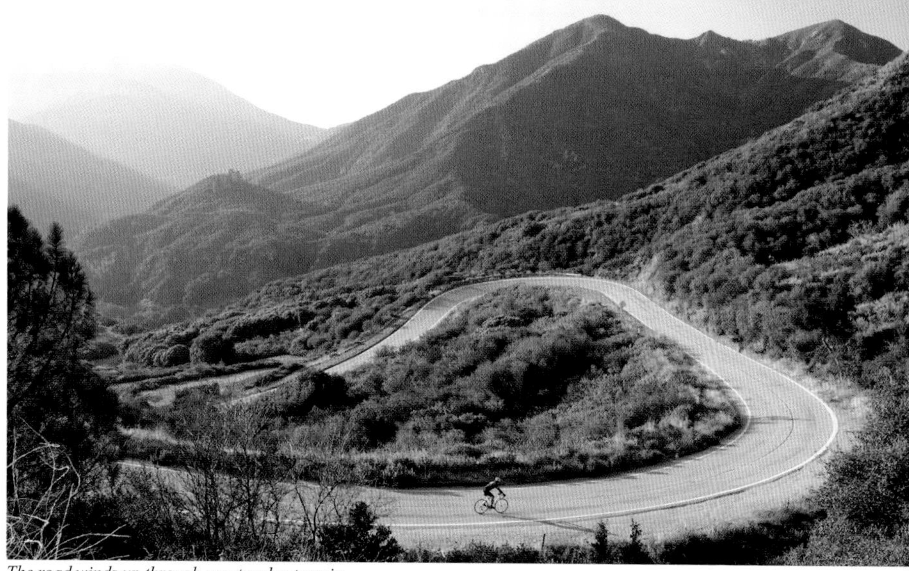

*The road winds up through spectacular terrain.*

## At a Glance

**Distance** 45.9 miles **Elevation Gain** 3,750 feet

### Terrain

This route has rolling-hills, steep mountains and twisting canyon roads, with approximately 11 flat miles mid-ride along riverfront bike paths. The pavement quality is good.

### Traffic

Little Tujunga Canyon Road sees very little traffic, and the river bike paths are, of course, car-free. The remaining roads have moderate traffic. Another bike path you'll ride parallels San Fernando Road from Roxford to the Metrolink station.

### How to Get There

Exit the 5 or 405 Freeway onto San Fernando Mission Boulevard. Continue northeast to the T and turn left onto Truman Street. After five blocks, make a right onto Hubbard Avenue and then, an immediate left to Metrolink parking.

### Food and Drink

The Saugus Café (Place of Interest 4) is one of the oldest cafés in Southern California. Even Teddy Roosevelt ate here. Food's okay, but the history is priceless.

### Side Trip

Placerita Canyon Road makes an excellent side trip (or a shortcut to Newhall). This canyon road is narrower and closer to the cottonwoods and sycamores throughout Placerita Canyon State Park. The nature center merits a visit too. From the park, continue west through a gated community, turn left onto Railroad Avenue, right onto Lyons Avenue and rejoin the main route at Wiley Canyon Road.

**Links to** 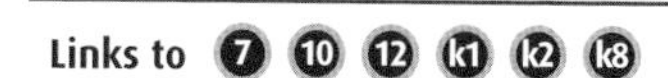


**Where to Bike Rating** 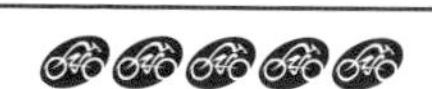

# About...

If you define an epic as something surpassing the usual or the ordinary, particularly in scope or size, then Little Tujunga Canyon Road is an epic ride. Rising from the alluvial plains of the San Fernando Valley, this little-used mountain passage winds up switchbacks, over summits and through a remote, tree-shaded valley through the San Gabriel Mountains to high desert. But the drama does not end there. After arcing through Santa Clarita, this ride returns via the woodland-fringed Newhall Pass, following a former stagecoach route.

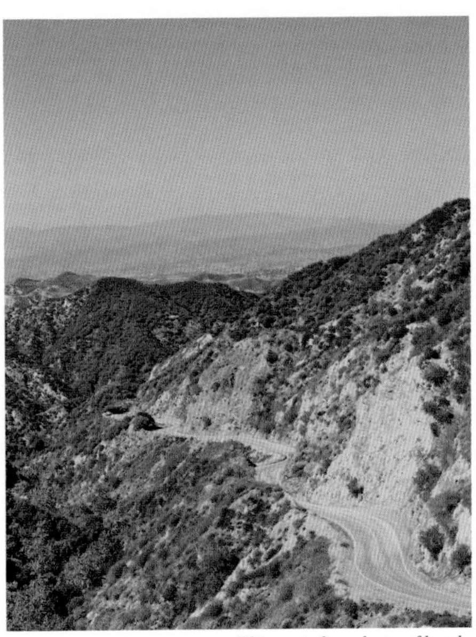

*This route has plenty of bends.*

From Sylmar, the warm-up goes through downtown San Fernando, past Whiteman Airport to Little Tujunga Canyon Road, just north of Hansen Dam (Ride 12). This country road rolls past ranches, equestrian schools, a few houses and then, along a wash hemmed in by steepening hillsides. Just as the climbing begins, around mile 11, you might wonder: Am I hearing monkeys squealing and lions roaring? You are not suffering climbing-induced hallucinations—those sounds come from denizens of the Wildlife Waystation, a non-profit sanctuary that rescues hundreds of animals.

The next 2.5 miles of switchbacks gain about 1,200 feet to the first summit. As you cross this ridgeline notch, you'll catch glimpses of the valley—mountain meadows dotted with stands of pine and oak. Descending into the lowlands, down many shaded switchbacks, you'll feel the temperature grow cooler. The San Gabriel peaks, to the south, shorten daily sun exposure here. From the valley floor, the terrain pitches upward again, about 650 feet, to the second highpoint. Just past this saddle, the Santa Clarita Valley opens beneath you. Down below to the right, you'll see the road unfurling, seven miles downhill, to the Santa Clara River. You make that descent.

After a flat, urban interlude through Santa Clarita, another open space awaits at Newhall Pass. The Old Road, which totally deserves its name, dates from the1850s, when the pass along the Butterfield Overland Stagecoach road was called Beale's Cut. Even with an interstate looming nearby on higher ground, the Newhall terrain remains relatively unspoiled, with the 4,000-acre Santa Clarita Woodlands Park to one side and steep hillsides to the other. Except for the hum of interstate traffic, the pass feels remarkably rural. Once over the crest and under a freeway interchange, The Old Road becomes San Fernando Road. From there, it's a short ride through Sylmar to the Metrolink station.

Advisories: For a ride like this, with lots of climbing early on, a bailout plan for the second half is wise, should the legs refuse to listen. Metrolink offers a perfect escape hatch. There's a station in Santa Clarita on Soledad Canyon Road at mile 30.6. The train ride back to Sylmar takes about 20 minutes. Also, because Little Tujunga Canyon Road is remote with sparse traffic, be sure to bring along at least one companion, plus flat-fixing supplies, ample water and snacks.

# Ride Log

**0.0** From the Metrolink parking lot, ride southeast a short distance, turn right onto Hubbard Ave, cross Truman St and make a left onto San Fernando Rd.

**1.3** Continue straight on San Fernando Rd as it merges with Truman St.

**3.6** Pass Whiteman Airport and turn left onto Osborne St.

**5.3** Pass Hansen Dam Recreation Area and turn right onto Foothill Blvd.

**6.1** Cross under the 210 Freeway and turn left onto Osborne St, which becomes Little Tujunga Canyon Rd.

**11.6** Pass the Wildlife Waystation.

**13.4** Cross the first summit.

**17.7** Cross the second summit at the road leading to the Camp 9 fire station.

**20.7** Pass Placerita Canyon Rd. Little Tujunga Canyon Rd becomes Sand Canyon Rd.

**24.0** Turn left onto Soledad Canyon Rd, joining its bike lane.

**25.0** Turn left onto Lost Canyon Rd.

**25.1** Turn right onto the Santa Clara River Trail.

**27.4** Angle to the right at the Y onto the Chuck Pontius Commuter-Rail Trail, parallel to Soledad Canyon Rd (do not pass under Soledad Canyon Rd).

**29.8** Cross Soledad Canyon Rd at Santa Clarita Bowling Lanes. The trail resumes on the north side, parallel to the sidewalk.

**30.6** If you choose to return to the San Fernando Valley via Metrolink, cross Soledad Canyon Rd to the station.

**31.3** The trail curves behind several street-front businesses, then passes under Bouquet Canyon Rd.

**32.0** Angle to the right at the Y just before the Mercedes Benz dealership.

**32.5** Turn right and continue on the trail running along Valencia Blvd.

**32.6** Turn right, descend a short ramp, make a U-turn onto the South Fork Trail and then pass under Valencia Blvd.

**35.0** South Fork Trail ends. Turn right onto Orchard Village Rd.

**35.1** Turn left onto Wiley Canyon Rd joining its bike lane.

**36.2** Cross Lyons Ave.

**37.3** Turn right onto Calgrove Blvd, which then becomes The Old Rd.

**41.3** Cross under the 5 Freeway/14 Freeway interchange. The Old Rd becomes San Fernando Rd at Sierra Hwy.

**44.0** Cross Roxford Rd, join the bike path along the northeast side of San Fernando Rd.

**45.9** Arrive at the Sylmar/San Fernando Metrolink station. End of ride.

B
- *B1* Pedalers West Bike Shop
  412 Maclay Ave, San Fernando
- *B2* Willy's Bikes
  11968 Foothill Blvd, Lake View Terrace
- *B3* Canyon Bicycles
  18833 Soledad Canyon Rd, Canyon Country
- *B4* Bicycle John's
  26635 Valley Center Dr, Santa Clarita
- *B5* Performance Cyclery
  23360 Cinema Dr, Santa Clarita
- *B6* Valley Bicycles
  24727 Railroad Ave, Santa Clarita
- *B7* Newhall Bicycle Co
  24261 Main St, Santa Clarita
- *B8* Bicycle Den, 16908 San Fernando Mission Road, Grenada Hills

## Little Tujunga Canyon Road

*Please note: the profile for Ride 11 is depicted in 500ft vertical increments due to unusually high elevation.*

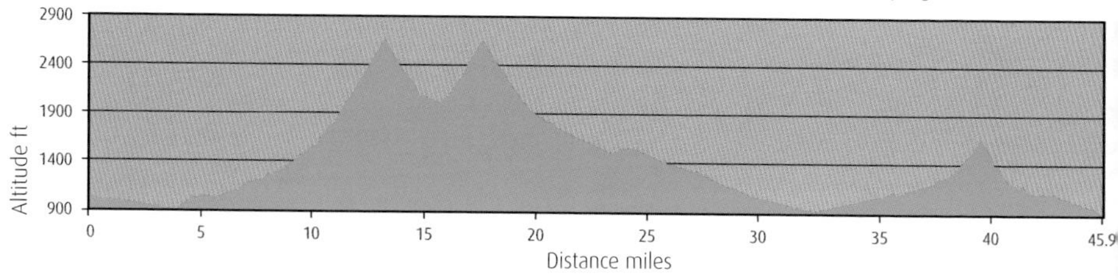

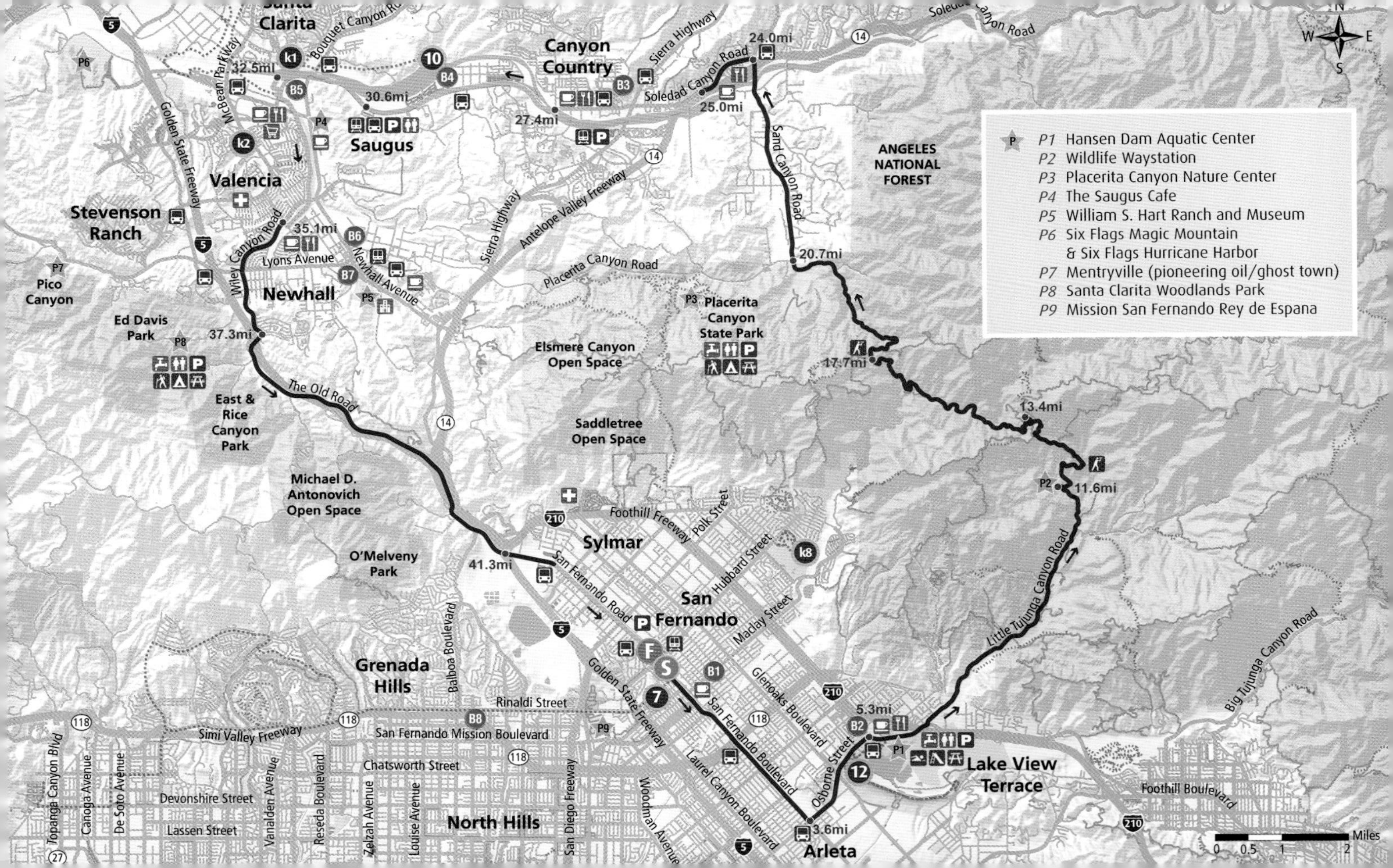

P1 Hansen Dam Aquatic Center
P2 Wildlife Waystation
P3 Placerita Canyon Nature Center
P4 The Saugus Cafe
P5 William S. Hart Ranch and Museum
P6 Six Flags Magic Mountain & Six Flags Hurricane Harbor
P7 Mentryville (pioneering oil/ghost town)
P8 Santa Clarita Woodlands Park
P9 Mission San Fernando Rey de Espana
ANGELES NATIONAL FOREST
Canyon Country
Saugus
Valencia
Stevenson Ranch
Newhall
Pico Canyon
Ed Davis Park
East & Rice Canyon Park
Michael D. Antonovich Open Space
O'Melveny Park
Elsmere Canyon Open Space
Saddletree Open Space
Placerita Canyon State Park
Sylmar
San Fernando
Grenada Hills
North Hills
Lake View Terrace
Arleta
Golden State Freeway
McBean Parkway
Bouquet Canyon Road
Sierra Highway
Soledad Canyon Road
Sand Canyon Road
Antelope Valley Freeway
Placerita Canyon Road
Wiley Canyon Road
Lyons Avenue
Newhall Avenue
The Old Road
Foothill Freeway
Polk Street
Hubbard Street
Maclay Street
San Fernando Road
Glenoaks Boulevard
San Fernando Boulevard
Laurel Canyon Boulevard
Osborne Street
Little Tujunga Canyon Road
Big Tujunga Canyon Road
Foothill Boulevard
Balboa Boulevard
Rinaldi Street
Simi Valley Freeway
San Fernando Mission Boulevard
Chatsworth Street
Devonshire Street
Lassen Street
Topanga Canyon Blvd
Canoga Avenue
De Soto Avenue
Vanalden Avenue
Reseda Boulevard
Zelzah Avenue
Louise Avenue
San Diego Freeway
Woodman Avenue
3.6mi
5.3mi
11.6mi
13.4mi
17.7mi
20.7mi
24.0mi
25.0mi
27.4mi
30.6mi
32.5mi
35.1mi
37.3mi
41.3mi
Miles
0
0.5
1
2

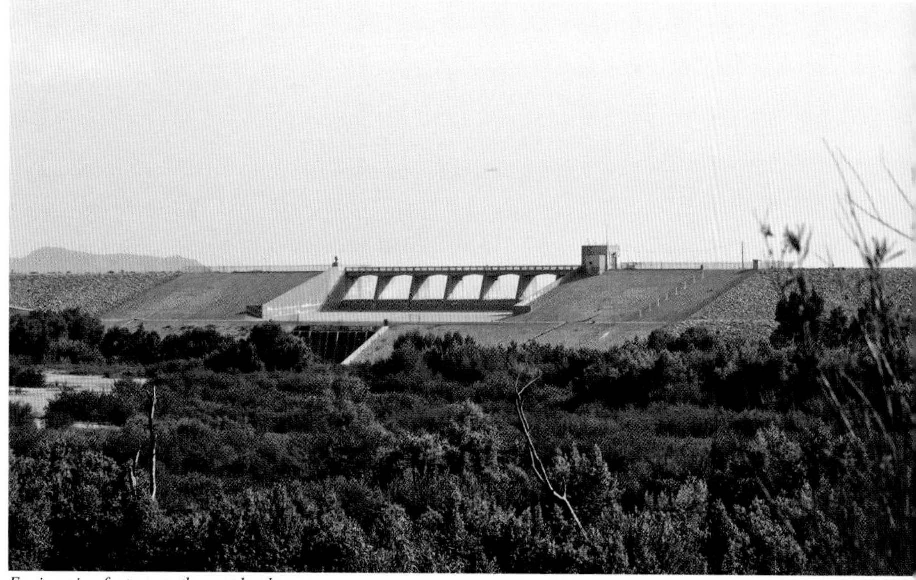

*Engineering feats span the vast landscape.*

## At a Glance

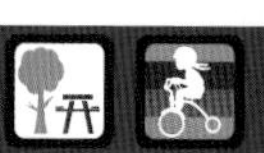

**Distance** 6.3 miles **Elevation Gain** 200 feet

### Terrain

This short ride is flat, except for the slope up or down at each end of the dam. Overall, the pavement is pretty good.

### Traffic

The path across the dam is car-free. The recreation area's interior access roads can be busy, though traffic is usually slow moving, regulated by frequent speed bumps.

### How to Get There

Exit the 210 Freeway onto Foothill Boulevard heading south. At Dronfield Avenue, turn left and enter the Hansen Dam Recreation Area.

### Food and Drink

You'll find convenience stores west of the dam, along Foothill Boulevard and south of it, on Osborne Street. On weekends, truck and pushcart vendors throughout the park sell ice cream, cold drinks and snacks.

### Side Trip

For extra miles, turn left at the park's Wentworth Street gate. Take Wentworth to Foothill Boulevard, turn left and follow it back to the recreation area. While this is a utilitarian road outside of the recreation area, it does offer close-ups of the San Gabriel Mountains and Tujunga Wash.

**Links to** 

**Where to Bike Rating** 

 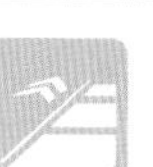 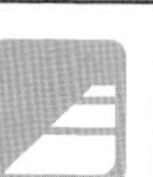 

# About...

Twenty-five miles northwest of Downtown, where Tujunga Wash snakes out from the San Gabriel Mountains, the Hansen Dam spans the alluvial plain, protecting downstream communities from winter rains and spring thaws. The rest of the year, the dam offers a fun, short, scenic ride across its top. In summer, when temperatures soar, bring along a swimsuit for a dip in Hansen Dam Aquatic Center's mega-pool —1.5 acres of water with a twisting waterslide. Bike racks and changing rooms are provided. This has the makings of a leisurely family ride.

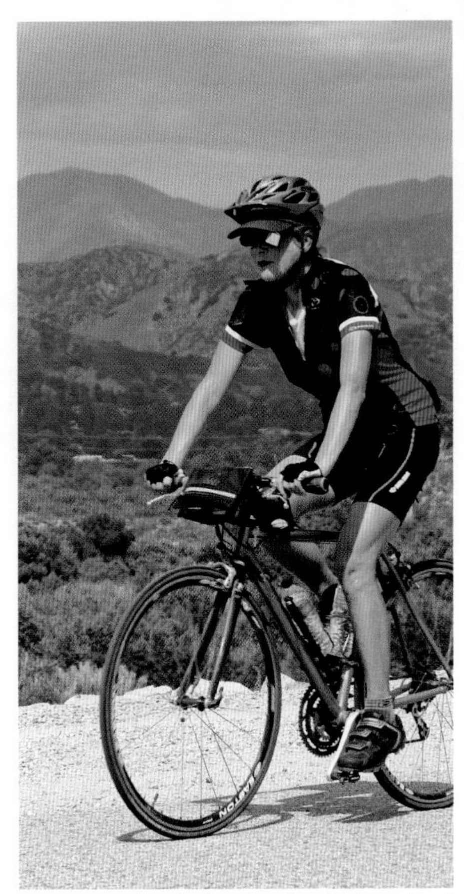

*Over the dam: the path and vistas are broad. (The rider's "eye patch" is a rearview mirror.)*

Hansen Dam's existence has everything to do with the extreme lifecycle of its surrounding landscape. Just to its north, the San Gabriel Mountains jut up at a radically sharp angle. Across this steep terrain, a sparse drama plays out almost annually in a cycle of fire and flood. In the rainy season, the area's creeks and rivers, the Big and Little Tujunga Washes, can change almost instantly from parched arroyos to raging, debris-filled torrents. In the hot summer and fall, brush fires, whipped up by canyon-accelerated Santa Ana winds, can ravage the hillsides. Once stripped bare of vegetation, the terrain only amplifies flood-producing runoff when the rains finally arrive.

Battling this devastating cycle, the United States Army Corps of Engineers seized this land in 1939 via eminent domain from a ranching family—Homer and Marie Hansen—and built the dam. It reins in the Tujunga Wash, which combines the Big and Little Tujunga, draining a watershed of some 225 square miles. The dam is roughly two miles long and rises about 97 feet from the ground plane below it.

In the 1980s, the dam gained a bike path across its top—transforming this engineering intervention into a short, interesting cycling route that integrates other paths and roads within the recreation area. Rolling across the spine of this flood barrier, you can take in views of the San Gabriel Mountains, the expansive San Fernando Valley, a scenic golf course just below you and the recreation area itself. Midway across, you can peer straight down a spillway of the Tujunga Wash. Its crisp edges converge to a vanishing point, approaching the waterway's union with the Los Angeles River in Studio City.

In summer months, you can end your ride with a plunge in the Aquatic Center's vast pool, or, for another kind of splash, the park's nine-acre recreation lake offers fishing, small-craft boating, bird watching and pedal boat rentals.

# Ride Log

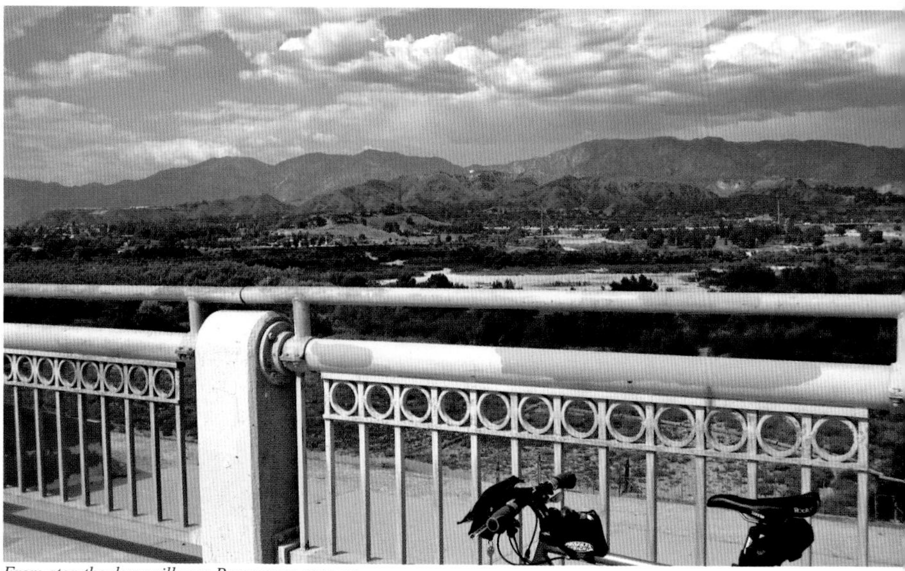

*From atop the dam spillway: Panoramas open up.*

**0.0** Begin in the park's main parking area adjacent to Kagel Canyon St. Ride toward the dam on the bike path on the east side of the same access road.

**0.3** Turn right onto the bike path.

**0.5** Turn left, passing through a gate onto the dam.

**1.6** Pass over the dam's spillway.

**2.6** Short descent.

**2.8** Arrive at the Wentworth St gate. Make a U-turn.

**4.0** Pass over the dam's spillway again.

**5.1** Pass through a gate, then turn right and descend toward the recreation area.

**5.6** Arrive back near the parking area, continue straight on the bike path.

**5.7** Turn right onto the access road.

**5.8** Turn left at the roundabout.

**6.0** Make a U-turn at the fishing pier, then return to ward the parking area.

**6.1** Turn right onto the access road.

**6.2** Turn left, continuing on the access road.

**6.3** Arrive back at the parking area. End of ride.

P *P1* Little Tujunga Canyon
*P2* Hansen Dam Swim Lake (seasonal)
*P3* Hansen Dam Recreational Lake (year round)

B *B1* Willy's Bikes
11968 Foothill Boulevard, Lake View Terrace

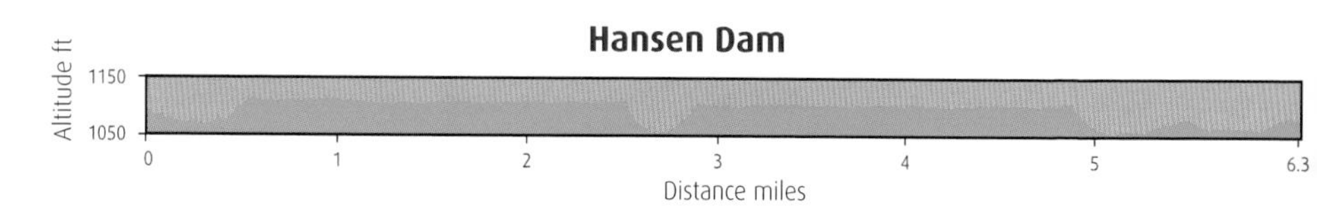

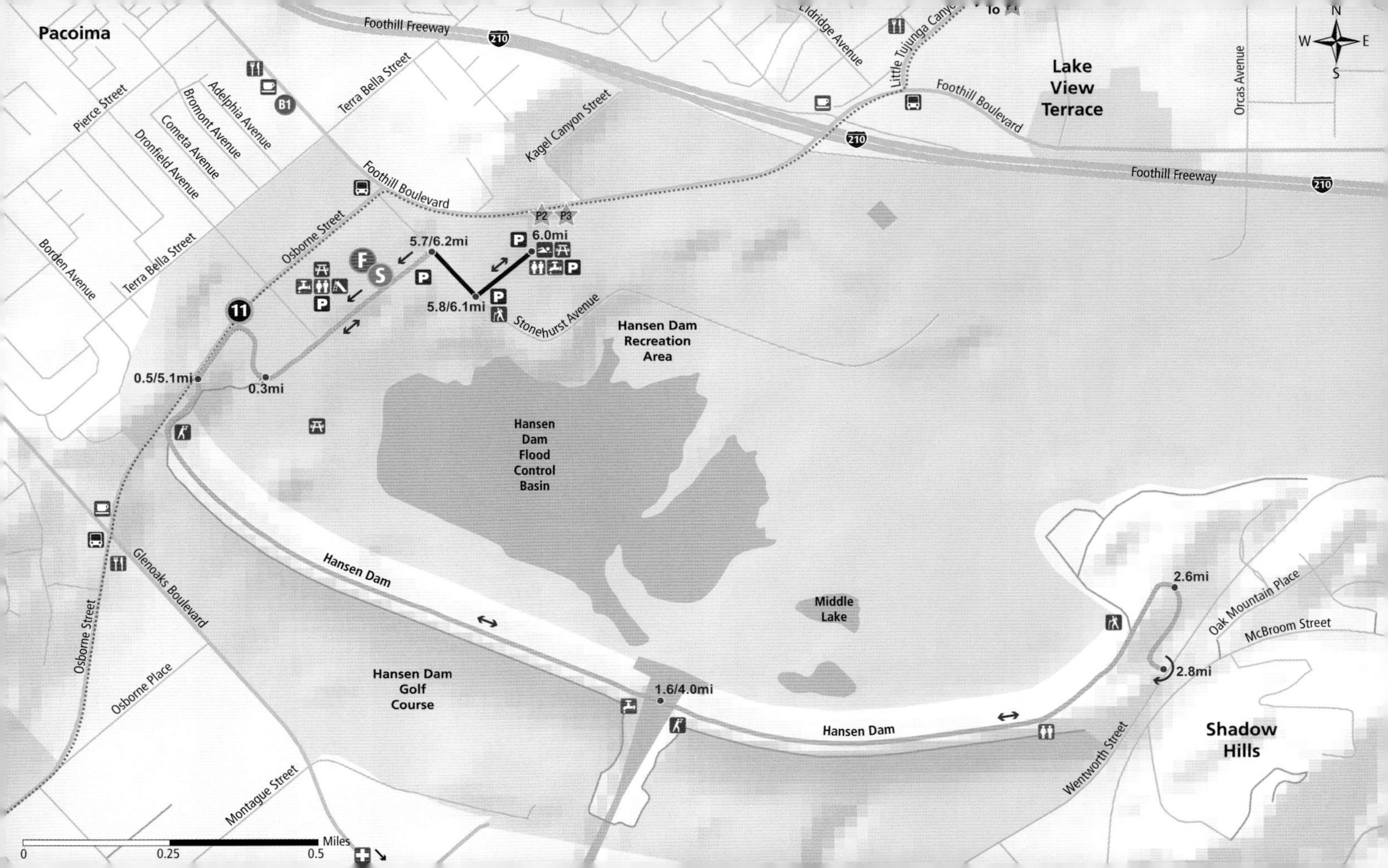

Pacoima
Lake View Terrace
Shadow Hills
Foothill Freeway
210
Foothill Boulevard
Little Tujunga Canyon
Eldridge Avenue
Orcas Avenue
Terra Bella Street
Pierce Street
Adelphia Avenue
Bromont Avenue
Cometa Avenue
Dronfield Avenue
Borden Avenue
Osborne Street
Kagel Canyon Street
Stonehurst Avenue
Glenoaks Boulevard
Osborne Place
Montague Street
Wentworth Street
Oak Mountain Place
McBroom Street
B1
11
F
S
P2
P3
5.7/6.2mi
6.0mi
5.8/6.1mi
0.5/5.1mi
0.3mi
1.6/4.0mi
2.6mi
2.8mi
Hansen Dam Recreation Area
Hansen Dam Flood Control Basin
Middle Lake
Hansen Dam
Hansen Dam Golf Course
N
S
E
W
Miles
0
0.25
0.5

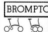

# The San Gabriel Valley

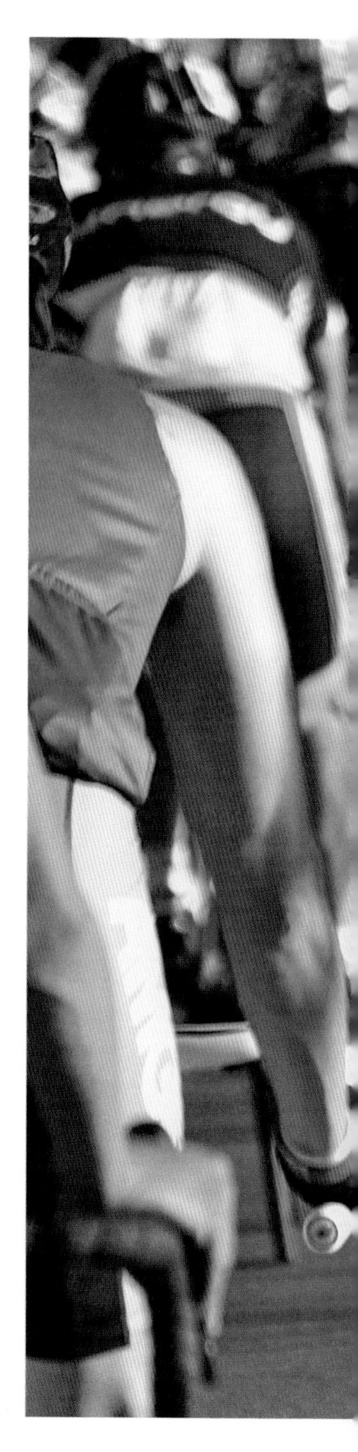

The San Gabriel Valley extends east from the Verdugo Mountains, through Pasadena and Sierra Madre, out past Azusa to Glendora. Along with the mountains, this northeastern region's distinguishing geological features are its rivers, flowing (when they actually contain water) from the highlands south toward the ocean. As the San Gabriel River cuts across the valley on a bias, the shorter Rio Hondo roughly parallels it, feeding into the L. A. River.

Decades ago, the Army Corps of Engineers strong-armed L.A.'s rivers, encasing much of their length in concrete as (now-controversial) flood-control measures. Fortunately, you can still experience rare natural stretches of the San Gabriel and Rio Hondo in their wild, soft-bottomed, forested state as you ride the San Gabriel's West Fork, Glendora Mountain Road and the lower Rio Hondo. The easy, tranquil West Fork ride—amid sheer rock walls, sycamore, scrub oak, fragrant chaparral and a flowing stream—is unquestionably one of the best short jaunts we know. You can picnic or even camp there, just a 20-minute ride into the beautiful Angeles National Forest. In the same forest is Glendora Mountain Road, a remote alpine route amid rugged high peaks; a spectacular ride but one of this book's most challenging.

Where the rivers have been channelized, the upside of such aggressive engineering is the network of bikeways atop the concrete levees. The long, uninterrupted car-free paths contribute nearly 100 miles to this chapter: In the Three Rivers, Upper San Gabriel (from Whittier Narrows to the San Gabriel Mountains) and Rio Hondo rides. Incidentally, if you're feeling highly energetic and ambitious, you could cycle the entire length of the San Gabriel River—by connecting the Upper San Gabriel to the San Gabriel River segments of our Three Rivers and Long Beach Periferico rides—38 miles each way from mountains to ocean.

Near the San Gabriel-San Fernando Valley border are three Pasadena rides, arrayed along the leafy Arroyo Seco: the Rose Bowl Circuit, a three-mile lap (over and over) around this landmark stadium, where you may be chased by a couple hundred other cyclists; the Descanso Gardens spin, up into the San Rafael Hills, with panoramic views into the San Fernando Valley and an optional visit to the burgeoning Descanso Gardens; and the Tour of Pasadena, a leisurely ride that takes in Old Pasadena, Caltech, the Rose Bowl, Pasadena City Hall, the Huntington Gardens and more.

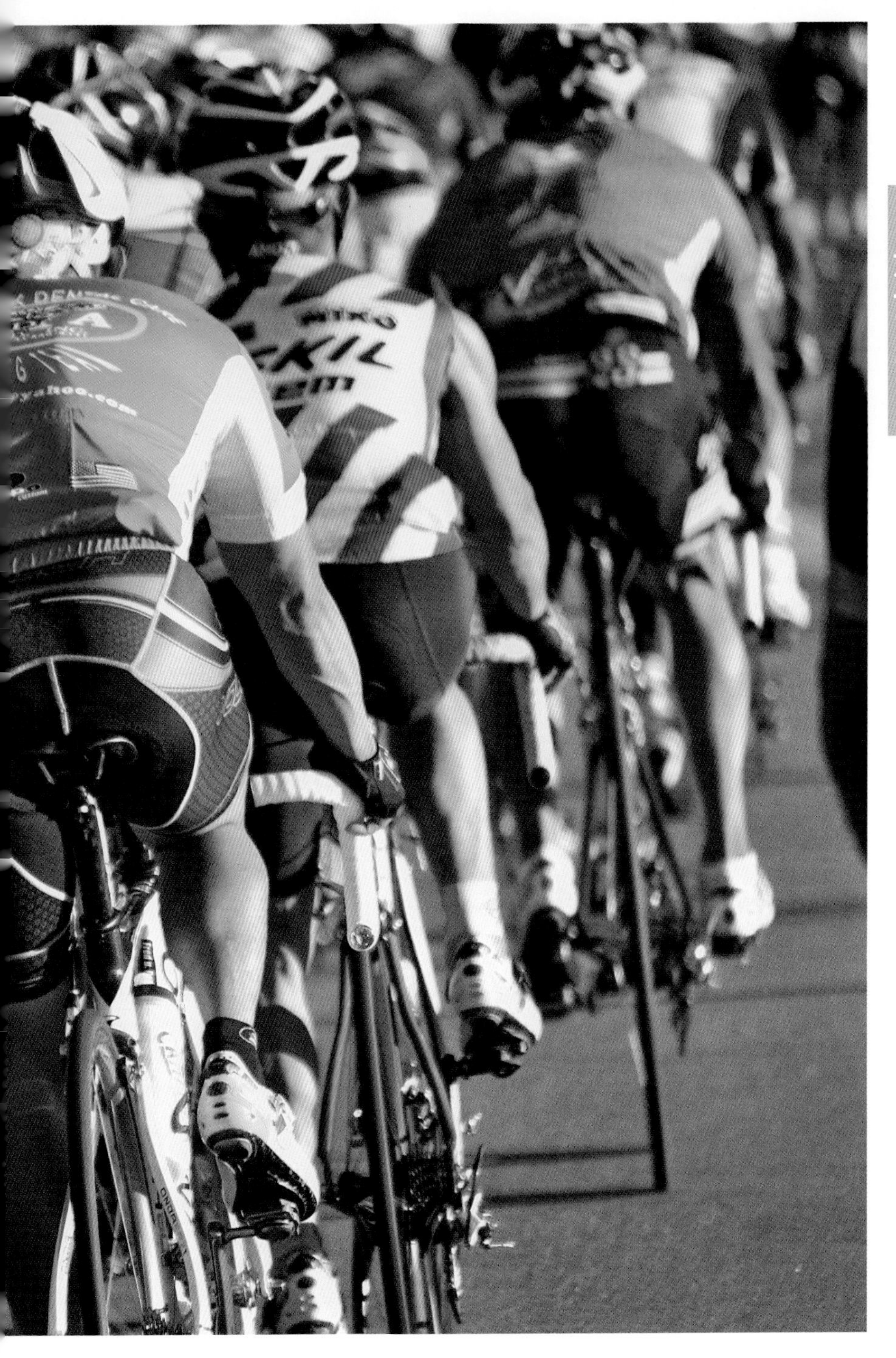

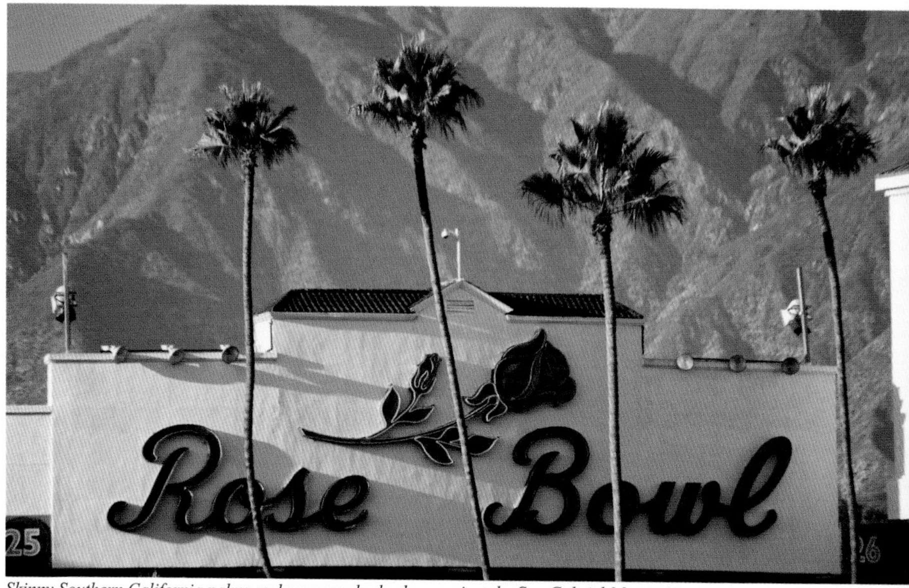

*Skinny Southern California palms and neon rosebuds glow against the San Gabriel Mountains.*

## At a Glance

**Distance** 3.1 miles (per circuit)
**Elevation Gain** 160 feet (per circuit)

### Terrain

The entire course was resurfaced in 2010, so road conditions are excellent. A small gradient rises gently from south to north.

### Traffic

The course—a circuit of city streets—is not 100 percent car-free, but traffic tends to be light, with most drivers respecting bicyclists and other athletes. A wide pedestrian lane (popular with joggers) borders the road to the right, so be mindful not to hit, or veer beyond, the white-plastic separation poles.

### How to Get There

In and near Pasadena, multiple exits off the 110, 210 and 134 freeways lead to the Rose Bowl. Follow the signs from the exit. Park in Lots F or I, at the intersection of North Arroyo Boulevard and Seco Street.

### Food and Drink

Be prepared: there are no regular refreshment outlets on the Rose Bowl grounds (except for an occasional vendor selling cut fruit and drinks from a cart on Seco Street).

### Side Trip

Ride into scenic Old Pasadena for refreshments at the eateries along Colorado Boulevard. To get there, ride east on Seco Street, turn right on Lincoln Avenue, then right on Orange Grove, followed by a left at Colorado Boulevard. Continue a few blocks down Colorado to check out the many snacking and dining options.

**Links to** 14 15

**Where to Bike Rating** 

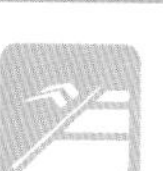

## About...

This ride traces an elongated circuit around the famous Rose Bowl, a National Historic Landmark, dating back to 1922. Most famous for its New Year's Day Tournament of Roses—the "granddaddy" of all college football games—the Rose Bowl is home to the UCLA Bruins.

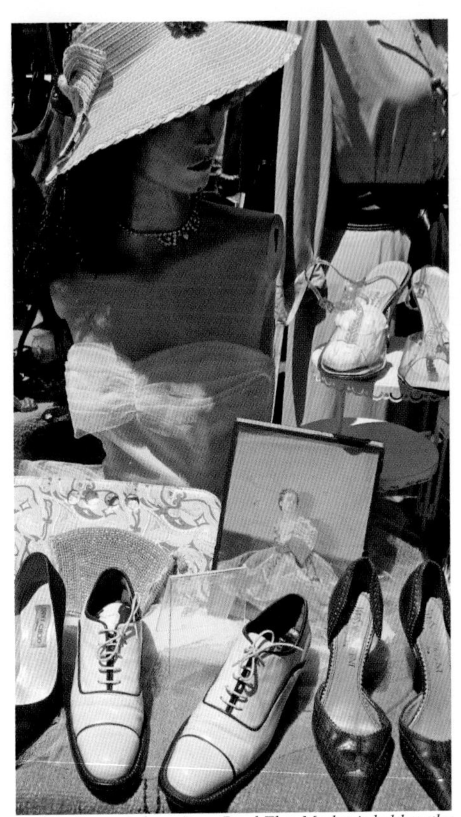

*The famously huge Rose Bowl Flea Market is held on the second Sunday of each month.*

Except during games, this 3.1-mile circuit is open for riding. Cyclists pass under a canopy of oak and eucalyptus trees as the road proceeds along the sides of a broad arroyo. North of the stadium, the manicured green and lush landscaping of the Brookside golf course borders the right side of the road. This setting, combined with the uncomplicated repetition of relatively short laps makes it a nearly perfect place to spin your gears, or perhaps train for your next circuit race or criterium.

The Rose Bowl figures prominently in the history of bicycle racing in Los Angeles. During the 1932 Olympics, this was the site of track-cycling events. (Just imagine one of the quirkier events: a 1,000-meter time trial contested with tandem bikes on a wooden track.) Though no U.S. rider placed here, on native soil, competitors from Italy, France, the Netherlands and Australia took home gold. In the 60-plus years since, cyclists have flocked to the Rose Bowl, joining one of the longest-standing group rides in the United States.

The joy of this course is in its simplicity. From the unofficial start/finish line at Seco Street and North Arroyo Boulevard, the circuit makes exactly four turns, all to the right, as riders gradually ascend the west side of the arroyo toward Washington Boulevard and then gain back a little speed on the run down the east side. Heading clockwise almost completely neutralizes any cross-traffic hazards and the need to stop at intersections. You can just enjoy the ride and hone your technique. If your legs are willing, you can boost the distance simply by increasing the number of circuits. You'll find riders here almost every day, except during games.

Experienced or accomplished cyclists in the mood for a hammerfest might want to join the Rose Bowl Peloton Ride on Tuesday or Thursday evenings. From mid-March to the last day of Pacific Standard Time in October, these training sessions kick off about an hour before sundown. The 10-lap, 30-mile ride starts from the north side of Seco Street at North Arroyo. After an initial half-lap or so of warm-up, you can expect some fast riding. Though not a race, this group spin tends to be competitive, so be sure to learn the established peloton etiquette and be considerate of others. If the pace heats up too much, don't be afraid to ease your way to the back for a while.

# Ride Log

0.0 Begin along Seco St riding in the clockwise direction.

0.1 Turn right on West Dr.

1.4 Turn right on West Washington Blvd.

1.7 Turn right on Rosemont Ave.

2.9 Turn right on Seco St.

3.1 Cross the "finish line" at North Arroyo Blvd.

Repeat as desired.

P1 Rose Bowl
P2 Rose Bowl Flea Market
(2nd Sunday every month)
P3 Bose Bowl Aquatics Center
P4 Gamble House
P5 Old Pasadena

B1 Incycle *(Rentals available)*
175 South Fair Oaks Avenue, Pasadena
B2 Pasadena Cyclery
1670 E Walnut Street, Pasadena

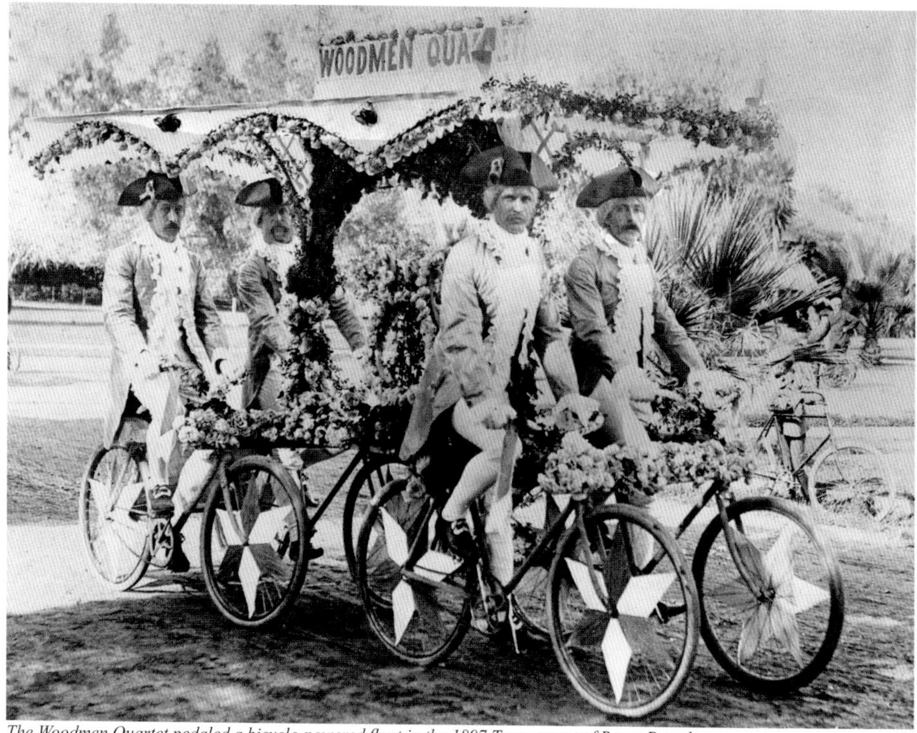


*The Woodmen Quartet pedaled a bicycle-powered float in the 1897 Tournament of Roses Parade. (Photo courtesy of the Archives, Pasadena Museum of History.)*

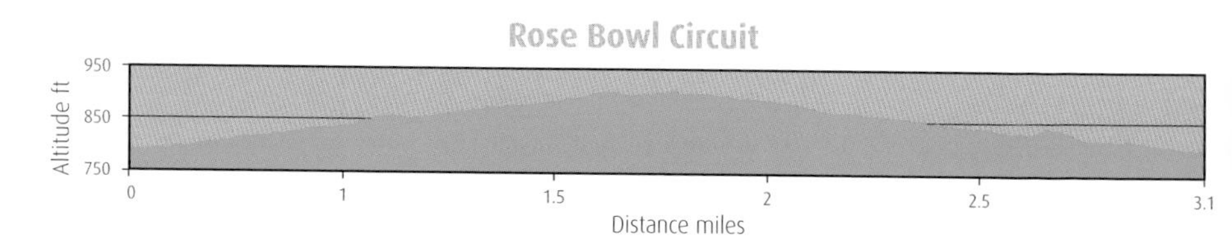

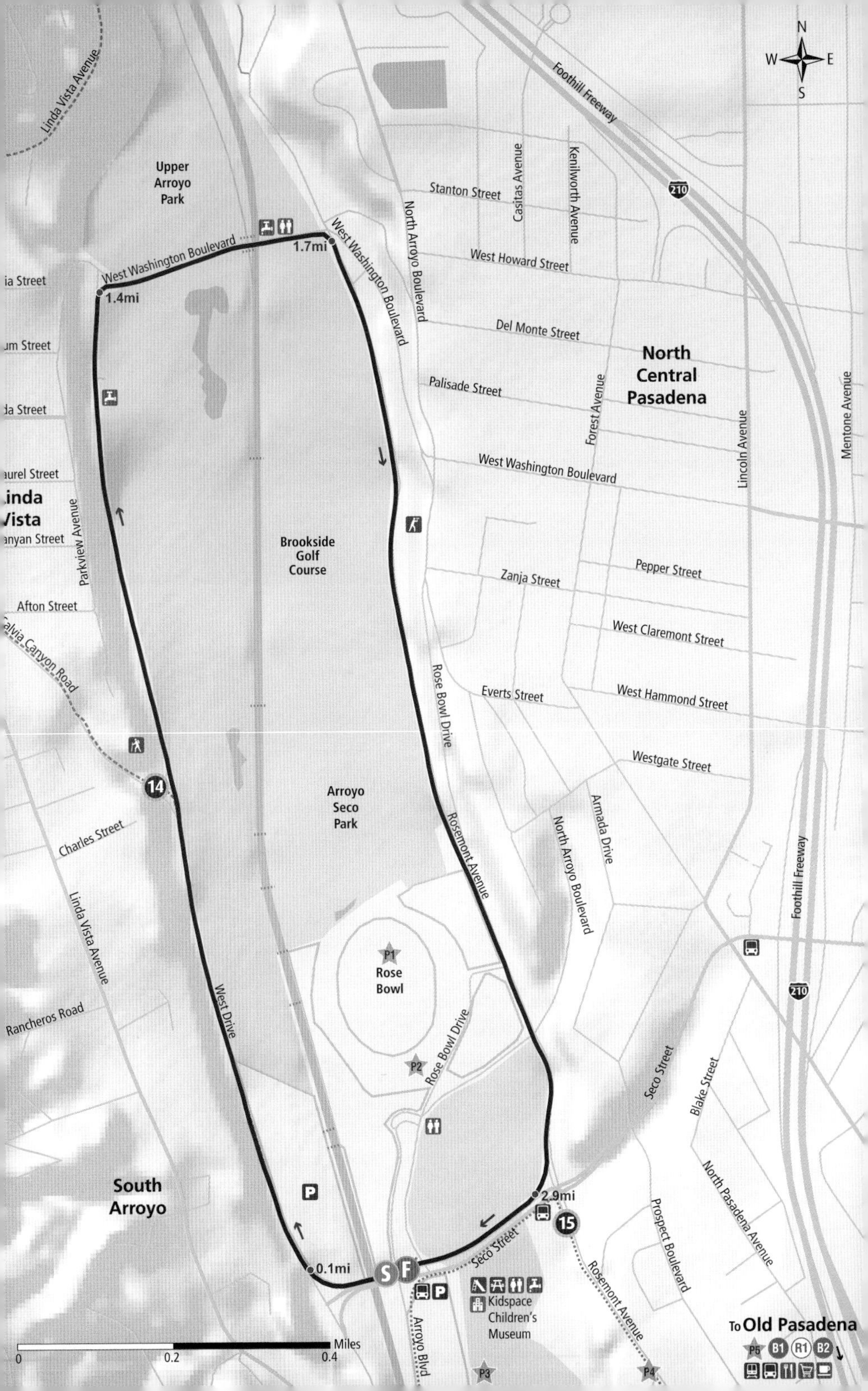

N
W
E
S
Linda Vista Avenue
Foothill Freeway
210
Upper Arroyo Park
Stanton Street
Casitas Avenue
Kenilworth Avenue
North Arroyo Boulevard
West Washington Boulevard
1.7mi
West Washington Boulevard
West Howard Street
West Washington Boulevard
1.4mi
Del Monte Street
North Central Pasadena
Palisade Street
Forest Avenue
Lincoln Avenue
Mentone Avenue
Linda Vista
Parkview Avenue
West Washington Boulevard
Brookside Golf Course
Pepper Street
Zanja Street
Afton Street
West Claremont Street
Salvia Canyon Road
Rose Bowl Drive
Everts Street
West Hammond Street
Westgate Street
14
Arroyo Seco Park
Armada Drive
North Arroyo Boulevard
Rosemont Avenue
Charles Street
Foothill Freeway
Linda Vista Avenue
P1
Rose Bowl
210
Rancheros Road
West Drive
Rose Bowl Drive
P2
Seco Street
Blake Street
South Arroyo
2.9mi
15
North Pasadena Avenue
Prospect Boulevard
Seco Street
0.1mi
S
F
Rosemont Avenue
Kidspace Children's Museum
Arroyo Blvd.
Miles
0
0.2
0.4
P3
P4
To Old Pasadena
P5
B1
R1
B2

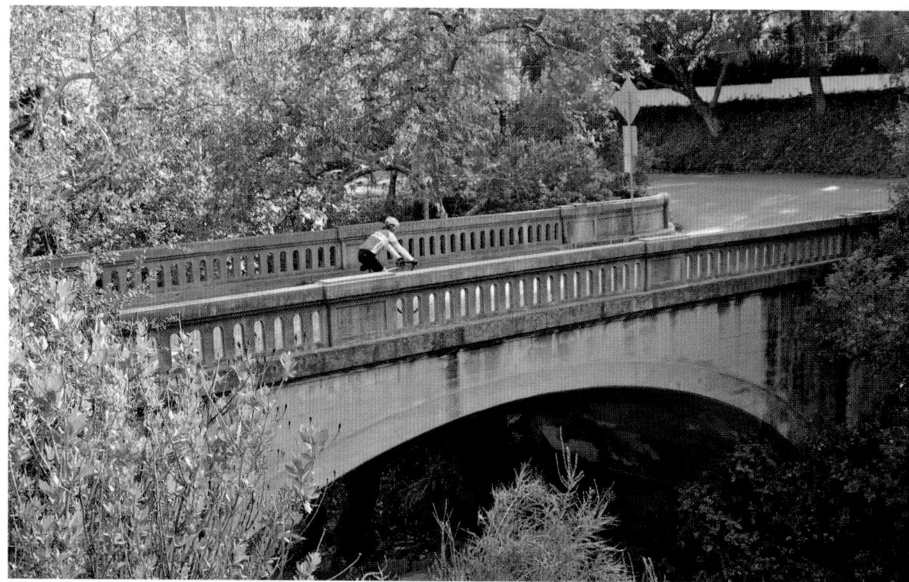
*A 1924 bridge spans the Flint Canyon Creek in La Cañada.*

## At a Glance

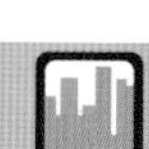

**Distance** 12.2 miles **Elevation Gain** 900 feet

### Terrain

The route to Montrose and back along the eastern and northern slopes of the San Rafael Hills has an undulating profile with no steep, prolonged climbs and descents. The optional "High Road" has more dramatic grade changes. The roads are in good condition.

### Traffic

These semi-rustic residential streets see little traffic. Chevy Chase Drive, part of the High Road option, tends to be a little more trafficked. Old Town Montrose is a bustling commercial district.

### How to Get There

Around Pasadena, the 110, 210 and 134 freeways offer multiple exits to the Rose Bowl. Follow the signs from the exit and park in Rose Bowl Lot F or I, at the intersection of North Arroyo Boulevard and Seco Street.

### Food and Drink

The Black Cow, a breakfast, lunch and dinner café in Montrose definitely rates a stop. Excellent store-baked goods, Fosselman's Ice Cream and outstanding coffees are just part of the extensive menu.

### Side Trip

Hahamongna Watershed Park is a 300-acre oak woodland with a network of paved roads that double as bike paths. It's also home to the world's first Frisbee-golf course. Turn left onto Berkshire Place, then left onto Oak Grove Drive to the park entrance.

**Links to**  

**Where to Bike Rating** 

  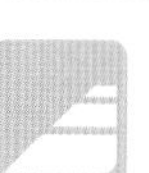 

## About...

This short ride heads up into the San Rafael Hills, a low peripheral range of the Verdugo Mountains, which separate the San Gabriel and San Fernando valleys. With two variations on the route—a fairly flat, low road and a higher one that climbs into more rustic reaches—you'll leave the Rose Bowl and cycle northwest through tranquil, tree-lined residential streets in south La Cañada Flintridge, past Descanso Gardens, home of an extensive botanical collection, to the turnaround in Old Town Montrose.

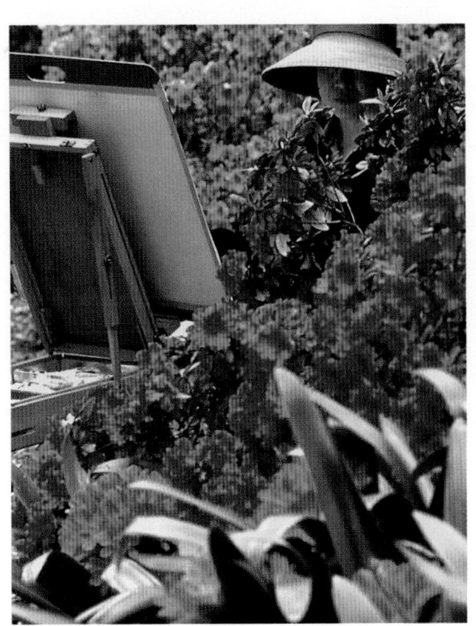

*An artist paints amid Descanso's azalea blossoms.*



The Rose Bowl parking area can be remarkably vélo-centric, a place where cyclists congregate before tacking the Rose Bowl criterium circuit (see Ride 13) or pair up for long excursions toward Angeles Crest Highway or shorter loops into the San Rafael Hills. From that launch site, this ride heads into the hills, to the Descanso Gardens and Old Town Montrose.

To reach our destinations, you'll have a couple of options along leafy wooded slopes and mellow residential neighborhoods. Our "Low Road" follows a relatively level contour around the hills. Instead of turning onto Lida Street, it continues north on Linda Vista Avenue, running parallel to the Arroyo Seco toward Devil's Gate Dam. A tree canopy shades nearly the entire route.

The "High Road" adds roughly two miles and 500 feet of climbing. It diverges from the Low Road with a left onto Lida Street, leaving the arroyo as it crosses the hills into the Chevy Chase neighborhood. The High Road takes on almost a saw-toothed profile—with a climb of about 350 feet over a mile, followed by a descent of similar magnitude and another six percent climb with a more gradual ride down. The journey then levels out, but the roads remain serpentine with many dead-ends branching off. So, make sure to follow the double yellow centerline, and you shouldn't get lost. The high and low routes reconnect at Berkshire Avenue and Chevy Chase Drive, near Descanso Gardens.

"Descanso," meaning restful, is a relaxing place to dismount—once the estate of E. Manchester Boddy, the feisty *Los Angeles Daily News* owner and publisher, who died in 1967. Across its 150 acres, a series of vivid gardens bloom: one Japanese; another exhibiting California natives; and some devoted to a particular flower, such as the camellia (Boddy was in the boutonniere business for a while), rose, iris, lilac and tulip. Just as impressive is Descanso's forest of native Live Oaks, some centuries old. Pathways, as well as a ride-able 1/8-size replica of a diesel train, meander through the estate. Bike racks are at the visitors center.

After you've inhaled rose aromas, but before you head back to the Rose Bowl, the ride swings by Old Town Montrose, a historic shopping row—a Main Street USA that's actually called Honolulu Street—with cafés, eateries, a Sunday farmers' market and retail, including a bike shop.

# Ride Log

## The Low Road Option

0.0 From the Rose Bowl's parking, begin riding west along Seco St.
0.1 Merge onto West Dr.
0.7 Angle to the left onto Salvia Canyon Rd.
1.1 Angle to the right onto Linda Vista Ave.
1.3 Continue straight past Lida St.
2.4 Linda Vista Ave becomes Highland Dr at the stop sign.
2.7 At the fork, angle to the right onto Berkshire Ave.
4.0 Turn right onto Chevy Chase Dr.
4.3 Turn left onto Descanso Dr, joining the bike lane.
4.9 Descanso Gardens.
5.1 Turn left onto Verdugo Blvd. Join its bike lane.
5.9 Cross Verdugo Rd/Montrose Ave. Verdugo Blvd becomes Honolulu Ave.
6.1 Arrive in Old Town Montrose for a snack and rest stop.
6.3 On the return, cross Verdugo Rd/Montrose Ave. Honolulu Ave becomes Verdugo Blvd. Join the bike lane.
7.0 Turn right onto Descanso Dr.
7.9 Bike lane ends. Turn right onto Chevy Chase Dr.
8.2 Turn left onto Berkshire Ave.
9.5 Merge onto Highland Dr.
9.8 Highland Dr becomes Linda Vista Ave at the stop sign.
10.8 Cross Lida St.
11.1 Angle to the left onto Salvia Canyon Rd.
11.4 Turn right onto West Dr at the Rose Bowl.
12.1 Turn left onto Seco St.
12.2 Arrive at Arroyo Blvd. End of ride.

B1 Incycle
175 South Fair Oaks Avenue, Pasadena
B2 Pasadena Cyclery
1670 E Walnut Street, Pasadena
B3 Montrose Bike Shop, 2501 Honolulu Avenue, La Cresenta-Montrose
B4 Bicycle Land
422 Glendale Avenue, Glendale
B5 Budget Pro Bicycles
2750 Colorado Boulevard, Eagle Rock

(R) R1 Incycle
175 South Fair Oaks Avenue, Pasadena

## The High Road Option

1.3 Turn left onto Lida St.
2.1 Pass Art Center College of Design.
2.6 Cross Figueroa St.
3.5 Turn right onto Chevy Chase Dr at the stop sign.
4.4 Cross Emerald Isle Dr. Emerald Isle Park, with pic nic tables, water and restrooms, is 0.3 miles further, o the left.
4.7 Continue straight on Chevy Chase Dr when i merges with Figueroa St.
6.0 Continue straight where Chevy Chase Dr recon nects with the Low Road route at Berkshire Ave.
6.3 Turn left onto Descanso Dr and join its bike lane.
6.9 Pass Descanso Gardens.
7.1 Turn left onto Verdugo Blvd. Continue along it bike lane.
7.9 Cross Verdugo Rd/Montrose Ave. Verdugo Blv becomes Honolulu Ave.
8.1 Arrive in Old Town Montrose for a snack and res stop. Return via the Low Road.

### Descanso Gardens - The Low Road Option

*Please note: the profile for Ride 14 (Low Road) is depicted in 200ft vertical increments due to unusually high elevation.*

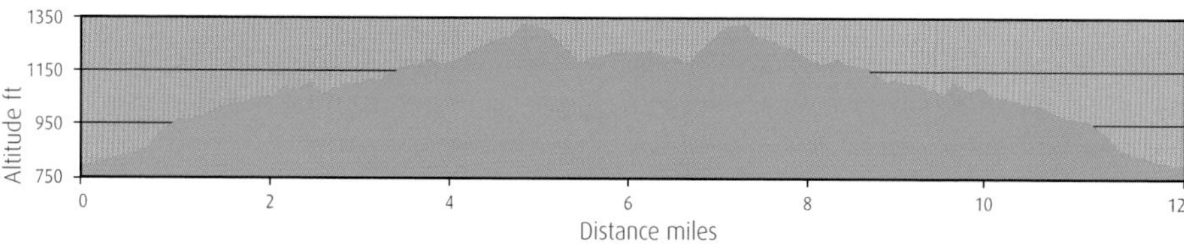

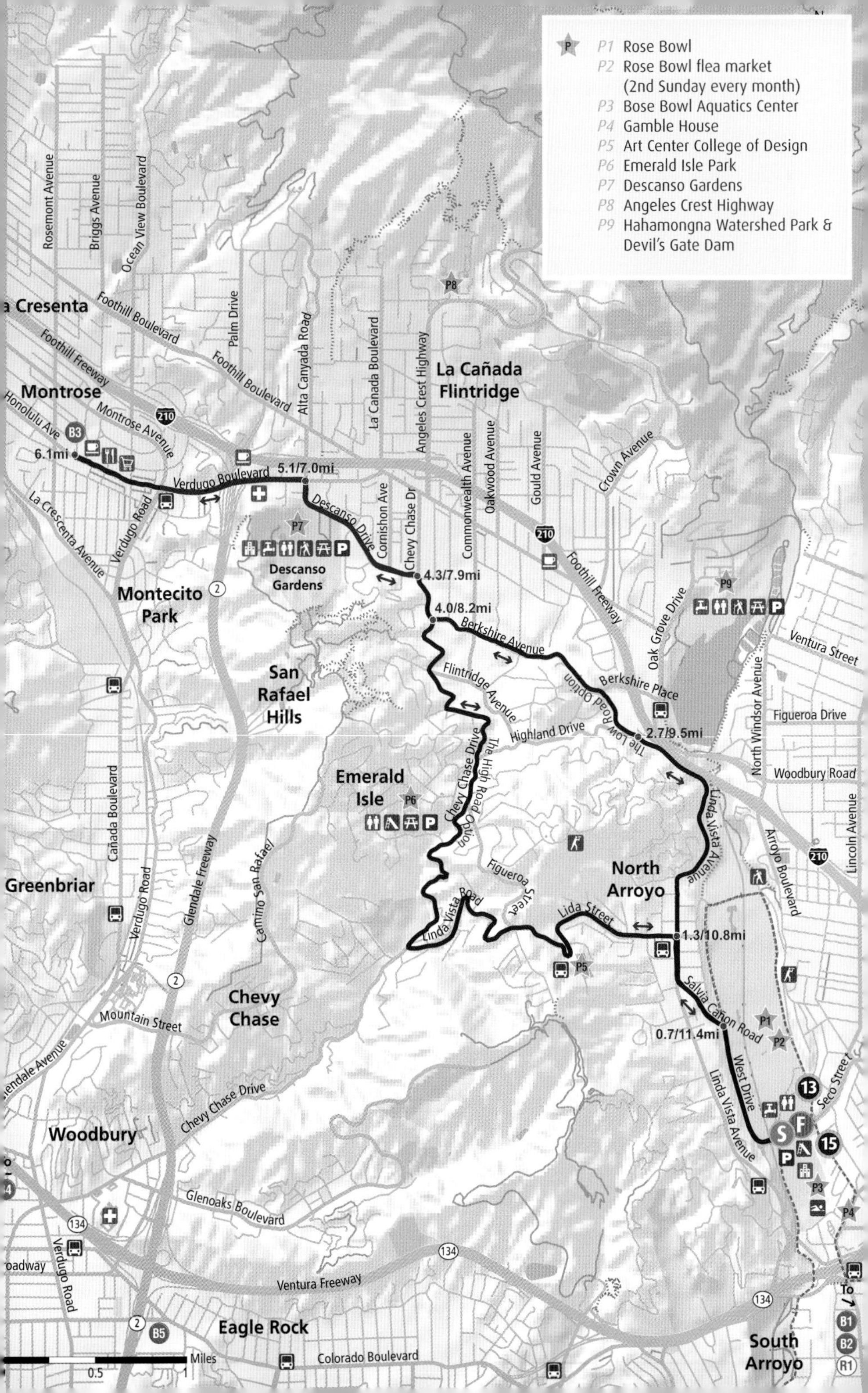

P1 Rose Bowl
P2 Rose Bowl flea market (2nd Sunday every month)
P3 Bose Bowl Aquatics Center
P4 Gamble House
P5 Art Center College of Design
P6 Emerald Isle Park
P7 Descanso Gardens
P8 Angeles Crest Highway
P9 Hahamongna Watershed Park & Devil's Gate Dam
La Cresenta
Montrose
La Cañada Flintridge
Montecito Park
Descanso Gardens
San Rafael Hills
Emerald Isle
North Arroyo
Greenbriar
Chevy Chase
Woodbury
Eagle Rock
South Arroyo
6.1mi
5.1/7.0mi
4.3/7.9mi
4.0/8.2mi
2.7/9.5mi
1.3/10.8mi
0.7/11.4mi
Foothill Boulevard
Foothill Freeway
Verdugo Boulevard
Descanso Drive
Berkshire Avenue
Flintridge Avenue
Chevy Chase Drive
The High Road Option
The Low Road Option
Linda Vista Road
Linda Vista Avenue
Lida Street
Figueroa Street
Salvia Canon Road
West Drive
Ventura Freeway
Colorado Boulevard
Glenoaks Boulevard
Glendale Freeway
Mountain Street
Miles
0.5
1

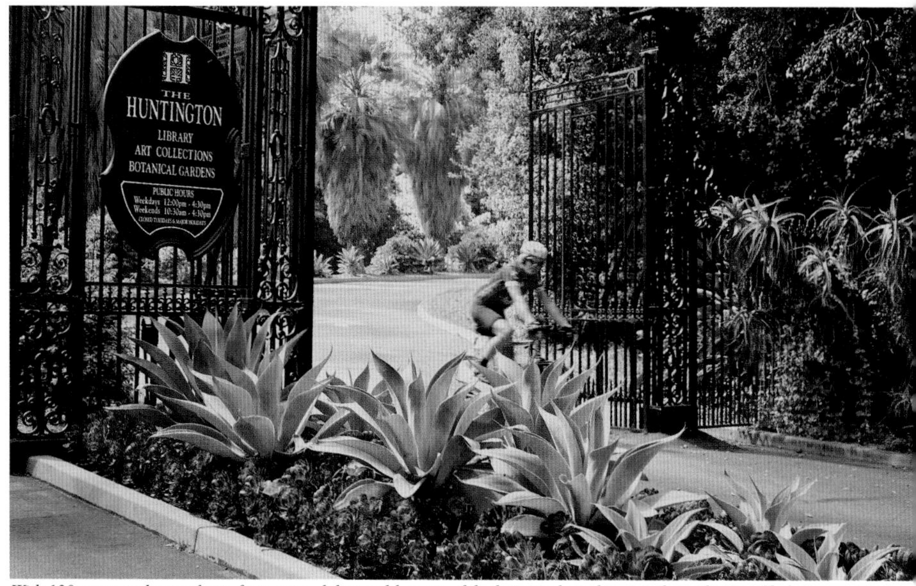


*With 120 acres and rare plants from around the world, many of the botanical gardens are themed—Zen, Shakespeare, Australian and others.*

## At a Glance

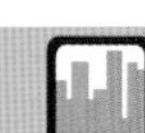

**Distance** 13.4 miles **Elevation Gain** 800 feet

### Terrain

Though varied in its streetscapes, this city route is mostly flat, with just a few short uphills.

### Traffic

This ride is a combo of bike lanes and many wide, quiet residential streets.

### How to Get There

Start at Metro's Mission station in South Pasadena, accessible via Gold Line trains from Downtown L.A. Or, by car, take the 110 Freeway north; after it becomes Arroyo Parkway, exit at Orange Grove Avenue. Go two blocks south, turn right onto Mission and then, left to Orange Grove Park where on-street parking is available.

### Food and Drink

Old Pasadena has plenty of eateries clustered on Colorado Boulevard. In South Pasadena, the Fair Oaks Pharmacy and Soda Fountain, on old Route 66 (at Fair Oaks Avenue and Mission), features a vintage soda fountain serving up sundaes and floats (plus burgers and fries).

### Side Trip

Listed on the National Register of Historic Places, El Molino Viejo is Southern California's oldest surviving commercial building. Originally a mill for the San Gabriel Mission, the 1816 structure combines adobe, brick and volcanic tuff. Visits to El Molino and its gardens are free (1120 Old Mill Road, San Marino; open 1 to 4 p.m., Tuesday through Sunday).

**Links to** 13 14 38 k7

**Where to Bike Rating** 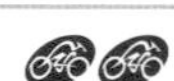

## About...

This leisurely spin through South Pasadena, Pasadena and San Marino takes in a bounty of local landmarks and destinations, including the Rose Bowl, Gamble House, City Hall, Caltech Campus and the Huntington Library and Botanical Gardens. While the route includes many gracious, tree-lined streets—posh enclaves with grand, old houses—you'll also pedal through (or near) such shopping, dining and entertainment districts as Old Pasadena, the area's vintage commercial center.

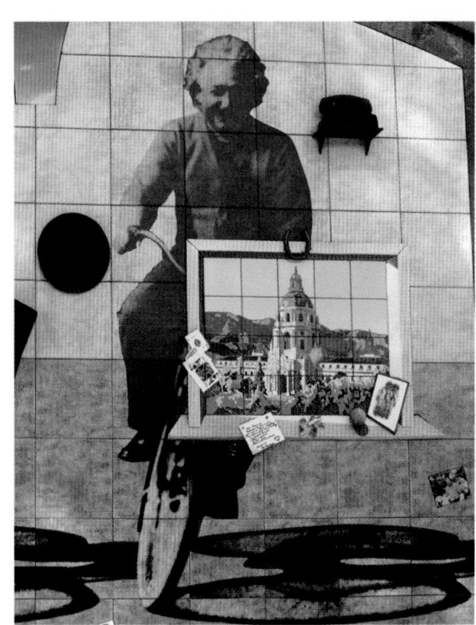

*Our fellow cyclist Albert Einstein was a visiting professor at Caltech, where his papers now reside.*

Pasadena's early boom years—the 1880s through the Great Depression—were fueled by strong rail connections, bringing tourists from across the country. This leafy city, with its San Gabriel Mountain backdrop, became a fashionable winter retreat for wealthy Easterners, who commissioned architecturally notable homes and patronized grand resort hotels here. Around 1940, the first U.S. freeway was built, connecting Pasadena to Downtown Los Angeles. Our leisurely spin hits landmarks from those days, as well as other eras in the city's evolution.

Early in the journey, you'll reach Arroyo Boulevard, a curving, tree-canopied residential way, overlooking the arroyo. The route soon passes under the 1913 Colorado Street Bridge (listed on the National Register of Historic Places) a span with elegant structural arches.

Downhill is the Rose Bowl, with its 1922 stadium and surrounding soccer fields, golf course, Olympic-caliber aquatic center and vast monthly flea market (for more about the Rose Bowl, see Ride 13).

Up a short hill is the 1908 Gamble House, an outstanding example of Arts & Crafts-style architecture, designed by Greene & Greene for Cincinnati-native David Gamble of the Proctor & Gamble Company. Currently owned by the city of Pasadena and the University of Southern California, this National Historic Landmark is open for visits, Thursday through Sunday (**www.gamblehouse.org/tours**).

The ride continues into Old Pasadena, the city's original commercial center, now a shopping and dining district, where every January 1, the Tournament of Roses Parade passes, its rose-festooned floats, marching bands and equestrian units welcome the New Year.

Next: Pasadena City Hall, a majestic, domed palace of government, from 1927, followed by a breeze through the California Institute of Technology (Caltech) campus. This lush oasis with fountains and gracious cloistered walkways belies the institution's scientific intensity—with many Nobel laureates in its ranks, Caltech is a virtual research crucible. Nearby is the Huntington Library, with its Art Collections and Botanical Gardens. This 207-acre institution, founded in 1919 by railroad-utility-and-real-estate baron Henry Huntington, is well worth a visit, if only for its diverse gardens—or such rare holdings as a Gutenberg Bible or the Gainsborough painting *Blue Boy*.

After wending through the enclave of San Marino and back to more urban territory, you might be ready for refueling at the vintage Fair Oaks Pharmacy and Soda, en route to the South Pasadena Metro station, where this odyssey began.

# Ride Log

0.0 From Orange Grove Park or Metro's Mission station, cross Mission St and begin riding west.
0.5 Turn right onto Arroyo Dr, which becomes Arroyo Blvd at San Rafael Ave.
2.8 Pass under the famous and picturesque Colorado Blvd Bridge and the 134 Freeway.
3.7 Turn right onto Seco St at the Rose Bowl.
3.9 Turn right onto Rosemont Ave.
4.3 Turn right onto Orange Grove Blvd and then, right into the drive leading to Gamble House.
4.4 Turn right onto Orange Grove Blvd.
4.8 Turn left onto Colorado Blvd.
5.6 Turn left onto Arroyo Pkwy. Use the crosswalk if traffic conditions warrant.
5.7 Turn right onto Holly St.
5.9 Arrive at Pasadena City Hall. Circle it by turning left onto Garfield Ave, right onto Ramona St, right onto Union St and right onto Garfield.
6.2 Return along Holly St.
6.4 Turn left onto Marengo Ave.
6.7 Turn left on Cordova St.
7.8 Turn right on Wilson Ave.
8.1 Turn left onto the Caltech campus just past the Braun Laboratories building (across from San Pasqual St).
8.5 Leave the Caltech Campus, cross Hill Ave and continue on San Pasqual St.
9.0 Turn right onto Allen Ave.
9.3 Arrive at the Huntington Library, Art Collections, and Botanical Gardens. If you are visiting the Huntington, you will locate the bicycle racks in the main parking lot. Ask the gate attendant for directions. If you are just passing by, you might see if the attendant will let you ride through the parking area to the Oxford Rd exit, otherwise, turn right onto Orlando Rd.
9.5 Turn right onto Oxford Rd.
10.0 Turn right onto Euston Rd.
10.8 Turn right onto Virginia Rd at Lacy Park.
11.1 Turn left onto Mill Ln.
11.3 Turn right onto Old Mill Rd.
11.9 Turn left onto El Molino Ave.
12.1 Turn right onto Mission St.
12.7 Pass Garfield Park (which has restrooms, drinking fountain, picnic area).
12.9 Cross Fair Oaks Ave.
13.4 Arrive back at Metro's Mission station or Orange Grove Park. End of ride.

P1 Rose Bowl & the flea market
P2 Gamble House
P3 Pasadena History Museum
P4 Norton Simon Museum
P5 Tournament of Roses House
P6 Old Pasadena
P7 Pasadena Memorial Park
P8 Pasadena City Hall
P9 Pacific Asia Museum
P10 Pasadena Museum of California Art
P11 California Institute of Technology
P12 Huntington Library, Art Gallery & Botanical Garden
P13 Lacy Park
P14 El Molino Viejo

A Tour of Pasadena

Altitude ft: 950, 850, 750, 650, 550
Distance miles: 0, 2, 4, 6, 8, 10, 12, 13.4

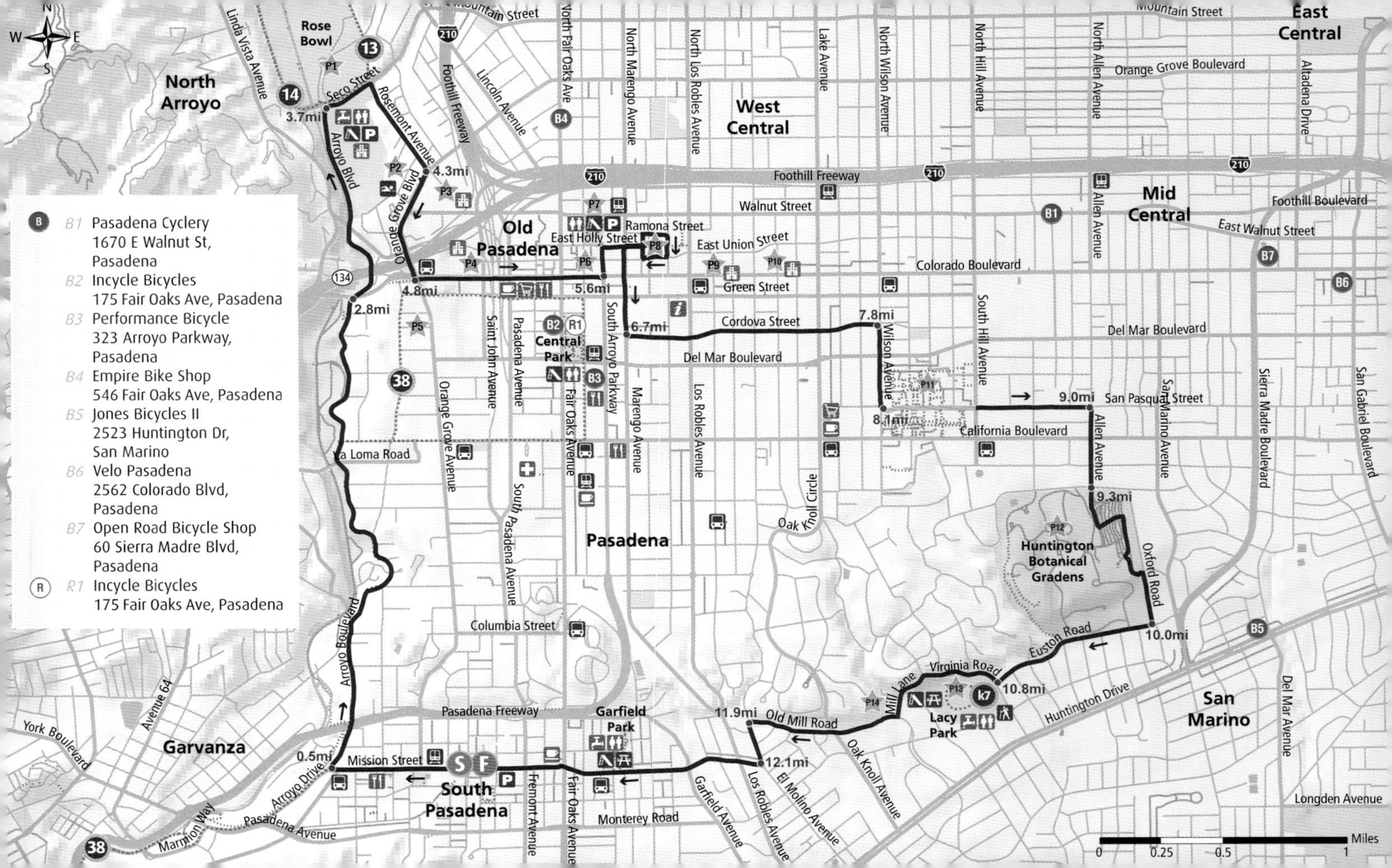

B1 Pasadena Cyclery
1670 E Walnut St, Pasadena
B2 Incycle Bicycles
175 Fair Oaks Ave, Pasadena
B3 Performance Bicycle
323 Arroyo Parkway, Pasadena
B4 Empire Bike Shop
546 Fair Oaks Ave, Pasadena
B5 Jones Bicycles II
2523 Huntington Dr, San Marino
B6 Velo Pasadena
2562 Colorado Blvd, Pasadena
B7 Open Road Bicycle Shop
60 Sierra Madre Blvd, Pasadena
R1 Incycle Bicycles
175 Fair Oaks Ave, Pasadena
North Arroyo
Rose Bowl
West Central
Mid Central
East Central
Old Pasadena
Central Park
Pasadena
Garfield Park
South Pasadena
Garvanza
Lacy Park
Huntington Botanical Gradens
San Marino
Foothill Freeway
Pasadena Freeway
Colorado Boulevard
Del Mar Boulevard
Cordova Street
California Boulevard
Arroyo Boulevard
Mission Street
Oxford Road
Euston Road
Virginia Road
Mill Lane
Old Mill Road
Huntington Drive
0.5mi
2.8mi
3.7mi
4.3mi
4.8mi
5.6mi
6.7mi
7.8mi
8.1mi
9.0mi
9.3mi
10.0mi
10.8mi
11.9mi
12.1mi
Miles
0
0.25
0.5
1

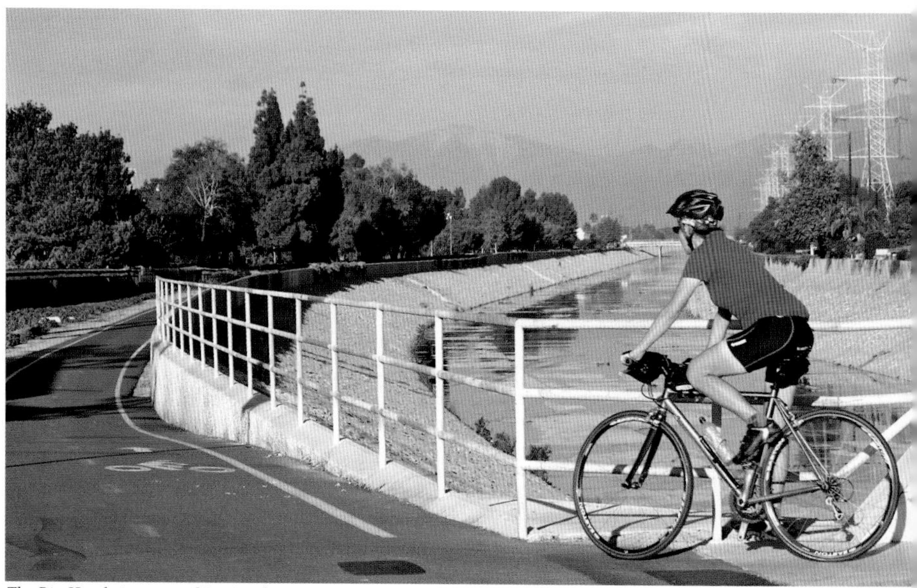

*The Rio Hondo is among this trio of rivers.*

## At a Glance

**Distance** 43.3 miles **Elevation Gain** 1,900 feet

### Terrain

While seemingly flat, this ride gradually gains elevation, mostly going north. (And afternoon winds from the coast can make southbound riding feel like a mild climb.)

### Traffic

The river paths are closed to vehicular traffic. The city streets connecting them have bike lanes or are quiet residential ways.

### How to Get There

To reach the start, at John Anson Ford Park, exit the 710 Freeway onto Florence Avenue eastbound. After about one and 1.5 miles, turn right onto Scout Avenue to the park.

### Food and Drink

The river paths have no refreshment stops. To fuel up, you'll need to venture into the adjacent neighborhoods. Long Beach Towne Center—with cafés, snack shops and a supermarket—makes a good mid-ride stop, just north of El Dorado Park.

### Side Trip

Old town Whittier's business district, along Greenleaf Avenue, has plenty of good places to eat and vintage signage everywhere (apparently they just never updated it, which adds a certain charm). To get there, exit the San Gabriel River path onto Beverly Boulevard. Turn right onto Frontier Boulevard, left onto the Whittier Greenway Trail (Ride 17) and then, left onto Philadelphia Street. Go several blocks to Greenleaf.

**Links to** 17 18 19 42 46 47 51 k9 k11 k12 k23

**Where to Bike Rating** 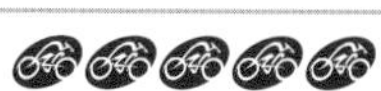

## About...

With stretches on the Los Angeles, San Gabriel and Rio Hondo rivers, this is the second longest spin in the book. Almost entirely on protected bike path, it's the ride with the most car-free miles. From the Rio Hondo, you'll head south along the L.A. River before traversing Long Beach's midsection on quiet residential streets. A northward turn leads to flat, easy riding along the San Gabriel River, where urban and industrial landscapes gradually give way to vital wetlands, particularly near the Whittier Narrows Dam, at the ride's northern end.

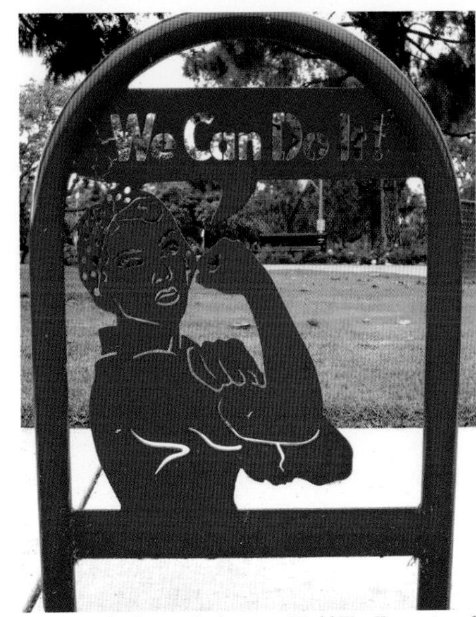


*At Rosie the Riveter Park, near a World War II-era aircraft plant, bike racks celebrate strong women.*



Three rivers flow from the San Gabriel Mountains toward the Pacific Ocean: the Los Angeles River to the west, the San Gabriel to the east, and the Rio Hondo in between, joining with the Los Angeles River near Southgate. But, channelized in concrete with the source waters trapped in flood-control reservoirs, they are, for much of their length, rivers in name only. For cyclists, the upside of these engineering interventions are the long, smooth, virtually uninterrupted bikeways. Such channels provide more than 80 miles of bike path across L.A., about half the rivers' total length.

On the Three Rivers ride, the first turn takes you onto the LARIO Trail, a path partly on the L.A. River and partly on the Rio Hondo. It's easy, car-free riding, past foundries, factories and warehouses. Further south, small residential backyards also come into view. Path-side parks—Hollydale, Ralph C. Dills, DeForest and Wrigley Greenbelt—also punctuate the journey, offering pockets of greenery (plus handy amenities, such as restrooms and drinking fountains).

Bixby Road, Conant Street and Wardlow Road, three Long Beach bikeways, provide a route across northern Long Beach, connecting the L.A. River path to the San Gabriel River Bikeway. En route, you'll pass an abandoned aircraft factory where the Douglas Aircraft Company built propeller-driven fighters, bombers and transport planes used during World War II. Successor companies McDonald Douglas and Boeing made passenger and cargo jets here until 2011. Rosie the Riveter Park, where this ride turns, honors the contributions women made to the war effort here.

After navigating a sequence of turns from Wardlow Road through El Dorado Park (Ride 47), the journey continues north along the San Gabriel River Bikeway. Spanning more than 39 miles from the beach to the mountains, it is L.A.'s single longest, continuous bike path. After miles of laid-back riding past small horse paddocks, back yards and industrial settings, you'll reach more natural parts of the river, where willow trees and wetland thickets have taken root. After the Whittier Narrows Dam, the highest point of the ride, the track turns south on the LARIO Trail, looping back to Bell Gardens. No guarantees about wind direction, but it's definitely downhill (slightly) from here to the start.

*While Ride 16 has not been deemed kid-friendly in its entirety, it does include substantial sections which are entirely safe for family use.*

# Ride Log

0.0 From the parking area, ride through the park toward the river. After you pass through the gate to the bike path, turn right.
0.6 Via the bike bridge at Crawford Park, cross to the Rio Hondo's east bank.
2.5 Merge with the Los Angeles River Bikeway at Imperial Hwy.
5.0 Pass Ralph C. Dills Park.
10.7 Turn left and exit the bike path at the Wrigley Greenbelt—just after you've passed under the 405 Freeway and Wardlow Rd. Descend the ramp and continue east on 34th St.
11.0 Merge with Wardlow Rd.
11.4 Turn left onto Pacific Ave, just after the Metro Blue Line station. Use the crosswalk at the station if traffic conditions warrant.
11.9 Turn right onto Bixby Rd, joining the bike lane.
13.6 Turn left onto Industry Ave.
13.7 Turn right onto Cover St, joining its bike lane.
14.8 Turn right onto Worsham Ave at the Douglas Park roundabout.
15.0 Turn left onto Conant St.
15.6 Pass Rosie the Riveter Park and Interpretive Center.
16.6 Turn right onto Woodruff Ave, joining the bike lane.
17.0 Turn left onto Wardlow Rd. Use the crosswalk.
18.6 Cross the San Gabriel River.
18.8 Enter El Dorado Park through the pedestrian gate (at the right end of the fence blocking automobile access). Follow the access road, joining the San Gabriel River Bikeway at Wardlow Rd.
27.6 Pass Wilderness Park (which has restrooms and drinking water).
33.8 Cross under the San Gabriel River Pkwy, make a U-turn and cross the river. The ramp up to San Gabriel River Pkwy is extremely steep, so be prepared to dismount.
33.9 Resume riding north on the San Gabriel River Bikeway.
34.6 Ride over the Whittier Narrows Dam.
34.9 Turn left onto the Rio Hondo Bikeway.
35.7 Cross Durfee Ave and Rosemead Blvd using the crosswalks.
36.1 Cross San Gabriel Blvd at Lincoln Ave, rejoining the Rio Hondo Bikeway.
37.4 Descend from the top of the dam.
37.9 Pass Grant Rea Park (which has restrooms and drinking water).
43.3 Arrive back at John Anson Ford Park. End of ride.

B
B1 J & M Bike Shop
6305 Florence Ave, Bell Gardens
B2 Junky Rusty Bikes
9555 Cherry Ave, Long Beach
B3 Frank's Bicycles, 3255 South St, Long Beach
B4 Lakewood Cyclery, 4313 Carson St, Lakewood
B5 California Cycle Sport
6759 Carson St, Lakewood
B6 Performance Bicycle
7611 Carson St, Long Beach
B7 Lakewood Bicycles
5930 Del Amo Blvd, Lakewood
B8 Big Wheel Bicycles
17314 Pioneer Blvd, Artesia
B9 Pats 605 Cyclery
12310 Studebaker Rd, Norwalk
B10 Russell's Bicycles
8027 Firestone Blvd, Downey
B11 Franks Bike Shop
10335 Lakewood Blvd, Downey
B12 G's Cyclery & Wheels
6713 Greenleaf Ave, Whittier

Three Rivers: Rio Hondo, San Gabriel & Los Angeles

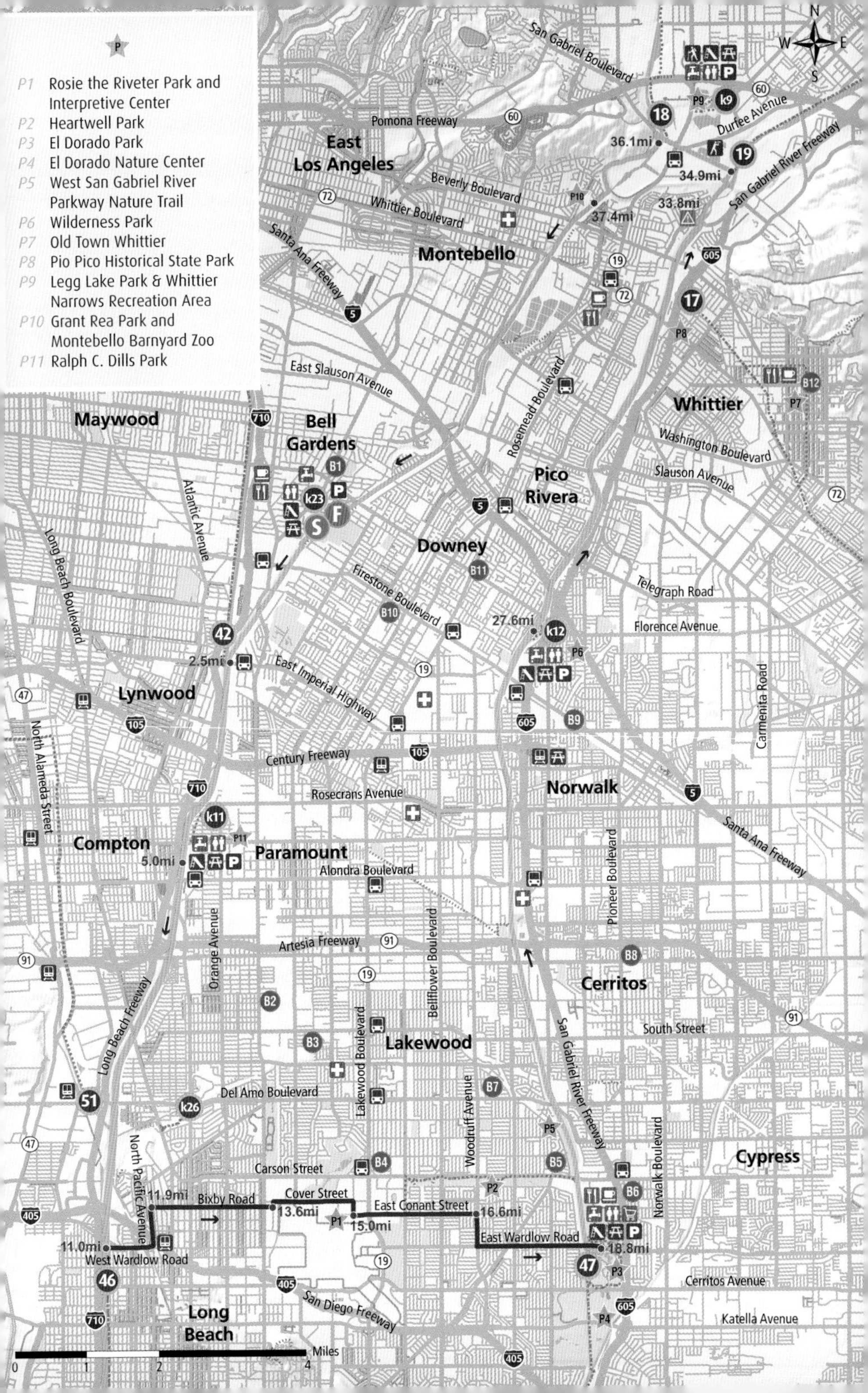

P1 Rosie the Riveter Park and Interpretive Center
P2 Heartwell Park
P3 El Dorado Park
P4 El Dorado Nature Center
P5 West San Gabriel River Parkway Nature Trail
P6 Wilderness Park
P7 Old Town Whittier
P8 Pio Pico Historical State Park
P9 Legg Lake Park & Whittier Narrows Recreation Area
P10 Grant Rea Park and Montebello Barnyard Zoo
P11 Ralph C. Dills Park
East Los Angeles
Montebello
Whittier
Maywood
Bell Gardens
Pico Rivera
Downey
Lynwood
Norwalk
Compton
Paramount
Cerritos
Lakewood
Cypress
Long Beach
San Gabriel Boulevard
Pomona Freeway
Durfee Avenue
San Gabriel River Freeway
Beverly Boulevard
Whittier Boulevard
Santa Ana Freeway
East Slauson Avenue
Rosemead Boulevard
Washington Boulevard
Slauson Avenue
Atlantic Avenue
Long Beach Boulevard
Firestone Boulevard
Telegraph Road
Florence Avenue
East Imperial Highway
Carmenita Road
North Alameda Street
Century Freeway
Rosecrans Avenue
Alondra Boulevard
Orange Avenue
Bellflower Boulevard
Pioneer Boulevard
Artesia Freeway
Long Beach Freeway
Lakewood Boulevard
South Street
Del Amo Boulevard
Woodruff Avenue
North Pacific Avenue
Norwalk Boulevard
Carson Street
Bixby Road
Cover Street
East Conant Street
East Wardlow Road
West Wardlow Road
San Diego Freeway
Cerritos Avenue
Katella Avenue
36.1mi
34.9mi
33.8mi
37.4mi
27.6mi
2.5mi
5.0mi
11.9mi
13.6mi
15.0mi
16.6mi
18.8mi
11.0mi
Miles
0
1
2
4

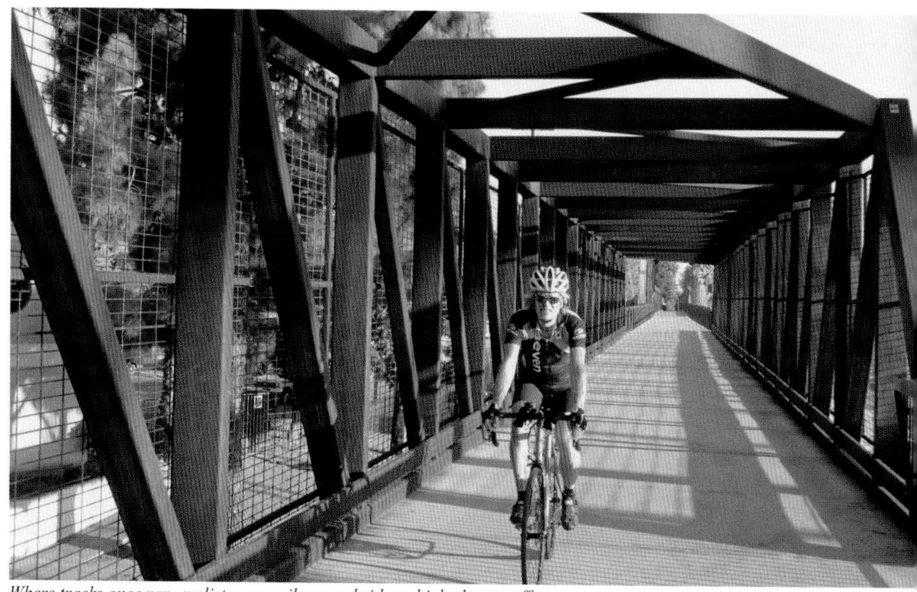


*Where tracks once ran, cyclists now sail across bridges, high above traffic.*

## At a Glance

**Distance** 10.3 miles **Elevation Gain** 400 feet

### Terrain

The path is mostly at grade and flat, except for the modest ascent to a pair of bridges.

### Traffic

The Greenway is car-free. At street crossings, respect traffic signals. Greenleaf Avenue and Broadway are moderately busy city streets.

### How to Get There

Exit the 605 Freeway onto Whittier Boulevard heading east. Turn left onto Lockheed Avenue, then left onto Orange Drive and, finally, right onto Pioneer Boulevard. Park in the lot at Guirado Park.

### Food and Drink

You'll find plenty of eateries on both Greenleaf Avenue and Whittier Boulevard in downtown Whittier. Greenleaf Avenue merits a detour if only because, apparently, no one got around to replacing the sometimes amusing 1950s signage on many of its commercial establishments.

### Side Trip

Jonathan Bailey House, circa 1869, is the city's oldest building and former home to its first settlers, Jonathan and Rebecca Bailey, who held Quaker meetings on the front porch. (To reach the house, at 13421 Camilla Street, turn east from the Greenway onto Broadway and right onto Camilla. Call 562- 945-3871 for guided tours.) The 1892 Whittier Train Depot has been relocated to Greenleaf Avenue, near Penn Street in Whittier's historic downtown district.

**Links to** 16

**Where to Bike Rating** 

  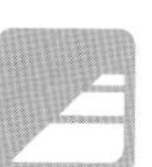 

## About...

This rails-to-trails spin, just under five-miles long, gives you a rolling glimpse of Whittier's past as a citrus-and-walnut-growing center, fueled by active rail connections. Part of the fun of this ride is the variety of neighborhoods en route—residential, light industrial and commercial areas, interspersed with parks and vintage relics. The north end of this ex-rail spur does not yet connect readily with the (tantalizingly close) San Gabriel River Bikeway, though hopefully it will soon. The south end's turnaround is at Mills Avenue.

A lot of transformation happened in Whittier around the turn of the 20th century. Founded by Quakers in the 1880s, the town became a booming citrus-growing area and the U.S.'s biggest walnut producer. Named for Quaker poet John Greenleaf Whittier, it's also where Richard Nixon—Whittier's most famous and controversial figure—grew up and attended college. In 1904, nine years before Nixon's birth, the Pacific Electric Railway launched a popular trolley route, about 12-miles long, connecting Whittier to Downtown L.A. via the company's signature "Red Cars."

But just as the region's commercial orange and lemon groves are now history (mostly subdivided into housing tracts after World War II), the trolley route is long gone, as is its freight-train successor. This stretch lay idle for decades—until Whittier acquired 4.8 miles of the rail right of way and, by 2009, successfully turned it into a thriving bicycling-and-pedestrian greenway.

Though hardly a long rail-to-trails (Whittier has ambitions of extending it), the Greenway is exceptional in its well-tended landscaping—featuring drought-resistant, native plants and sycamore trees—integrated with spinning wind sculptures.

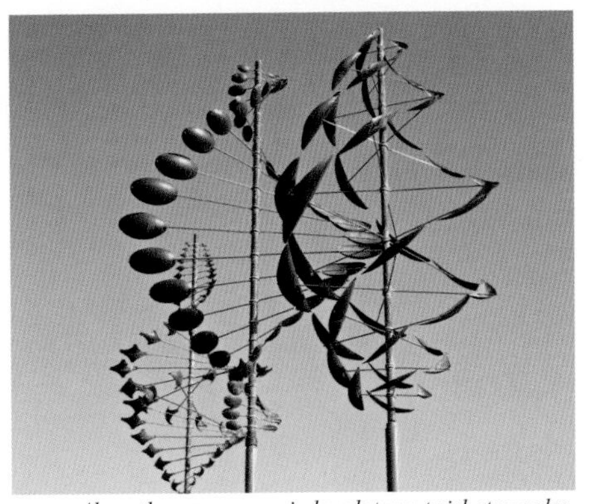

*Along the greenway, wind sculptures twirl atop poles.*



Beginning near Guirado Park, the journey later bisects Palm Park (a leafy green space with a community swimming pool and tennis courts) and passes through residential, light industrial and commercial areas—sparked with relics of Whittier's agricultural and railway past. Interpretive panels mark former rail stops: at Palm Station, within Palm Park; Citrus Station, south of Penn Street; Sycamore Station, near the Five Points traffic node; and Oak Station, west of Mills Avenue.

Though the path is mostly at grade, you can blissfully roll across an old rail bridge high above Five Points' clogged traffic arteries. Near Citrus Station is the cavernous old Sunkist orange-packing house (now King Richard's Antiques emporium). On Hadley Street's north side, watch for the Whittier Ice Cream building, an icy white Art Deco architectural confection, where the late and legendary chocolate-dipped Cool-a-Coo ice cream sandwich—a Dodgers Stadium favorite—was born. At Mar Vista Street, a few yards west of the route, visit the 1907 Paradox Hybrid Walnut Tree, a National Landmark and prodigious survivor of a formerly flourishing industry. The greenway is a leisurely path. Multiple, sometimes convoluted, street crossings keep the pace slow. It's a place where families ride or stroll, enjoying a quiet passage of Whittier where life once clanged and sped through.

*While Ride 17 has not been deemed kid-friendly in its entirety, it does include substantial sections which are entirely safe for family use.*

# Ride Log

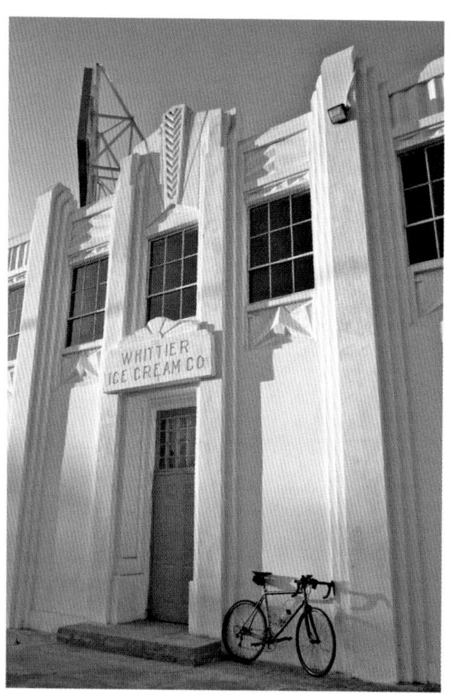


*Glacial Art Deco: Back in the day, Cool-A-Coo ice cream sandwiches were made here.*

0.0 From Guirado Park, ride north along Pioneer Blvd for about one block.

0.1 Turn right onto the Whittier Greenway Trail.

0.9 Pass Palm Park station and wind sculptures.

1.1 Cross Palm Ave.

1.3 Cross Broadway.

1.5 Cross the Camilla St-Magnolia Ave intersection.

1.6 Cross Hadley St.

1.8 Cross the Bailey St-Gregory Ave intersection.

1.9 Cross Philadelphia St.

2.2 Cross Penn St. Citrus Station with interpretive panels describing Whittier's agricultural history.

2.4 Cross Mar Vista St using the cross walk at Mar Vista and Whittier Blvd.

2.7 Sycamore Station with panels focused on native sycamores and transportation along the rail route.

2.8 Cross over the Five Points intersection (Washington Blvd, Whittier Blvd, Pickering Ave, La Cuarta St, and Santa Fe Springs Rd) on the steel-truss bridges (a vintage rail bridge and a modern, rusted-steel span).

3.2 Cross Greenleaf Ave using the crosswalk.

3.5 Cross Painter Ave using the crosswalk.

3.8 Cross Laurel Ave using the crosswalk.

4.2 Cross Calmada Ave using the crosswalk.

4.5 Cross Gunn Ave using the crosswalk.

4.8 Arrive at Mills Ave. End of the Whittier Greenway. Turn around and head back down the greenway to Greenleaf Ave.

6.5 Turn right onto Greenleaf Ave.

6.7 Cross Whittier Blvd.

8.1 Turn left onto Broadway.

9.0 Turn right onto the Whittier Greenway Trail.

9.4 Pass through Palm Park.

10.2 End of the Whittier Greenway Trail. Turn left onto Pioneer Blvd.

10.3 Arrive back at Guirado Park. End of ride.

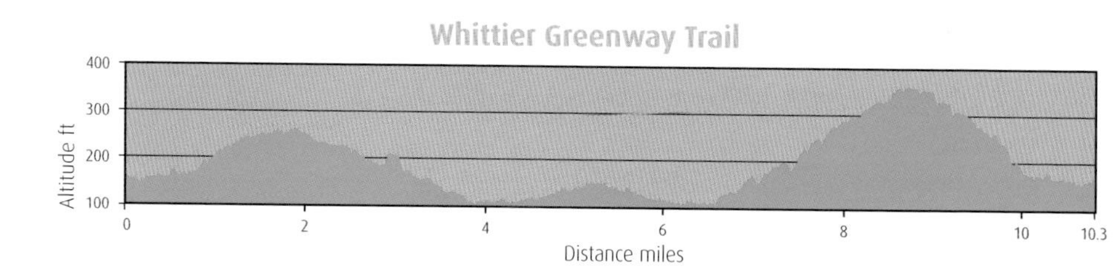

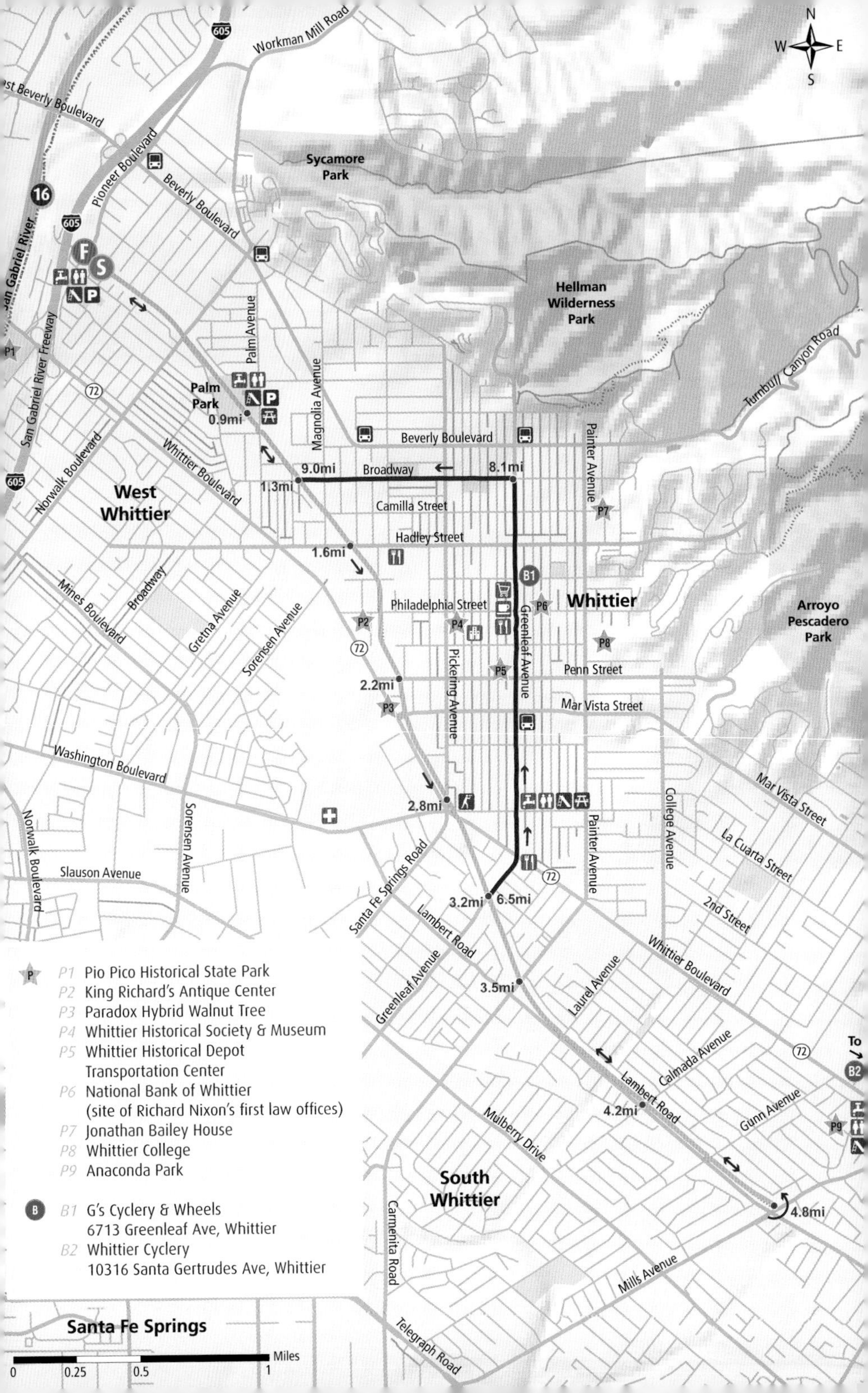

Workman Mill Road
605
East Beverly Boulevard
Pioneer Boulevard
Beverly Boulevard
Sycamore Park
16
605
San Gabriel River
F
S
Hellman Wilderness Park
San Gabriel River Freeway
P1
Palm Avenue
Magnolia Avenue
Turnbull Canyon Road
72
Palm Park
0.9mi
Beverly Boulevard
Painter Avenue
Norwalk Boulevard
605
Whittier Boulevard
9.0mi
Broadway
8.1mi
1.3mi
West Whittier
Camilla Street
P7
Hadley Street
1.6mi
B1
Broadway
Philadelphia Street
P6
Whittier
Arroyo Pescadero Park
Mines Boulevard
Gretna Avenue
Sorensen Avenue
P2
P4
P8
72
Greenleaf Avenue
P5
Penn Street
2.2mi
Pickering Avenue
P3
Mar Vista Street
Washington Boulevard
Mar Vista Street
College Avenue
2.8mi
La Cuarta Street
Norwalk Boulevard
Sorensen Avenue
Santa Fe Springs Road
Painter Avenue
Slauson Avenue
72
3.2mi
6.5mi
2nd Street
Lambert Road
Whittier Boulevard
3.5mi
Greenleaf Avenue
Laurel Avenue
Calmada Avenue
To B2
72
Lambert Road
4.2mi
Gunn Avenue
Mulberry Drive
P9
South Whittier
4.8mi
Carmenita Road
Mills Avenue
Santa Fe Springs
Telegraph Road
Miles
0
0.25
0.5
1
P1 Pio Pico Historical State Park
P2 King Richard's Antique Center
P3 Paradox Hybrid Walnut Tree
P4 Whittier Historical Society & Museum
P5 Whittier Historical Depot Transportation Center
P6 National Bank of Whittier (site of Richard Nixon's first law offices)
P7 Jonathan Bailey House
P8 Whittier College
P9 Anaconda Park
B1 G's Cyclery & Wheels 6713 Greenleaf Ave, Whittier
B2 Whittier Cyclery 10316 Santa Gertrudes Ave, Whittier

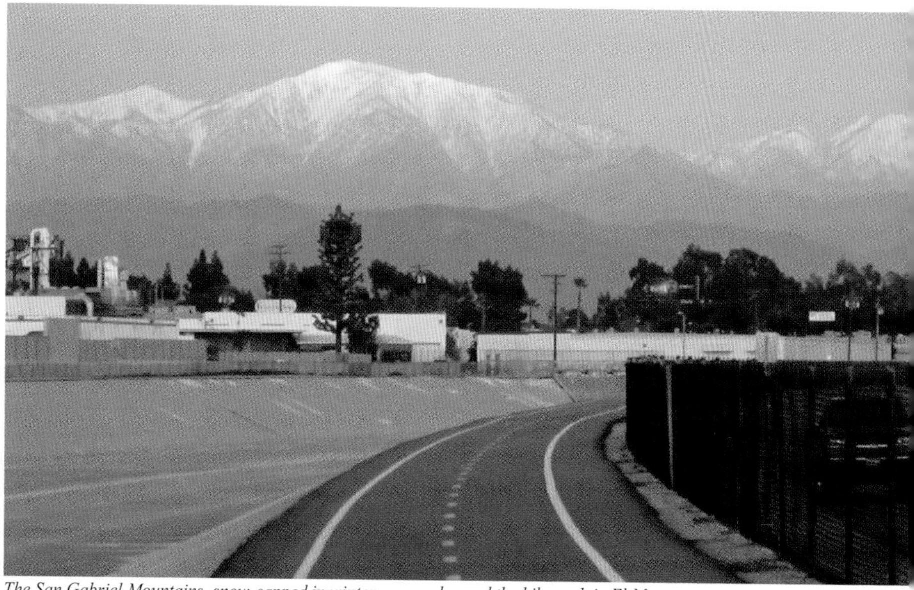
*The San Gabriel Mountains, snow-capped in winter, appear beyond the bike path in El Monte.*

## At a Glance

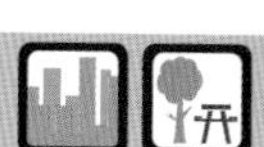

**Distance** 21.6 miles **Elevation Gain** 900 feet

### Terrain

This smooth, paved bike path runs from the trailhead to Peck Road, where the route shifts to city streets, slightly uphill to Monrovia.

### Traffic

The bike path is car-free. Peck Road and Myrtle Avenue, with traffic typical of a small municipality, offer wide shoulders.

### How to Get There

From the 60 Freeway, exit onto Rosemead Boulevard and continue south. Turn right onto San Gabriel Boulevard, followed by a right into Bosque Del Rio Hondo's parking area ($5.00 per car). Alternatively, from Rosemead, make a left onto Durfee Avenue, another left at Santa Anita Avenue and a final left into Legg Lake's parking lot (free).

### Food and Drink

Old Town Monrovia offers the best snacking and dining options: everything from restaurants to a bakeshop established in 1900. We like the Monrovia Coffee Company (Myrtle at Lemon Avenue) for coffee, teas, cookies, carrot cake, fresh sandwiches and more.

### Side Trip

Consider riding to Monrovia Canyon Park for a leisurely picnic. From Old Town continue north on Myrtle, turn right on Greystone Avenue for two blocks, turn left on Canyon Boulevard, and ride about two miles. An easy one-mile hike to a waterfall makes a great excursion within the park.

**Links to** 16 19 k9

**Where to Bike Rating** 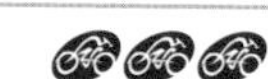

 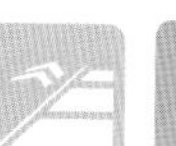 

San Gabriel Valley

# About...

Named for one of the three rivers flowing from the San Gabriel Mountains through the Los Angeles Basin to the ocean, this easy ride meanders along the Rio Hondo, from Whittier Narrows north to a vintage town near the headwaters. En route, the scene unfolds: from river wetlands to residential pockets and industrial areas before reaching Monrovia's tree-lined, old-time main street (along Myrtle Avenue), with the San Gabriel Mountains as its backdrop.

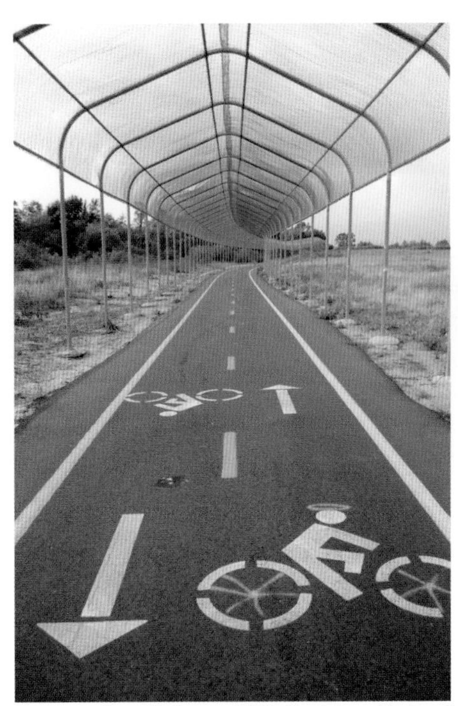

*Alongside Bosque del Rio Hondo's model aircraft field, the path (with angelic cyclists) ducks beneath a protective canopy.*

One turn from the Bosque del Rio Hondo parking lot, and you've suddenly left urban life. Bosque del Rio means "forest of the river," and this park celebrates one of Rio Hondo's last remaining natural streambeds. Along this short stretch, you'll see this river as it once was—with slow moving water, wildlife and brambly, overarching native trees. After about two miles, however, the ride continues along the Army Corps of Engineers' 1950s-era reincarnation of the river: a concrete-lined flood-control channel. Fortunately, the rim of this levee makes for a smooth, paved bike path, with miles of easy pedaling—past plant nurseries, a golf course and the small planes at El Monte's airfield—to the picturesque manmade lake at Peck Road Water Conservation Park. If you want just a short spin, this is a good turnaround point.

Of course, every good ride deserves a satisfying lunch stop, and the Rio Hondo is no exception. An ideal spot for a brief hiatus is Old Town Monrovia, along Myrtle Avenue. Just a few years ago, Monrovia wasn't much more than an aging bedroom community. But recently, the place has enjoyed a revival, especially its historic downtown area, where benign neglect has given way to nouveau-quaint. Here, you'll find an assortment of cyclist-friendly snack options, including cafés, neo-folksy food shops and newer English, French and Italian eateries. On Friday evenings, Old Town hosts a farmers' market and, in March through December, the Family Festival Street Fair on Myrtle Avenue.

By the way, lunch in Monrovia happens to have a great bit of history. In 1937, Patrick McDonald opened a successful burger joint at the now-vanished Monrovia Airport. A few years later, Patrick and his sons, Maurice and Richard, packed up their grills and moved the whole eatery to San Bernardino, California, where the MacDonald family's cutting-edge burger innovations were discovered (and ultimately bought out) by milkshake-machine salesman Ray Kroc. So the ubiquitous Golden Arches can trace their truest and deepest roots right here to Monrovia.

*While Ride 18 has not been deemed kid-friendly in its entirety, it does include substantial sections which are entirely safe for family use.*

# Ride Log

P1 Legg Lake
P2 Whittier Narrows Nature Center
P3 Monrovia Canyon Park
P4 Los Angeles County Arboretum & Botanic Garden

B1 RB Bicycle Shop
9533 Garvey Ave, South El Monte
B2 Pepe's Bicycle Shop
11426 Garvey Ave, El Monte
B3 2 Wheel Bikes
11688 Clark St # A, Arcadia
B4 Lloyd's Custom Bicycle Shop
816 Highland Ave, Duarte
B5 Stan's Monrovia Bikes
880 S. Myrtle Ave, Monrovia
B6 Bicycle Sam
503 W Duarte Rd #A, Monrovia
B7 Helen's Cycles
142 East Huntington Dr, Arcadia
B8 REI Co-op
214 N. Santa Anita Ave, Arcadia
B9 Temple City Bike Shop
9628 Las Tunas Dr, Temple City

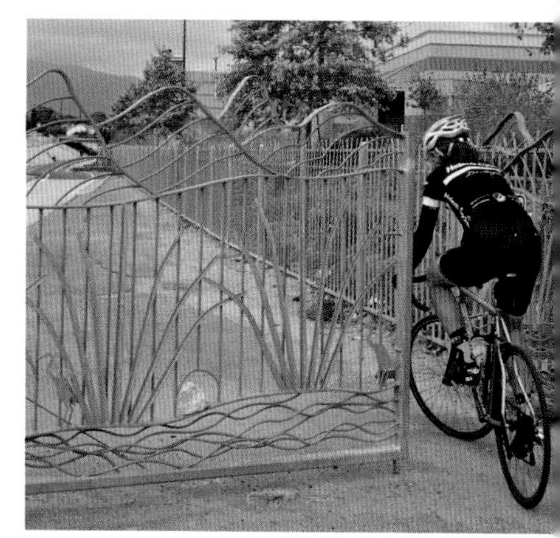

*Entry gates along the Rio Hondo evoke mountains, flowin waters, river rocks and reeds*

0.0 Bike out of Bosque del Rio Hondo's gate and turn right onto the Rio Hondo bike path. If you've parked at Legg Lake, a short warm-up ride will get you to the trailhead. Ride south on Santa Anita Ave to Durfee, turn right and, after about a mile, cross Rosemead to the Rio Hondo bike path.

1.1 Turn left, following the arrows directing you to the "Upper Rio Hondo Trail."

1.9 Leave the wetlands, begin riding along the top of the Rio Hondo on the paved bike path.

3.9 Fletcher and Pioneer parks.

4.4 El Monte Valley Mall (Valley Blvd and Santa Anita Ave, just east of Rio Hondo).

5.5 Pass the El Monte Airport.

7.0 Arrive at the Peck Road Water Conservation Par exit the park, then turn left on Peck Rd.

8.0 Peck Rd becomes Myrtle Ave at Live Oak Ave.

8.5 Stay to the left at the Y where Myrtle meets S Ca fornia Ave.

9.5 There are railroad tracks just north of Duarte Rd– be careful.

9.7 Pass under the 210 Freeway.

10.4 Pass under the "Myrtle Avenue Old Town Mo rovia" sign.

10.8 Arrive at Library Park. Reverse the route back Bosque del Rio Hondo.

21.6 End of ride.

Rio Hondo

Altitude ft: 200, 300, 400, 500, 600
Distance miles: 0, 4, 8, 12, 16, 20, 21.6

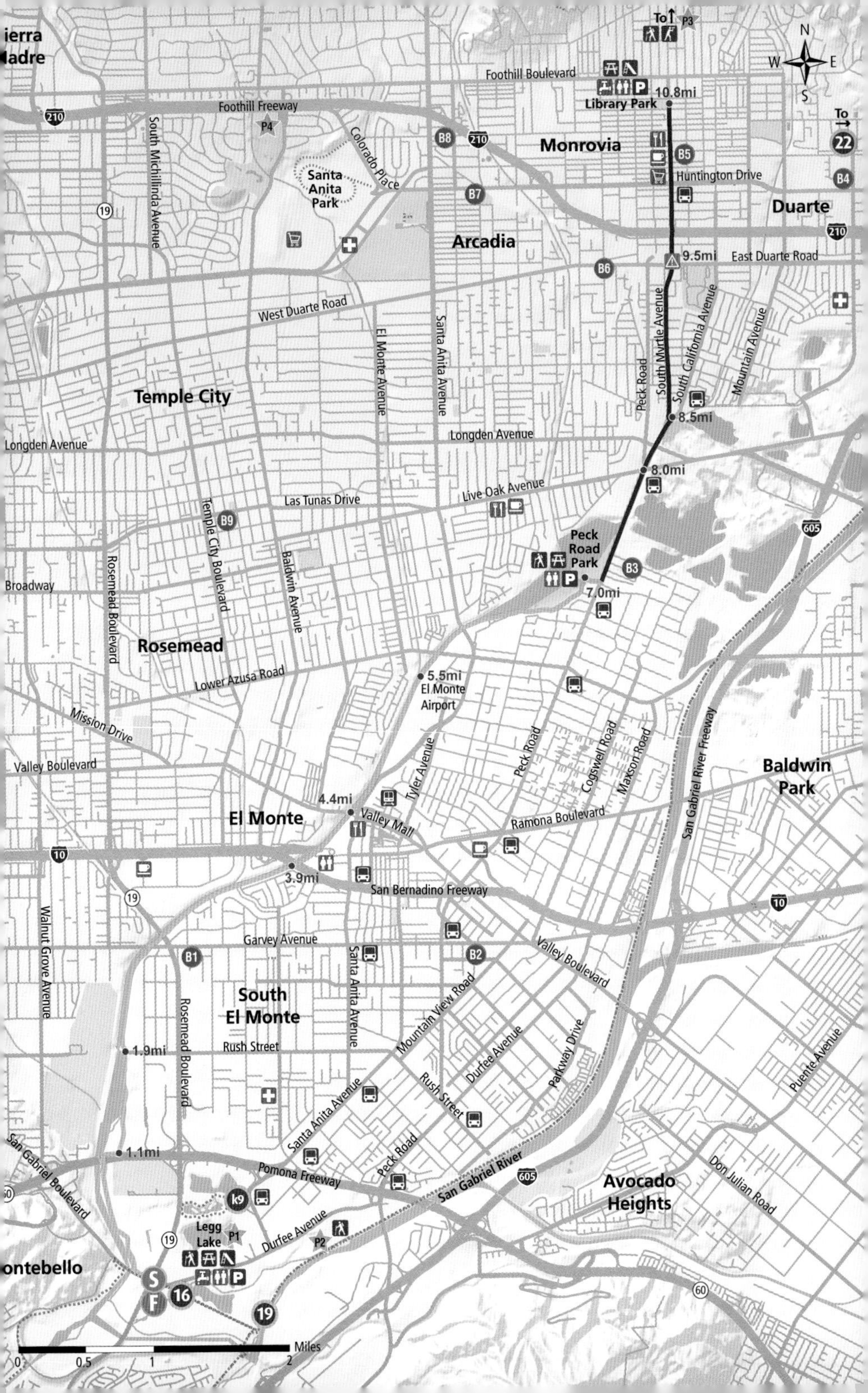

Sierra Madre
To P3
Foothill Boulevard
10.8mi
Library Park
Foothill Freeway
P4
Santa Anita Park
Colorado Place
B8
Monrovia
B5
Huntington Drive
To 22
B4
Duarte
B7
Arcadia
9.5mi
East Duarte Road
B6
West Duarte Road
South Michillinda Avenue
El Monte Avenue
Santa Anita Avenue
Peck Road
South Myrtle Avenue
South California Avenue
Mountain Avenue
Temple City
8.5mi
Longden Avenue
8.0mi
Live Oak Avenue
Las Tunas Drive
Temple City Boulevard
B9
Peck Road Park
B3
7.0mi
Broadway
Rosemead Boulevard
Baldwin Avenue
Rosemead
Lower Azusa Road
5.5mi
El Monte Airport
Mission Drive
Valley Boulevard
Tyler Avenue
Peck Road
Cogswell Road
Maxson Road
San Gabriel River Freeway
Baldwin Park
4.4mi
El Monte
Valley Mall
Ramona Boulevard
3.9mi
San Bernadino Freeway
Garvey Avenue
B1
B2
Valley Boulevard
Walnut Grove Avenue
Rosemead Boulevard
South El Monte
Santa Anita Avenue
Mountain View Road
1.9mi
Rush Street
Durfee Avenue
Parkway Drive
Puente Avenue
Rush Street
Santa Anita Avenue
San Gabriel Boulevard
1.1mi
Pomona Freeway
Peck Road
San Gabriel River
Avocado Heights
Don Julian Road
k9
Legg Lake
P1
Durfee Avenue
P2
Montebello
S
F
16
19
Miles
0
0.5
1
2

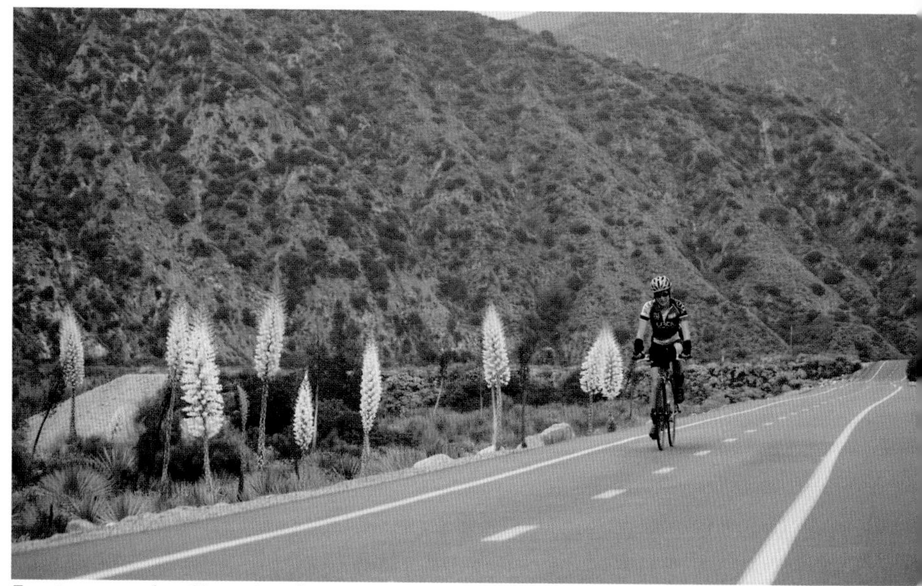

*Towering century plants blossom in early spring.*

## At a Glance

**Distance** 33.6 miles **Elevation Gain** 1,100 feet

### Terrain

The San Gabriel River Bike Trail has a newly paved, smooth surface. The only relatively steep incline is the short climb up the Santa Fe Dam.

### Traffic

The route is car-free, with only one street crossing, at Arrow Highway, just below the dam. Drivers are generally courteous here, but use caution.

### How to Get There

Exit the 60 Freeway at Rosemead Boulevard, travel south and turn right onto San Gabriel Boulevard to Bosque Del Rio Hondo's parking area ($5.00). Or make a left onto Durfee Avenue, then a left onto Santa Anita Avenue to Legg Lake's parking (free).

### Food and Drink

This route cuts across a broad urban landscape, but with surprisingly few "refueling" stops—just two convenience stores at Peck Road, near the start. So, bring water and snacks.

### Side Trip

Santa Fe Dam Recreation Area adjoins the bike path. (Turn downhill at mile 11.8, at the parking kiosk.) This 836-acre park includes picnic areas and a 70-acre fishing lake with non-motor boat rentals and a summertime swim beach. The park hosts an annual Renaissance Pleasure Faire, a historic re-enactment festival (Saturdays and Sundays, early April to late May).

**Links to** 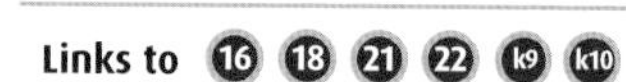


**Where to Bike Rating** 

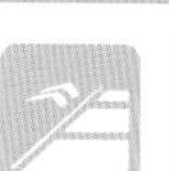
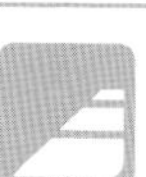

# About...

This ride covers the northern segment of the San Gabriel River Bike Trail: from Whittier Narrows, where the San Gabriel and Rio Hondo Rivers converge, up toward the San Gabriel Mountains. Miraculously, the path is not merely free of automobile traffic, but crosses only one street. After pedaling past many scruffy backyard stables—L.A.'s unofficial cowboy land—as well as quarries and school playing fields, you'll ascend the Santa Fe Dam and continue into the less inhabited terrain of high desert and San Gabriel foothills.

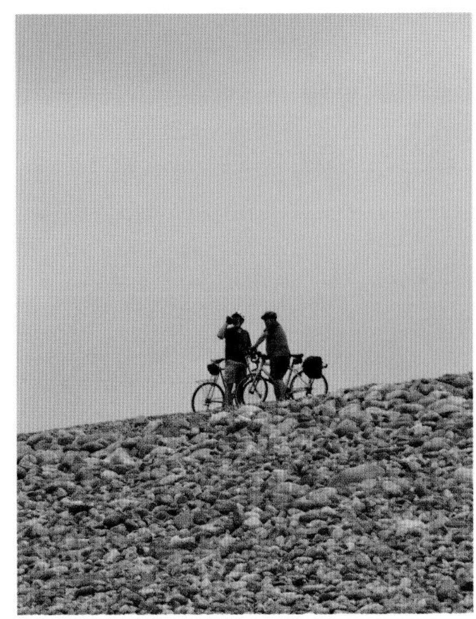

*The bike path crosses atop the Santa Fe Dam.*



The San Gabriel, like most rivers in Los Angeles, is often more of a dry riverbed than a gushing torrent. But after a wet and stormy winter, the upper San Gabriel cascades toward the lowlands through a series of waterfall-like spill basins. Here, seasonal change can be extreme. But—guaranteed year-round—the San Gabriel Bike Trail is always a great way to cross a vast swath of Los Angeles county, passing through urban territory and beyond, as the path extends car-free from ocean to mountains.

This ride, a 33-mile round-trip, is the northern segment of that long trail. We begin just above the Whittier Narrows, where the San Gabriel and Rio Hondo Rivers converge. Snaking through the city's urban cowboy terrain, the route borders small backyard stables with horses and, occasionally, ramshackle mini-rodeos with bleachers and loudspeakers booming mariachi music.

Beyond the gritty, homemade paddocks, a few community schools and a gravel quarry, you'll suddenly see the 92-foot-high Santa Fe Dam looming just ahead. The four-mile-long dam was built in 1949 to control catastrophic flooding. The region's typically arid climate, coupled with a strategic series of flood-control structures further upstream, however, makes a deep water-filled reservoir behind the dam extremely rare.

After crossing Arrow Highway, the route ramps up to the top of the dam. Here, striking views open toward the San Gabriel Mountains to the north and, on a clear day, L.A.'s Downtown skyline to the south. The path across the dam is gloriously wide and smooth. Past the parking kiosk, miles of tree nurseries extend over a narrow strip of land just below the trail. Beyond the Santa Fe Dam Nature Center, with the mountains directly ahead, the route becomes immersed in picturesque high desert—thick with seasonally blooming cacti, towering century plants and sage scrub. By the time you reach the turnaround, urban life begins to feel like the distant past.

If you arrive back at the trailhead still hungering for more pedaling, you can easily add on superb, equally car-free extensions. From Whittier Narrows, you might detour onto the Rio Hondo going north or south (Rides 16 and 18), or you can continue south on the San Gabriel River Trail all the way to Seal Beach (Rides 16 and 46) at ocean's edge.

*While Ride 19 has not been deemed kid-friendly in its entirety, it does include substantial sections which are entirely safe for family use.*

# Ride Log

Ride out of Bosque del Rio Hondo's front gate, turn left to the intersection, then cross both San Gabriel Blvd and Rosemead Blvd to the beginning of the bike path. If you've parked at Legg Lake, take a short warm-up ride to the trailhead: Ride south on Santa Anita Ave to Durfee Ave, turn right and continue about one mile. Cross San Gabriel Blvd to the bike path.

0.0 Head east, parallel to Durfee, following the sign pointing to "Rio Hondo Bike Trail."

0.1 Angle slightly to the right.

0.8 Continue straight at the intersection (don't turn right), follow the arrow to the San Gabriel River Trail and begin riding along the top of the levee.

2.1 Cross under Peck Rd (there's a sign on the highway bridge). The gas stations on Peck Rd, a short distance off the trail, have convenience stores.

4.6 Cross under Valley Blvd.

6.0 Cross under Ramona Blvd.

7.2 Cross under Lower Azusa Rd.

8.7 Cross under Live Oak Ave.

9.2 Cross Arrow Hwy at the crosswalk, exercising caution at the intersection with this active street. Turn left, continuing on the bike path.

9.6 Make a sharp right turn and climb to the top of the dam.

9.8 Continue riding along the top of the dam.

11.8 Pass the parking kiosk for the Santa Fe Dam Recreation Area.

12.3 Continue straight, cross Peckham Rd, at the stop sign.

12.6 Turn left towards the Santa Fe Dam Nature Center.

12.7 Follow the bike trail around the nature center, then turn right.

14.6 Pass the equestrian staging area (which has drinking fountains and restrooms).

16.9 Arrive at the junction of the bike trail and San Gabriel Canyon Rd. (The rangers' station across the road has restrooms.) Turn around and retrace the route back to Whittier Narrows.

33.6 Arrive back at Durfee Ave and San Gabriel Blvd.

P1 Legg Lake
P2 Whittier Narrows Nature Center
P3 Santa Fe Dam Recreation Area
P4 Santa Fe Dam Nature Center
P5 San Gabriel Canyon Gateway Center
P6 Fish Canyon Falls
P7 Monrovia Canyon Park
P8 Los Angeles County Arboretum & Botanic Garden

B1 RB Bicycle Shop
9533 Garvey Ave, South El Monte
B2 Pepe's Bicycle Shop
11426 Garvey Ave, El Monte
B3 2 Wheel Bikes
11688 Clark St # A, Arcadia
B4 Irwindale Cycles
15708 Arrow Hwy, Irwindale
B5 Lloyd's Custom Bicycle Shop
816 Highland Ave, Duarte
B6 Stan's Monrovia Bikes
880 S. Myrtle Ave, Monrovia
B7 REI Co-op
214 N. Santa Anita Ave, Arcadia
B8 Helen's Cycles
124 E. Huntington Dr, Arcadia
B9 Temple City Bike Shop
9628 Las Tunas Dr, Temple City

R1 Wheel Fun Rentals, Sante Fe Dam
15501 East Arrow Hwy, Irwindale

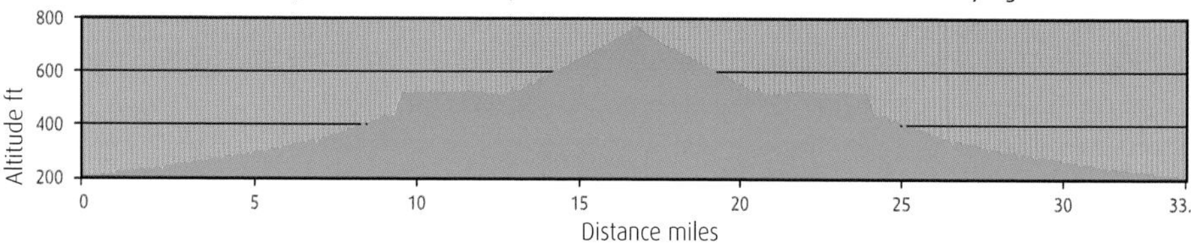

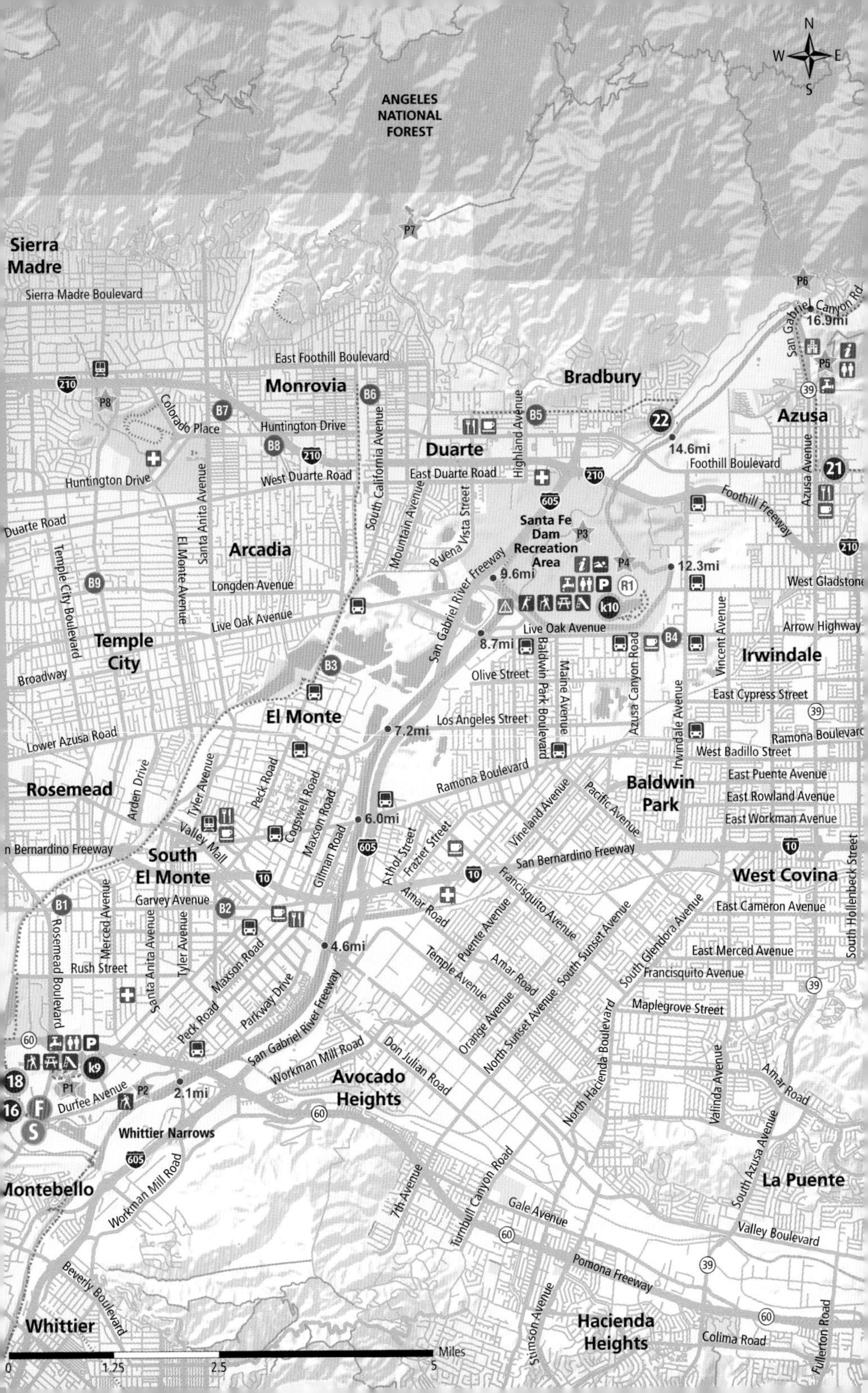

ANGELES NATIONAL FOREST
Sierra Madre
Sierra Madre Boulevard
East Foothill Boulevard
Monrovia
Bradbury
Azusa
Duarte
Arcadia
Temple City
El Monte
Rosemead
South El Monte
Irwindale
Baldwin Park
West Covina
Avocado Heights
Whittier Narrows
Montebello
Whittier
La Puente
Hacienda Heights
Santa Fe Dam Recreation Area
Colorado Place
Huntington Drive
West Duarte Road
East Duarte Road
Duarte Road
Foothill Boulevard
Foothill Freeway
San Gabriel Canyon Rd
16.9mi
14.6mi
12.3mi
9.6mi
8.7mi
7.2mi
6.0mi
4.6mi
2.1mi
Highland Avenue
Azusa Avenue
Buena Vista Street
Mountain Avenue
South California Avenue
Santa Anita Avenue
El Monte Avenue
Temple City Boulevard
Longden Avenue
Live Oak Avenue
Broadway
Lower Azusa Road
San Gabriel River Freeway
West Gladstone
Arrow Highway
Olive Street
Baldwin Park Boulevard
Maine Avenue
Azusa Canyon Road
Irwindale Avenue
Vincent Avenue
East Cypress Street
Los Angeles Street
Ramona Boulevard
West Badillo Street
East Puente Avenue
East Rowland Avenue
East Workman Avenue
Arden Drive
Tyler Avenue
Peck Road
Cogswell Road
Maxson Road
Gilman Road
Valley Mall
San Bernardino Freeway
Athol Street
Frazier Street
Vineland Avenue
Pacific Avenue
Francisquito Avenue
Amar Road
Puente Avenue
Temple Avenue
Orange Avenue
North Sunset Avenue
South Sunset Avenue
South Glendora Avenue
East Cameron Avenue
East Merced Avenue
Maplegrove Street
South Hollenbeck Street
Garvey Avenue
Rosemead Boulevard
Merced Avenue
Santa Anita Avenue
Rush Street
Parkway Drive
Durfee Avenue
Workman Mill Road
Don Julian Road
North Hacienda Boulevard
Valinda Avenue
South Azusa Avenue
Turnbull Canyon Road
7th Avenue
Gale Avenue
Valley Boulevard
Pomona Freeway
Beverly Boulevard
Stimson Avenue
Colima Road
Fullerton Road
Miles
0
1.25
2.5
5
N
S
E
W

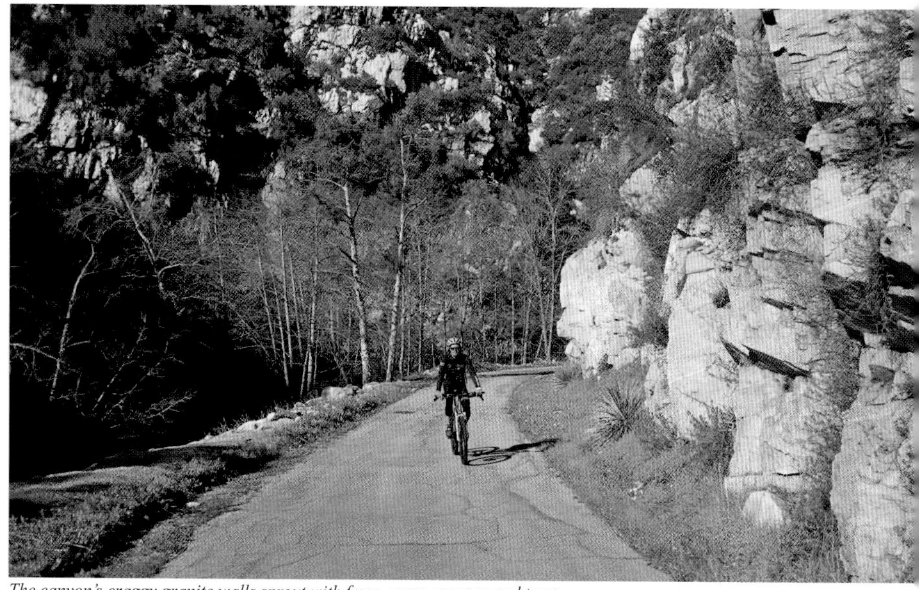

*The canyon's craggy granite walls sprout with ferns, moss, grasses and trees.*

## At a Glance

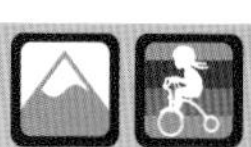

**Distance** 14.8 miles **Elevation Gain** 1,000 feet

### Terrain

This single-lane paved road meanders up a river canyon in the Angeles National Forest. Following a very gradual ascent to Glenn Camp, the road pitches steeply up to Cogswell Dam.

### Traffic

The route is closed to motorized vehicles. Bicycle and pedestrian traffic tends to be light, even on weekends.

### How to Get There

Take Highway 39/Azusa Avenue north from the 210 Freeway. Continue about 13.5 miles north to the parking lot on the left side of the road, right past the Rincon fire station. Before leaving the Azusa area, purchase a required Adventure Pass ($5) at the San Gabriel Canyon Gateway Center, or at the ARCO or Mobil gas stations, just north of the 210 Freeway.

### Food and Drink

Be sure to bring along enough water and food—they're not available in the West Fork area. The convenience store at Camp Williams Resort, six miles away on East Fork Road, sells drinks and some snacks on weekends (Friday to Sunday).

### Side Trip

To experience more of the Angeles National Forest, ride up Highway 39 towards Crystal Lake. Or lock up the bikes and take a hike on one of the trails from the West Fork area.

**Links to** 

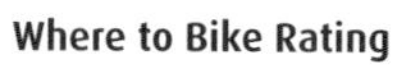

**Where to Bike Rating** 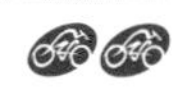

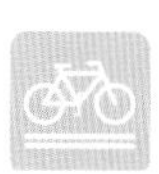 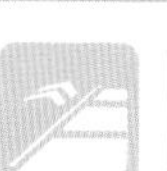 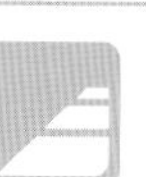 

# About...

West Fork is by far one of the best short rides around. Though barely 25 miles from Downtown L.A., it ventures into backcountry—the rugged, spectacular scenery of the Angeles National Forest. Sheer rock walls, fragrant chaparral and a flowing stream flank this tranquil, car-free route, shaded by sycamores and scrub oaks. Along the way, surrounding mountain peaks and occasional wildlife come into view

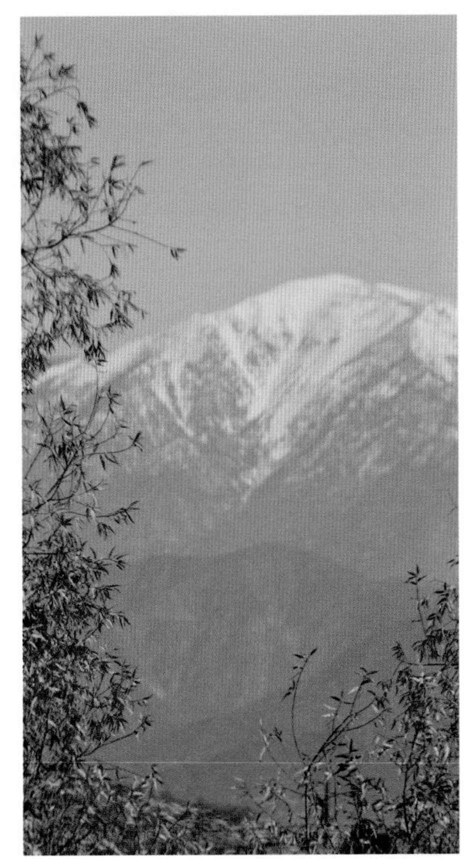

*At a few points along the path, Mount Baldy comes into view.*

This National Scenic Bikeway traces the course of the West Fork of the San Gabriel River upstream from its confluence with the North Fork, this route's trailhead. After passing through a small, open field, the bikeway enters a narrowing, tree-lined canyon. In the first mile or two, the route crosses the stream several times on rustic steel-beam bridges and then, meanders in a gradual ascent along the south bank. The river is never more than a pebble's throw away from the track, dappled in sunlight beneath a canopy of trees.

After a little more than six miles, you reach the small, sunny meadow of Glenn Camp. Here, you'll find picnic tables, plenty of shade along the stream and up a side canyon, plus restrooms. If you're feeling adventuresome, consider pedaling in with panniers or rucksacks packed with provisions for a night of camping under the stars (for information, or to make reservations with the Forest Service, call: 626-335-1251). The camp is also a good turnaround point if you opt for an easy, liesurely 13-mile ride, omitting the steep final, one-mile climb up to Cogswell Dam. But, if you choose to make the full ascent, you'll be rewarded by spectacular views back down the canyon toward Mount Baldy and a chance to see the rocky granite dam with its bridge and spillway, dating from the 1930s.

Changing with the seasons, this ride is enjoyable almost year round, except in the wake of big winter storms. In the early months, expect to see snow, particularly in the side canyons' shadowy depths. Through late spring, a few waterfalls flow into the West Fork (be careful crossing the open drainage channels that allow water, sometimes quite deep, to stream across the path). Springtime brings a short-lived array of wildflowers. In summer and fall, consider packing a swimsuit (and river sandals) for a dip into one of many swimming holes along the river. Plenty of large boulders provide excellent drying-off or sunbathing spots. During late fall you'll be treated to an array of colors with red and yellow leaves and golden grasses.

# Ride Log

0.0 Ride down Highway 39 a short distance from the parking lot to the West Fork Trailhead. Portage bikes around either end of the yellow gate.

4.0 Restrooms.

6.0 Glenn Camp.

7.4 Cogswell Dam. Don't attempt to cross the dam without permission. Use caution returning towards Glenn Camp because the descent is very steep and there can be sand and gravel on the roadway.

14.8 Arrive back at the trailhead. End of ride.

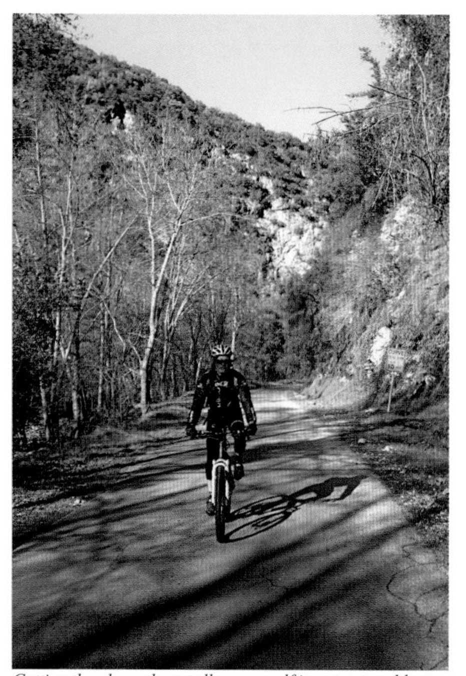

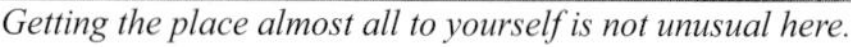

*Getting the place almost all to yourself is not unusual here.*

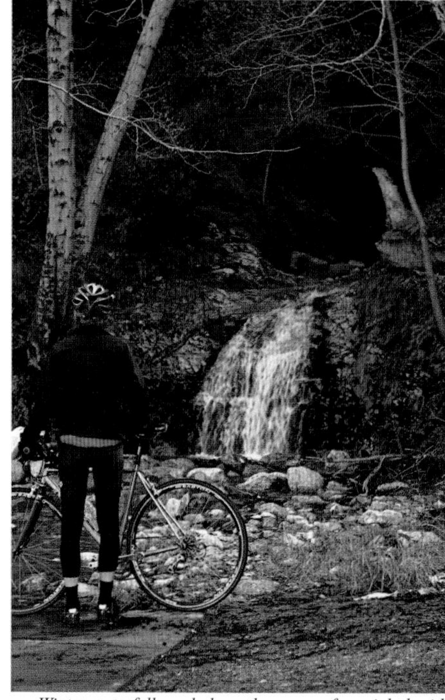

*Winter waterfalls rush down the canyon face right beside the bike trail.*

P1 San Gabriel Canyon Gateway Center
P2 Crystal Lake
P3 Mount San Antonio (Mt Baldy)

B1 Bicycle Central
942 S. Grand Ave, Glendora

## West Fork of the San Gabriel River

*Please note: the profile for Ride 20 is depicted in 300ft vertical increments due to unusually high elevation.*

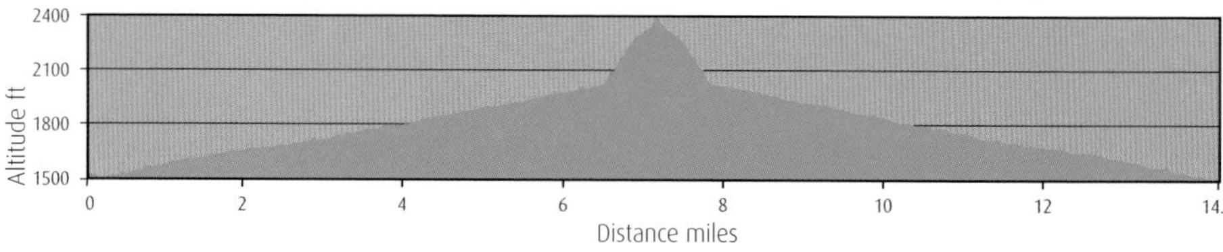

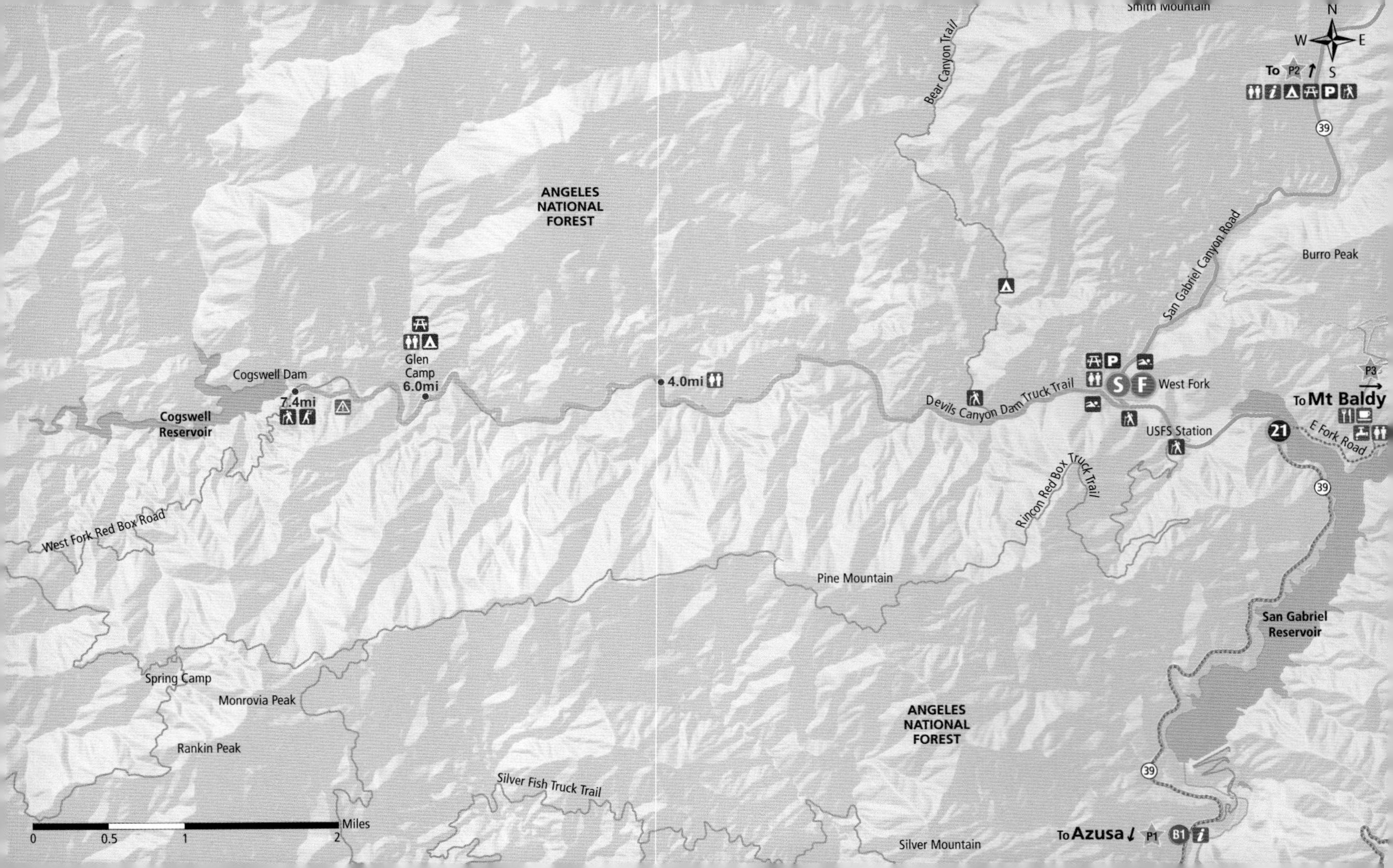

Smith Mountain
N
W
E
S
To P2
39
Bear Canyon Trail
ANGELES
NATIONAL
FOREST
Burro Peak
San Gabriel Canyon Road
Glen
Camp
6.0mi
Cogswell Dam
7.4mi
Cogswell
Reservoir
4.0mi
S F
West Fork
P3
To Mt Baldy
Devils Canyon Dam Truck Trail
USFS Station
21
E Fork Road
Rincon Red Box Truck Trail
West Fork Red Box Road
Pine Mountain
San Gabriel
Reservoir
Spring Camp
Monrovia Peak
Rankin Peak
ANGELES
NATIONAL
FOREST
Silver Fish Truck Trail
Miles
0
0.5
1
2
To Azusa
P1
B1
Silver Mountain

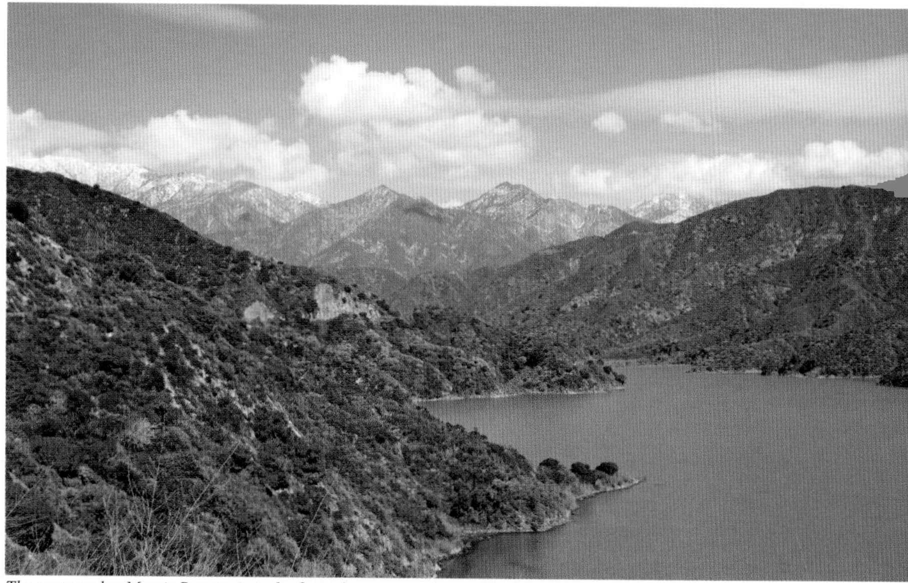

*The spectacular Morris Reservoir is the first of two reservoirs on this ride.*

## At a Glance

**Distance** 35.6 miles **Elevation Gain** 3,600 feet

### Terrain

Glendora Mountain Road features mountain riding on good pavement with two long, gradual climbs, separated by a rolling section. The descent to Glendora is nine-miles long and often twisting.

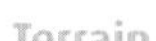

### Traffic

These mountain roads tend to have little traffic, but increased activity on weekends. Be attentive when approaching blind turns, especially those lacking center-line stripes.

### How to Get There

From the 201 Freeway, exit at Highway 39/Azusa Avenue. Go north, toward the mountains, about one mile. Turn right onto Foothill Boulevard for one block, followed by a left onto Alameda Avenue. Drive a half-block to free parking at Veterans Freedom Park.

### Food and Drink

There are no services en route, except at Camp Williams' café and convenience store (Friday to Sunday), so carry enough water and nourishment for a strenuous 35-mile ride. Afterwards, Glendora Village, with Classic Coffee and other options, is a great place to recover.

### Side Trip

Shoemaker Canyon Road, at mile 14, is another intriguing road to nowhere. Built with prison labor, this road was never completed, but left behind interesting artifacts. You can ride in about two miles and then, hike along the dirt path through a rough, never-used road and two tunnels.

**Links to**  19 20

**Where to Bike Rating** 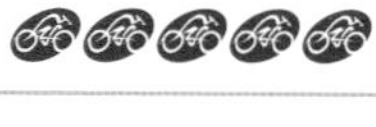 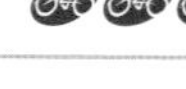

 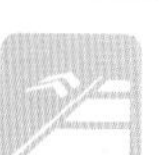  

## About...

Among avid Southern California cyclists, Glendora Mountain Road (GMR) is a classic ride, and it's one of Jon's favorites. Starting from the northeastern San Gabriel Valley, this beautiful and challenging route ventures into a remote end of the Angeles National Forest. The solitude of untraveled back roads and the up-close experience of the San Gabriel Mountains, in two of the river's main tributary canyons, gives this mini-epic great appeal. The rugged high peaks, visible en route, are magnificent—perhaps even more so after a springtime snowmelt.

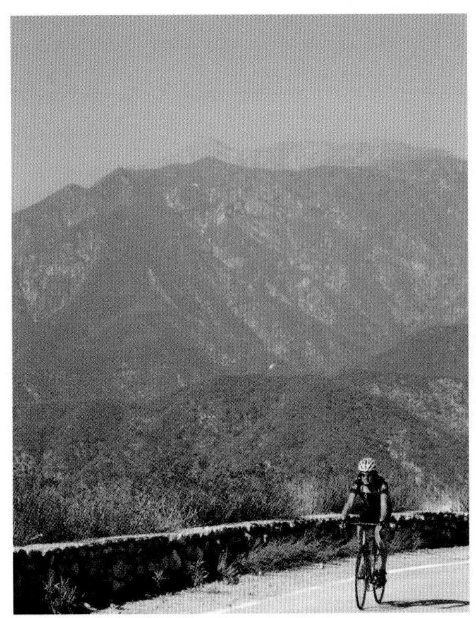

*Glendora Mountain Road: en route from East Fork to Horse Canyon Saddle.*



San Gabriel Canyon Road (Highway 39) once connected L.A.'s eastern end to Angeles Crest Highway at Islip Saddle. From there, you could proceed to the Wrightwood ski areas, the high desert or such distant getaways as Barstow and Las Vegas. But rockslides and forest fires have kept parts of Highway 39 closed for more than 30 years, turning the remaining route, through spectacular mountains, into a road to nowhere. Few people drive it, making it great for cyclists. Our ride begins with a couple of turns through Azusa's civic core, before 10-plus miles on San Gabriel Canyon Road, or Highway 39, to the "backdoor" of Glendora Mountain Road (GMR).

As you ascend Highway 39, you'll eventually pass two lakes, really, flood-control reservoirs. Soon after, turn right onto East Fork Road, along a tributary of the San Gabriel River. Gold prospectors and, later, developers of tourist and hunting camps explored and settled these banks in the latter half of the 19th century. Today, only Camp Williams, now a small hamlet survives, though remnants of Follows Camp and others of its ilk appear along this four-mile stretch on East Fork Road.

About a mile past Camp Williams, East Fork Road ends at Heaton Flats, a hiking and camping area. A tight, upward turn to the right leads onto GMR, a route of suffering and fun, in a beneficial ratio of 1:2 or better. After an ascent of just over four miles, averaging five percent grade, (and then, a well-deserved breather at Horse Canyon Saddle), you'll have the luxury of nine miles downhill through magnificent scenery.

The upper half of the descent has many graceful turns where you can safely, with exhilarating momentum, reap the fruits of your climbing labors. You will however, need to control your speed further down where the turns become sharper and closer together. Soon after, near the Glendora city limits sign, GMR levels out, ushering you into an historic town—and a welcome latte stop.

Words of advice: This ride is remote, so we recommend riding it with at least one companion and flat-fixing supplies. Drivers and sports motorcyclists love to slalom these roads too, and sometimes they crowd or cross the centerline, so, again, be vigilant around the turns.

# Ride Log

0.0 From the corner of Alameda Ave and Foothill Blvd, pedal west on Foothill one block to Azusa Ave, then turn north (toward the mountains).

0.9 Veer slightly to the left where Azusa Ave becomes San Gabriel Canyon Rd at Sierra Madre Ave.

2.0 Pass San Gabriel Canyon Gateway Center.

4.4 Pass Morris Reservoir Dam.

7.0 Pass San Gabriel Reservoir Dam.

10.9 Turn right on East Fork Rd and cross the late-1940s era bridge.

14.3 Pass Shoemaker Canyon Rd.

15.0 Pass Camp Williams Resort.

16.1 Make a sharp, upward right turn onto Glendora Mountain Rd.

21.1 Turn right at the T-intersection with Glendora Ridge Rd (Mt Baldy Village and ski resort are approximately 12 miles to the left) and continue on Glendora Mountain Rd. Next: approximately nine miles of continuous descending with many switchbacks. Watch your downhill speed.

30.7 Turn right onto Sierra Madre Ave.

32.3 Turn left onto Glendora Ave at the stop sign. Ride through the heart of Glendora Village. Take a breather here if you like.

33.1 Turn right onto Foothill Blvd.

34.5 Foothill turns to the left, becoming Citrus Ave just past Citrus College.

34.7 Turn right at the stoplight, continuing on Foothill Blvd.

35.6 Arrive at Alameda Ave in Azusa and turn right to Veterans Freedom Park.

P1 San Gabriel Canyon Gateway Center
P2 Shoemaker Canyon Road (also called the "road to nowhere")
P3 Heaton Flats trailhead
P4 Rubel Castle
P5 Glendora Historical Society Museum
P6 South Hills Park/Centennial Heritage Park
P7 Frank G Bonelli Regional Park
P8 Fairplex: Home of the Los Angeles County Fair

B1 Bicycle Central
942 S. Grand Ave, Glendora
B2 Sport Chalet—Bicycle department
940 S Grand Ave, Glendora
B3 Incycle
561 West Arrow Hwy, San Dimas
B4 Irwindale Cycles
15708 Arrow Hwy, Irwindale
B5 Covina Valley Schwinn
203 S. Citrus Ave, Covina

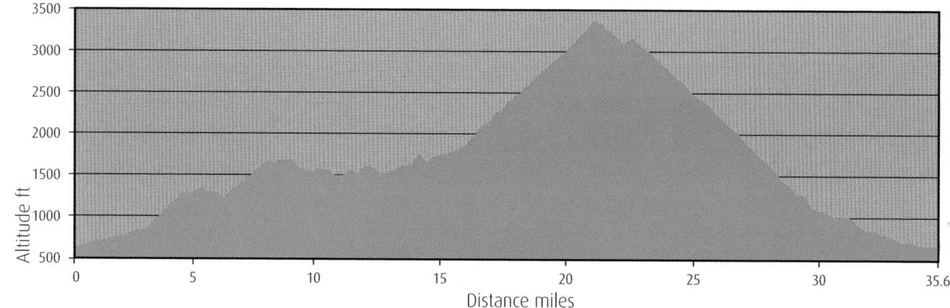

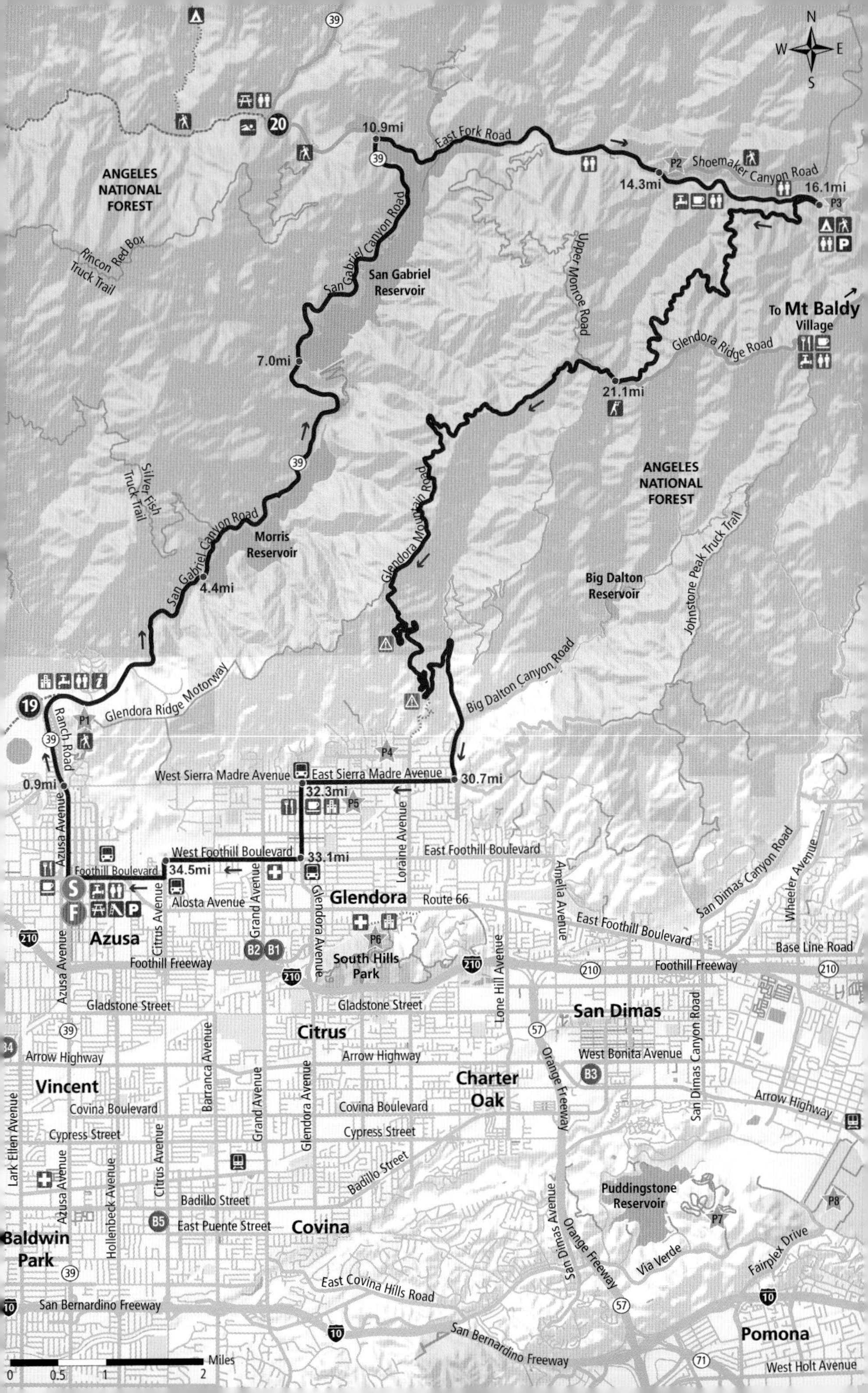

N
W
E
S
ANGELES NATIONAL FOREST
Rincon Red Box Truck Trail
20
10.9mi
East Fork Road
P2
Shoemaker Canyon Road
14.3mi
16.1mi
P3
San Gabriel Canyon Road
San Gabriel Reservoir
Upper Monroe Road
To Mt Baldy Village
Glendora Ridge Road
7.0mi
21.1mi
Silver Fish Truck Trail
ANGELES NATIONAL FOREST
Glendora Mountain Road
San Gabriel Canyon Road
Morris Reservoir
4.4mi
Big Dalton Reservoir
Johnstone Peak Truck Trail
Big Dalton Canyon Road
19
Glendora Ridge Motorway
Ranch Road
P1
P4
West Sierra Madre Avenue
East Sierra Madre Avenue
30.7mi
0.9mi
32.3mi
P5
Azusa Avenue
Loraine Avenue
West Foothill Boulevard
33.1mi
East Foothill Boulevard
Foothill Boulevard
34.5mi
Amelia Avenue
San Dimas Canyon Road
Wheeler Avenue
S
F
Alosta Avenue
Grand Avenue
Glendora Avenue
Glendora
Route 66
East Foothill Boulevard
Azusa
Citrus Avenue
P6
Base Line Road
B2
B1
South Hills Park
Lone Hill Avenue
Foothill Freeway
Foothill Freeway
Gladstone Street
Gladstone Street
San Dimas
Citrus
Arrow Highway
Arrow Highway
West Bonita Avenue
Vincent
Barranca Avenue
Charter Oak
B3
Covina Boulevard
Covina Boulevard
Orange Freeway
Arrow Highway
Lark Ellen Avenue
Cypress Street
Cypress Street
Badillo Street
Hollenbeck Avenue
Puddingstone Reservoir
P8
Badillo Street
P7
B5
East Puente Street
Covina
San Dimas Avenue
Baldwin Park
Orange Freeway
Via Verde
Fairplex Drive
East Covina Hills Road
San Bernardino Freeway
San Bernardino Freeway
Pomona
Miles
0
0.5
1
2
West Holt Avenue

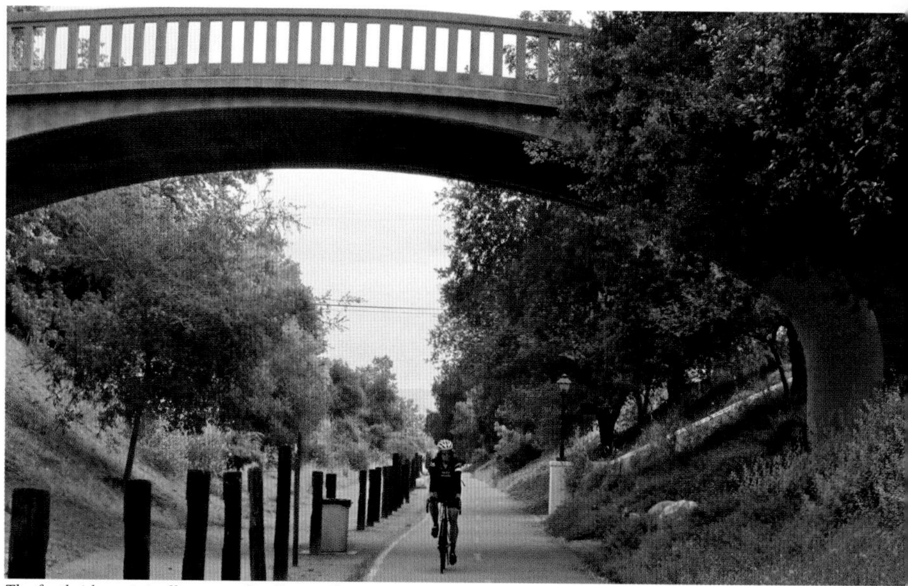

*The footbridge originally spanned trolley tracks.*

## At a Glance

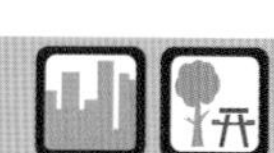

**Distance** 5.4 miles **Elevation Gain** 200 feet

### Terrain

Virtually flat, the bike path is concrete and asphalt paved, bordering a packed-dirt equestrian trail.

### Traffic

The bike trail is car-free. The ride's beginning and end include short stretches on quiet residential streets with very little traffic.

### How to Get There

From the 605 Freeway North, continue straight onto Mount Olive Drive, in Duarte. Turn right on Royal Oaks Drive for a little more that one mile, then right onto Encanto Parkway. Leave your car in Encanto Park's lot.

### Food and Drink

Each community en route—Monrovia, Bradbury and Duarte—offers clusters of eateries. Of note is Cuisine on the Green (Las Lomas Road in Duarte), tucked into a golf course and known for Lebanese kabobs and other Mediterranean fare.

### Side Trip

The four-mile round-trip Fish Canyon hike is legendary for its 80-foot-high, three-tiered waterfall and lush ferns. It's also blessed with a modest 400-foot elevation gain. But there's a catch. A quarrying company permanently impeded general access, back before environmental controls. So, to experience the old, easy trek, you need to schedule your hike on a day when the company, Vulcan Materials, provides shuttle service to the trailhead. It's worth the effort. (**www.asuzarock.com/fishcreek;** or call 323-474-3208.)

**Links to** 

**Where to Bike Rating** 

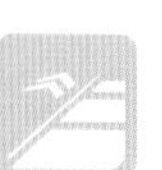
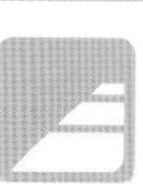

## About...

This flat, leisurely, relatively straight path follows a former trolley route through the residential and historic communities of Monrovia, Bradbury and Duarte. Against a backdrop of the nearby San Gabriel Mountains, the trail passes beneath shade trees and along a bridal path. A few blocks from the ride's eastern end, you can connect with the Upper San Gabriel River Trail and continue south to the Santa Fe Dam Recreation Area.

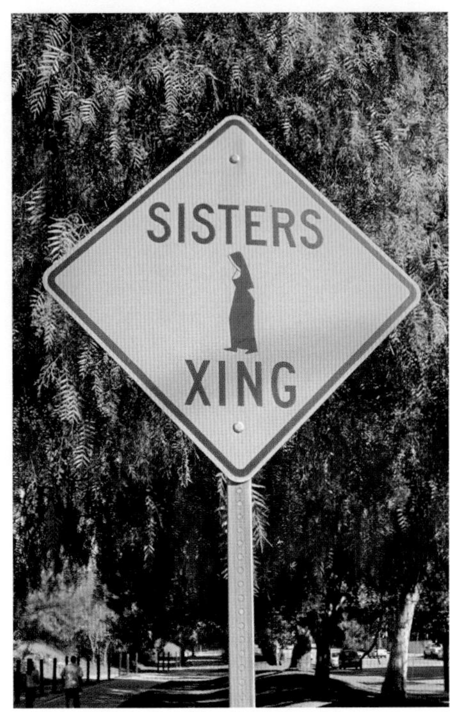


*Nuns in their habitat: The bikeway is right near a convent.*

Amid the foothills of the San Gabriel Mountains, the small cities of Monrovia, Bradbury, Duarte and Azusa once abounded with citrus groves. To link these farming communities, the Pacific Electric Railway created a trolley line across the San Gabriel Valley. The streetcars, which had their heyday in the first half of the 20th century, are long gone, as are the orange trees. But plenty of classic Craftsman-style houses and mountain scenery—including the protected Angeles National Forest—survive. The city of Duarte purchased the abandoned rail route, and ultimately the non-profit Rails to Trails Conservancy converted it into a pathway for biking, jogging and strolling. Graceful, fine-leafed pepper trees, fragrant with red pepper corns, form a canopy over the trail. Other shade trees thrive here, as do seasonally blooming wildflowers.

While connecting these foothill towns, the trail also runs by an elementary school and two modest parks: Royal Oaks Park and the somewhat larger Encanto Park, 12 acres with grassy fields, a kids' playground, tennis courts, picnic tables, restrooms and a nature walk along a bioswale. The Encanto Bioswale and Outdoor Nature Classroom, completed in 2010, feature a 1,500-foot-long, manmade stream with native plantings, an evolving habitat that cleans and conserves rainwater, filtering it back into the ground.

Near the path's east end, you'll find the Duarte Historical Museum (open Saturdays, 1 to 4 p.m., and on each month's first and third Wednesday, 1 to 3 p.m.). From there, it's a short spin to the San Gabriel River Bike Trail (pedal south on Encanto Parkway until the first turn-off on your right, a spur of the bike path that crosses the river on the old Pacific Electric Railway bridge). The river paths invite you to explore the Upper San Gabriel River or, to the south, the Santa Fe Dam Recreation Area. Alternatively, from the Royal Oaks path's west end, you can head into Old Monrovia, about 1.5 miles away (turn right on Buena Vista, immediately left on Orange, followed by a right on Bradbury Road. At Lemon, turn left and continue for about a mile to Myrtle Avenue in old town Monrovia).

*While Ride 22 has not been deemed kid-friendly in its entirety, it does include substantial sections which are entirely safe for family use.*

# Ride Log

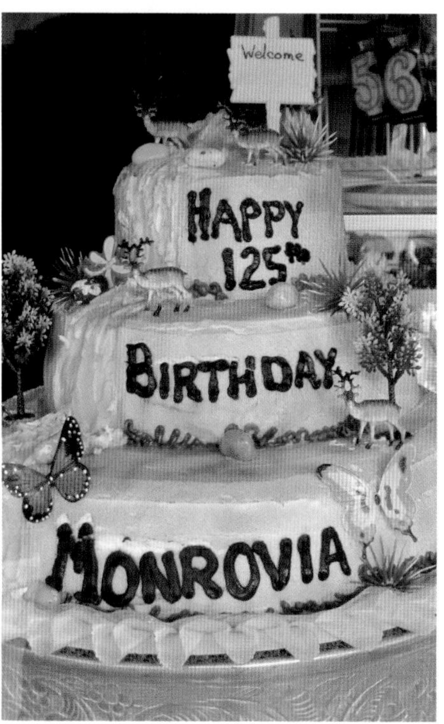


*Monrovia, still enriched today by waterfalls and wildlife, was incorporated in 1887.*

 P1 Fish Canyon Falls
P2 San Gabriel Canyon Gateway Center

 B1 Lloyd's Custom Bicycle Shop
816 Highland Ave, Duarte

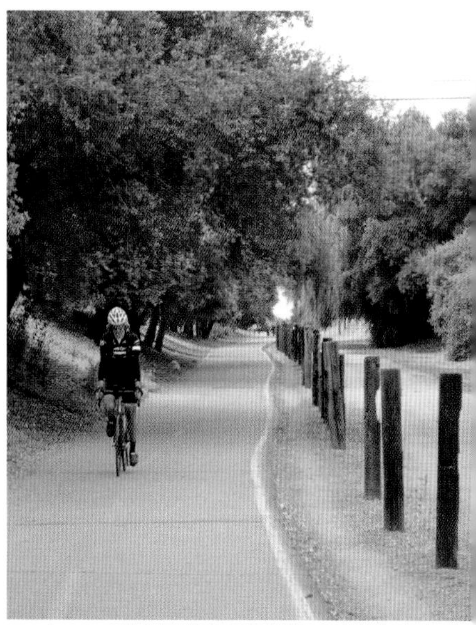

*Seasonal wildflowers border the trail along one side, with a bridal path along the other.*

0.0 From Encanto Park, turn left towards the mountains.

0.1 Turn left on Royal Oaks Dr.

1.0 Turn right on Vineyard Ave and begin the Royal Oaks Bike Path (Duarte Bike Trail).

1.2 Royal Oaks Elementary School.

1.4 Cross Mt. Olive Dr.

2.7 Arrive at Buena Vista St, then turn around for the return trip.

5.4 Arrive back at Encanto Park.

Royal Oaks Bike Path

Altitude ft: 650, 550

Distance miles: 0, 1, 2, 3, 4, 5, 5.4

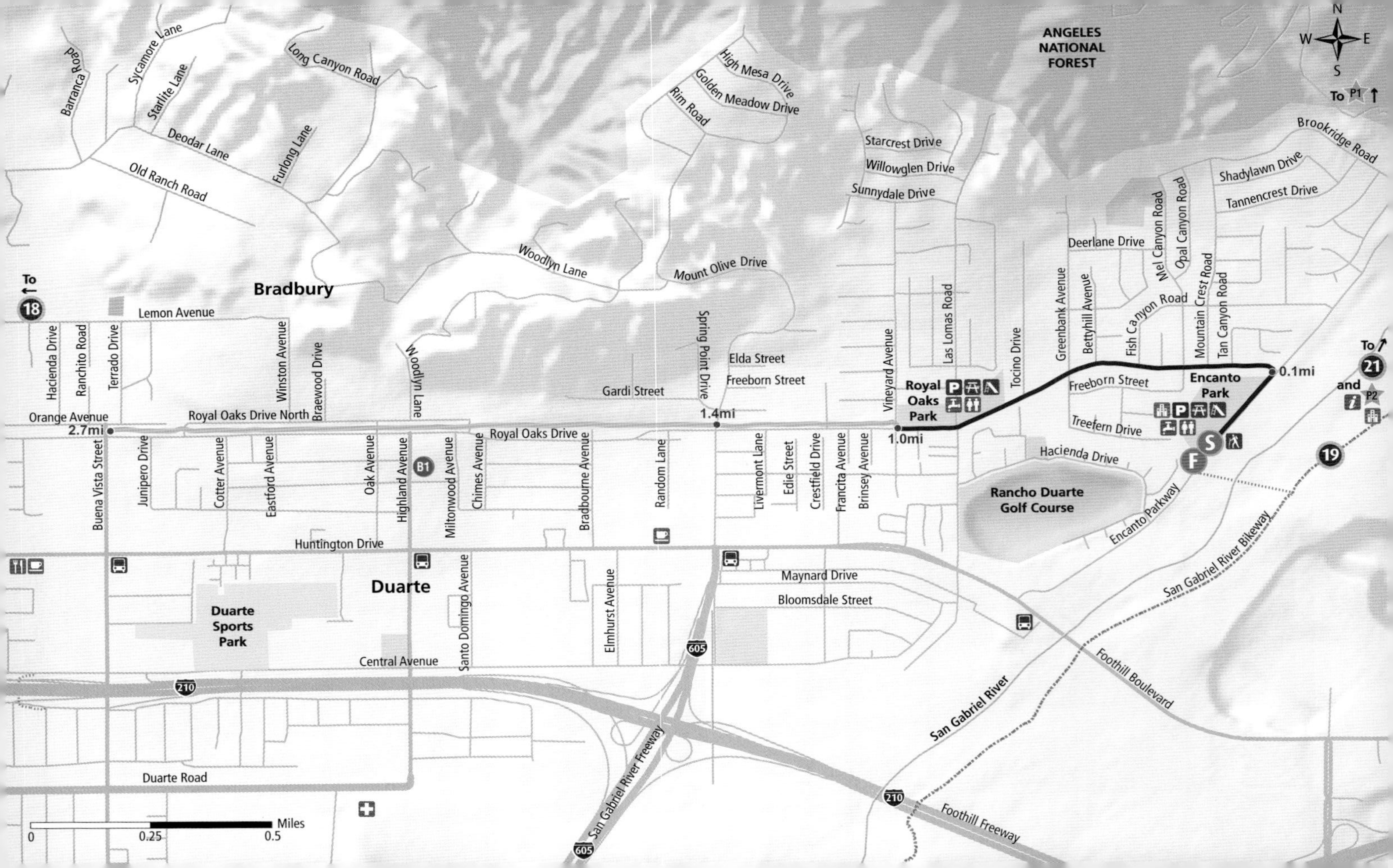

ANGELES NATIONAL FOREST
N
W
E
S
To P1
Bradbury
Duarte
To 18
Barranca Road
Sycamore Lane
Starlite Lane
Long Canyon Road
Deodar Lane
Furlong Lane
Old Ranch Road
High Mesa Drive
Golden Meadow Drive
Rim Road
Woodlyn Lane
Mount Olive Drive
Starcrest Drive
Willowglen Drive
Sunnydale Drive
Brookridge Road
Shadylawn Drive
Tannencrest Drive
Deerlane Drive
Mel Canyon Road
Opal Canyon Road
Mountain Crest Road
Tan Canyon Road
Fish Canyon Road
Greenbank Avenue
Bettyhill Avenue
Tocino Drive
Las Lomas Road
Vineyard Avenue
Lemon Avenue
Hacienda Drive
Ranchito Road
Terrado Drive
Winston Avenue
Braewood Drive
Woodlyn Lane
Spring Point Drive
Elda Street
Freeborn Street
Gardi Street
Royal Oaks Park
Encanto Park
Freeborn Street
Treefern Drive
0.1mi
To 21
and
P2
19
Orange Avenue
2.7mi
Royal Oaks Drive North
1.4mi
Royal Oaks Drive
1.0mi
Hacienda Drive
Rancho Duarte Golf Course
Encanto Parkway
S
F
Buena Vista Street
Junipero Drive
Cotter Avenue
Eastford Avenue
Oak Avenue
Highland Avenue
B1
Miltonwood Avenue
Chimes Avenue
Bradbourne Avenue
Random Lane
Livermont Lane
Edie Street
Crestfield Drive
Francita Avenue
Brinsey Avenue
Huntington Drive
Maynard Drive
Bloomsdale Street
San Gabriel River Bikeway
Foothill Boulevard
San Gabriel River
Duarte Sports Park
Santo Domingo Avenue
Elmhurst Avenue
Central Avenue
605
210
San Gabriel River Freeway
Foothill Freeway
Duarte Road
Miles
0
0.25
0.5

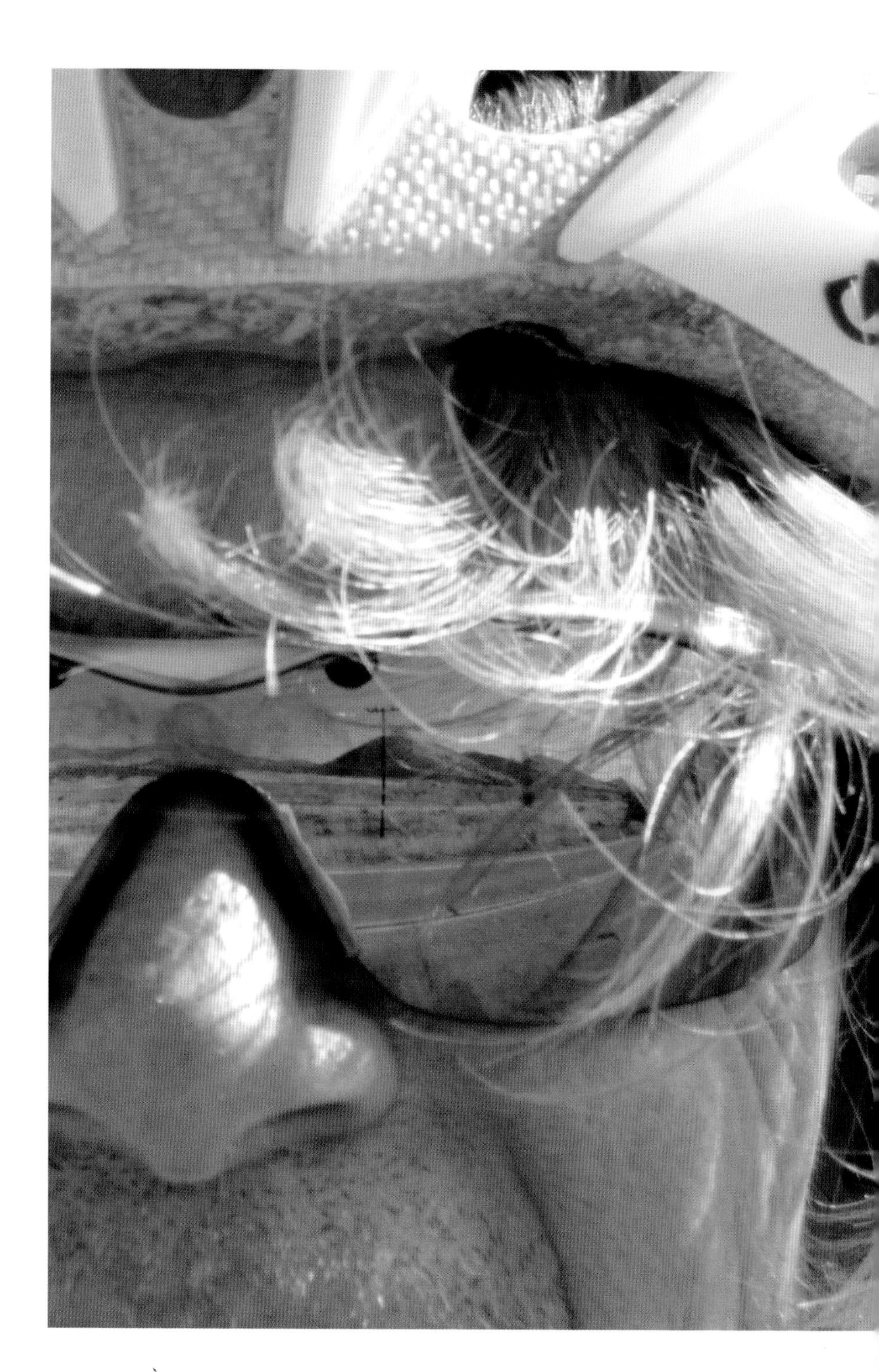

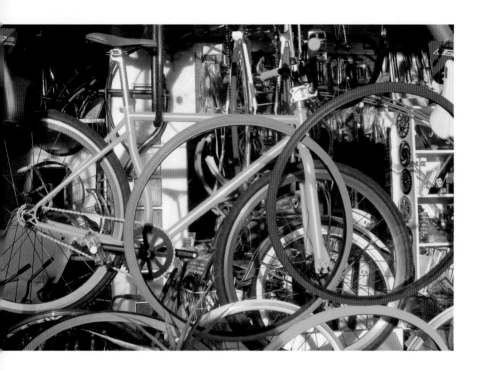

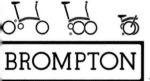

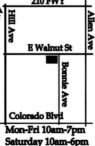

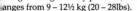

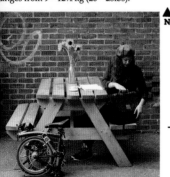

# The Westside

On the rare occasions when we're not on bikes, but airborne over coastal Los Angeles—taking off from LAX—we're always amazed to see, in one glance, the whole Westside, its texture of beach life extending in an arc from the Pacific Palisades, all the way south to the Palos Verdes Peninsula.

Directly beneath the ascending planes is the Marvin Braude Bike Trail, the best-known ride on the Westside, if not in all of Los Angeles. While treated as three separate segments in this book, the Santa Monica Bike Path, Marina del Rey Loop and South Bay Bike Path can be joined together for a beachside cruise stretching more than 45 miles round-trip.

On either end of this path, the narrow coastal strip gives way to hilly terrain and entirely different, though still incredibly popular, riding. On the southern end is the Palos Verdes Peninsula, with its rugged cliffs and coastal panoramas. Here, you'll find our two "fritter" rides: The Donut, around the peninsula (a virtual institution among local cyclists), and The Double Donut Holes, through upscale residential neighborhoods with vistas across the peninsula and, in the distance, to Downtown Los Angeles and Catalina Island.

At the opposite end of the great arc of beaches, our Pacific Coast Highway spin offers a flat excursion through the "Riviera of America" to Malibu—along a road between surf with sand to one side and mountains to the other.

Inland from the shore, the Ballona Creek and Tour of Santa Monica routes take you into lively communities with plentiful eating options, farmers' markets, hip shopping, art galleries and a Metro connection to many other parts of Los Angeles. Our canyon routes—San Vicente to Mandeville or up Topanga Canyon—lead the way into cool mountain clefts, including the wooded and chaparral-covered hillsides around Topanga's lightly traveled, scenic roadways.

Then, if you still hanker for more distance, you can continue from the Pacific Coast Highway along the coast to Zuma Beach, Trancas Canyon Road or the surf spot and seafood restaurant, Neptune's Net, a classic bikers' hang-out, right at the county line.

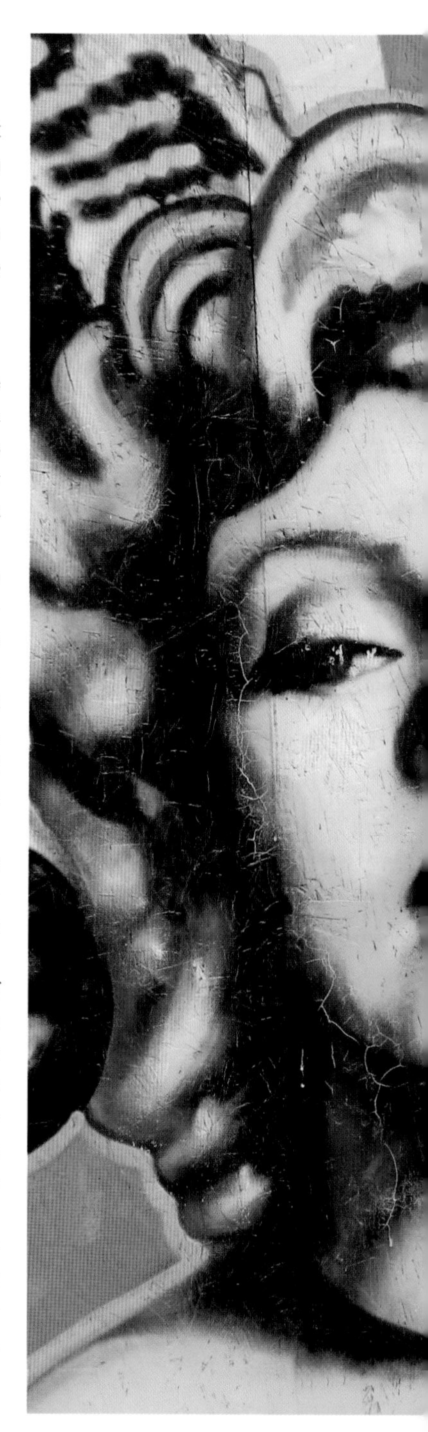

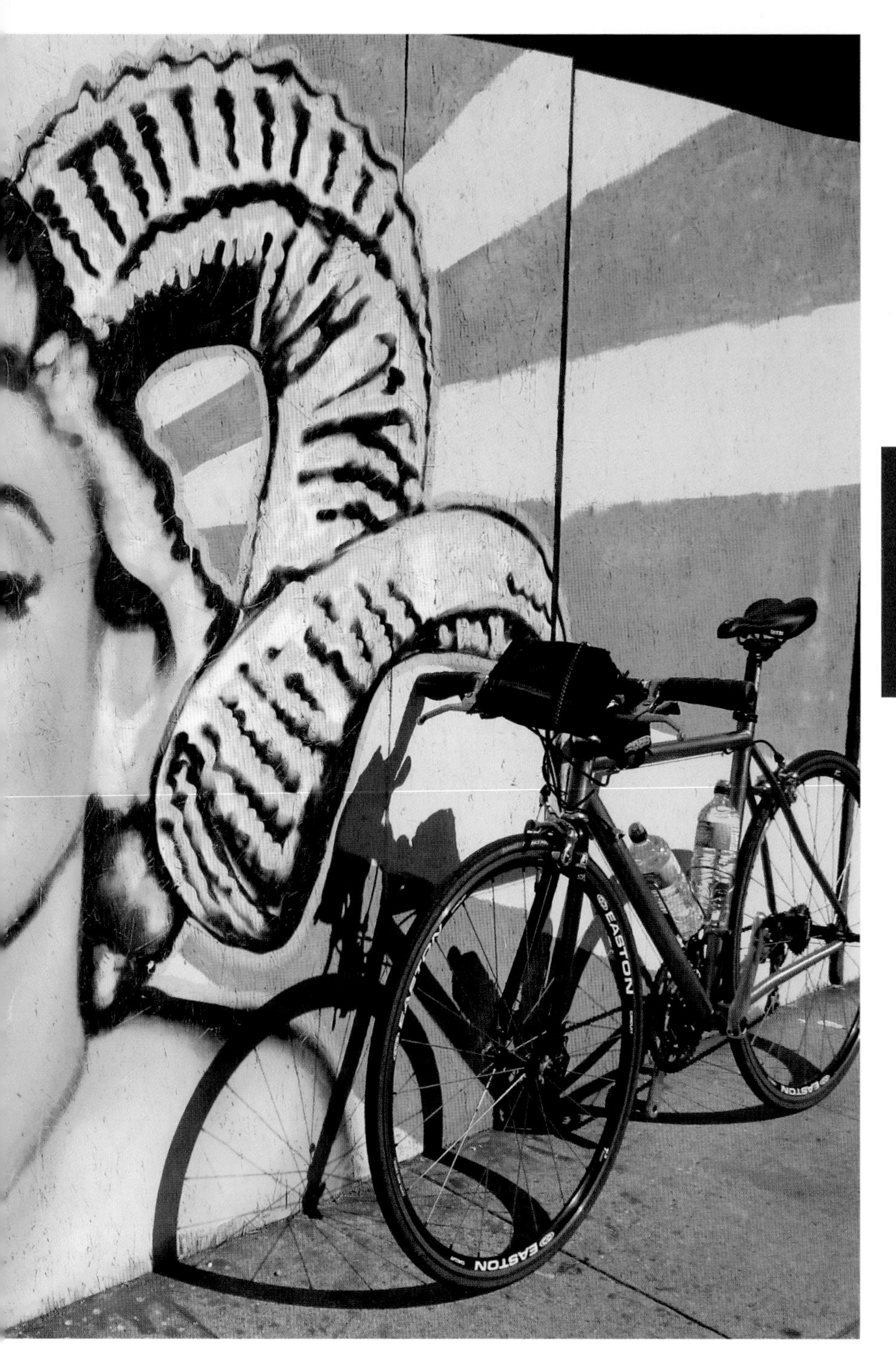
EASTON

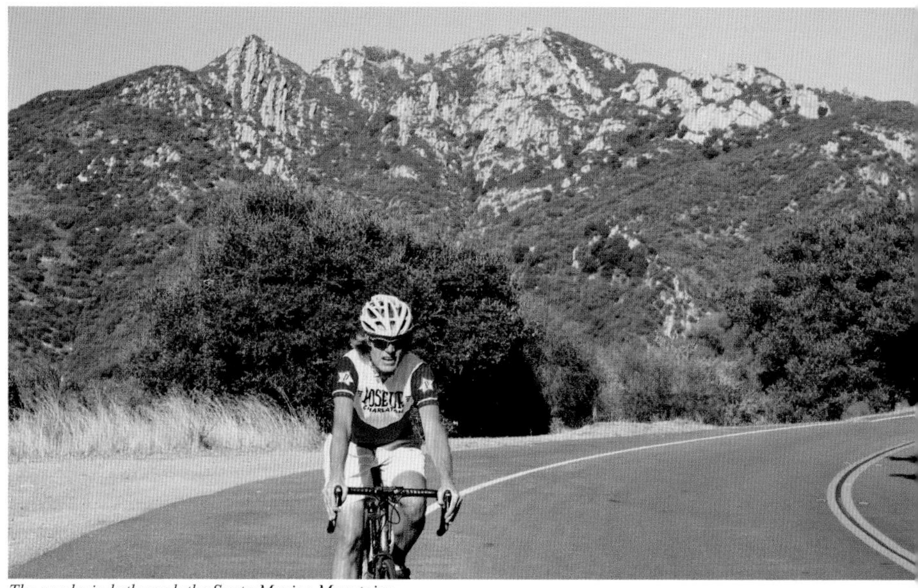


*The road winds through the Santa Monica Mountains.*

## At a Glance

**Distance** 26.8 miles **Elevation Gain** 3,800 feet

### Terrain

Sustained but gradual climbs, with a few steep pitches, lead up Mulholland Highway, Old Topanga Canyon, and Piuma and Schueren roads. Fast, curving descents intersperse these ascents. The surfaces are paved and generally good.

### Traffic

Traffic tends to be relatively light, except for moderately busy Mulholland Highway, which has wide shoulders that function as bike lanes.

### How to Get There

Drive all the way west on the 10 Freeway and continue 5.7 miles north on Pacific Coast Highway. Turn right onto Topanga Canyon Boulevard and travel about 4.3 miles to the community of Topanga. Park along Topanga Canyon Boulevard, just north of Old Topanga Canyon Road.

### Food and Drink

Topanga Creek General Store and Country Natural Food, on Topanga Canyon Boulevard, sell snacks, cold beverages and packaged sandwiches. Café Mimosa at Fernwood Pacific (open until 2 p.m. daily), is a laid-back spot for coffee, breakfast or light lunch.

### Side Trip

Explore the bohemian mountain enclave of Topanga, home of such funky stores as Hidden Treasures, with its trove of vintage clothes and trinkets. The building itself is a glittering, eclectic collage, encrusted with skulls, a life-size Captain Kidd, Tiki masks, a dinosaur and more.

**Links to** 

**Where to Bike Rating** 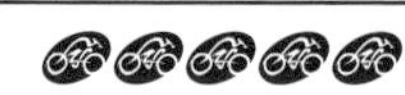

 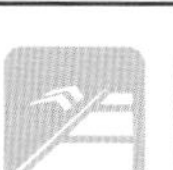  

# About...

In L.A.'s great rustic backyard, the Santa Monica Mountains National Recreation Area encompasses some 150,000 acres. Many miles of excellent cycling can be found here—on paved roads through lightly traveled wooded canyons, up chaparral-covered hillsides and along wide-open skylines. The ride starts from the canyon community of Topanga (whose native name aptly means "a place above") and transverses magnificent mountain scenery, ultimately reaching the area's high point: Saddle Peak summit with 360-degree views to distant horizons.

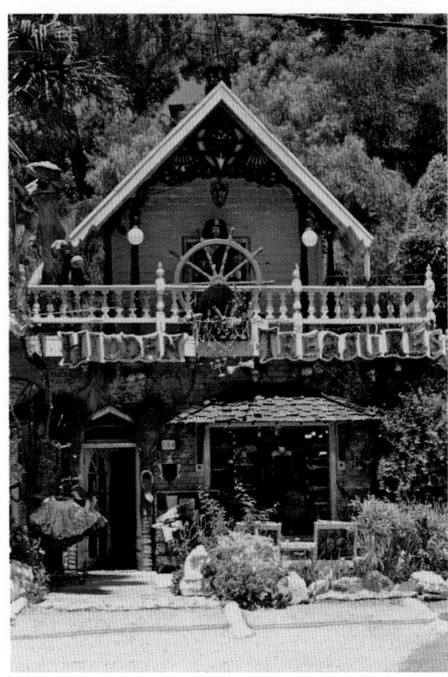


*Topanga Canyon has plenty of fun and funk.*



Leaving "downtown" Topanga, you'll cross a vintage truss bridge over Topanga Creek and continue a mile or two slightly uphill, virtually on flats. While it may be tempting to fly here, approach this stretch with moderation as a warm-up. Take time to enjoy this quiet country road beneath overarching coastal oaks. You'll soon be tackling a couple of steeper switchbacks and pushing to the first summit. A wide turnout just past the top reveals vistas of the mountains and valleys to the north. Two miles of sweeping descent follow, with some twisting passages (as well as cars on the road, so be attentive).

The next section of the ride is an interlude. Where Old Topanga flattens out, you'll turn left onto Dry Canyon-Cold Creek Road, which soon meets Mulholland Highway. After a short, sharp climb on this famous high roadway to the second summit, you'll rejoin Dry Canyon-Cold Creek Road, then Mulholland again, and finally Cold Canyon Road for winding descents amid country homes and sparse-to-nonexistent traffic. Next, onto Piuma Road, the ride's real climb (about 1,700 feet). Extremely popular among cyclists, this fairly gradual ascent, with only a couple of steep pitches, overlooks yet another spectacular series of unfolding views. The road's four switchbacks (plus a few minor turns) cover just over five miles. Right before the final switchback—leading to a lookout from which you can see Malibu Canyon cutting through the mountains from ocean to valley—you'll get the first of several progress markers, counting down to the third summit: 4 km, 3 km, 2 km, 1 km and finally 500 meters. A simple yellow line marks the apex.

A descent followed by a climb along Schueren Road leads to Saddle Peak where unparalleled panoramas open wide. From Saddle Peak, the ride's grand payoff begins: several miles of downhill, wending through the mountains back to Topanga. Be mindful of the many blind turns and hidden driveways along these narrow, twisting roads—hardly the route for cutting turns tight, crossing the centerline or indulging other feats of exuberance. So watch your speed. Midway down, you'll pass through a copse of fragrant pines and several places where, on a clear day, you can look down the canyon, all the way to East L. A., and beyond.

# Ride Log

*P1* Red Rock Canyon Park
*P2* Will Geer Theatricum Botanicum
*P3* Saddle Peak
*P4* The TV show M*A*S*H*'s filming location
*P5* Malibu Creek State Park
*P6* King Gillette Ranch Park
*P7* Tapia County Park

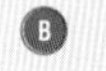

*B1* Topanga Creek Bicycles
1273 N. Topanga Canyon Blvd, Topanga
*B2* Wheel World Bike Shop
22718 Ventura Blvd, Woodland Hills
*B3* Santa Monica Mountains Cyclery
21526 Ventura Blvd, Woodland Hills

Ⓡ *R1* Topanga Creek Bicycles
1273 N. Topanga Canyon Blvd, Topanga

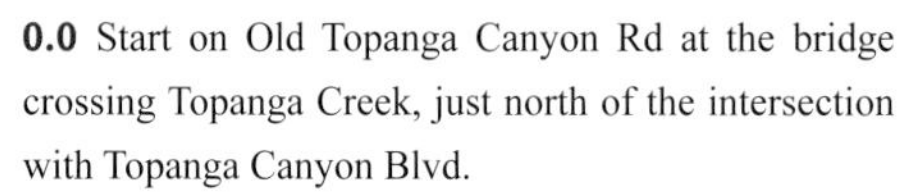

**0.0** Start on Old Topanga Canyon Rd at the bridge crossing Topanga Creek, just north of the intersection with Topanga Canyon Blvd.

**4.1** Summit.

**5.6** Turn left onto Dry Canyon-Cold Creek Rd. You'll be riding downhill and rounding a corner as you approach this turn. A fenced-off fragment of an old road will appear to your left and a big yellow and black directional sign directly ahead, pointing to the right, where Old Topanga turns in that direction. The turn to Dry Canyon-Cold Creek is just past the closed road and right before the arrow.

**6.4** Turn left onto Mulholland Hwy.

**7.2** Summit. Turn right onto Dry Canyon-Cold Creek Rd.

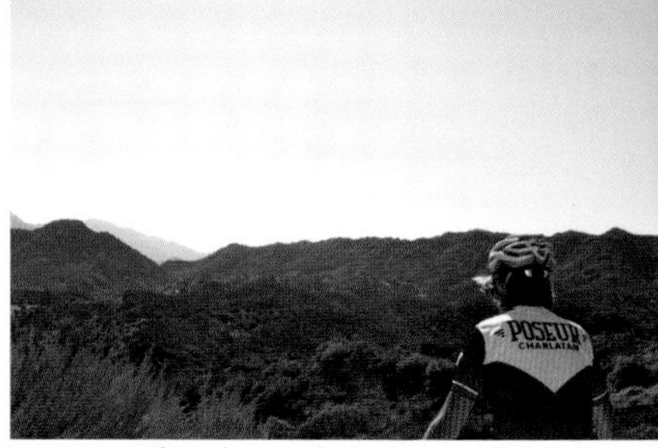


*Along the way, the landscape unfurls before you.*

**9.2** Turn right onto Mulholland Hwy.

**10.3** Turn left onto Cold Canyon Rd. Cold Canyon intersects Mulholland on the left two times before this turn. The first two instances lead back to Mulholland, so you can't get lost.

**12.4** Turn left onto Piuma Rd. There is a drinking fountain for a water stop at Los Angeles County Fire Station 67 in Monte Nido (just to the west of Saddle Peak Lodge).

**17.2** Summit. Continue straight on Piuma Rd.

**18.2** Turn left onto Schueren Rd.

**20.0** Summit. Continue east on Saddle Peak Rd (don't turn left or downhill onto Stunt Rd).

**23.4** Turn left onto Tuna Canyon Rd at the stop sign. Tuna Canyon becomes Fernwood Pacific Dr midway down the mountain.

**26.2** Turn left onto Topanga Canyon Blvd.

**26.8** Arrive at Old Topanga Canyon Rd.

## Topanga Canyon

*Please note: the profile for Ride 23 is depicted in 500ft vertical increments due to unusually high elevation.*

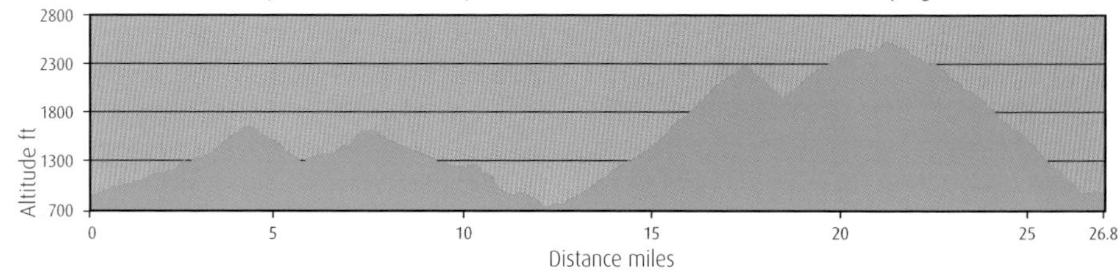

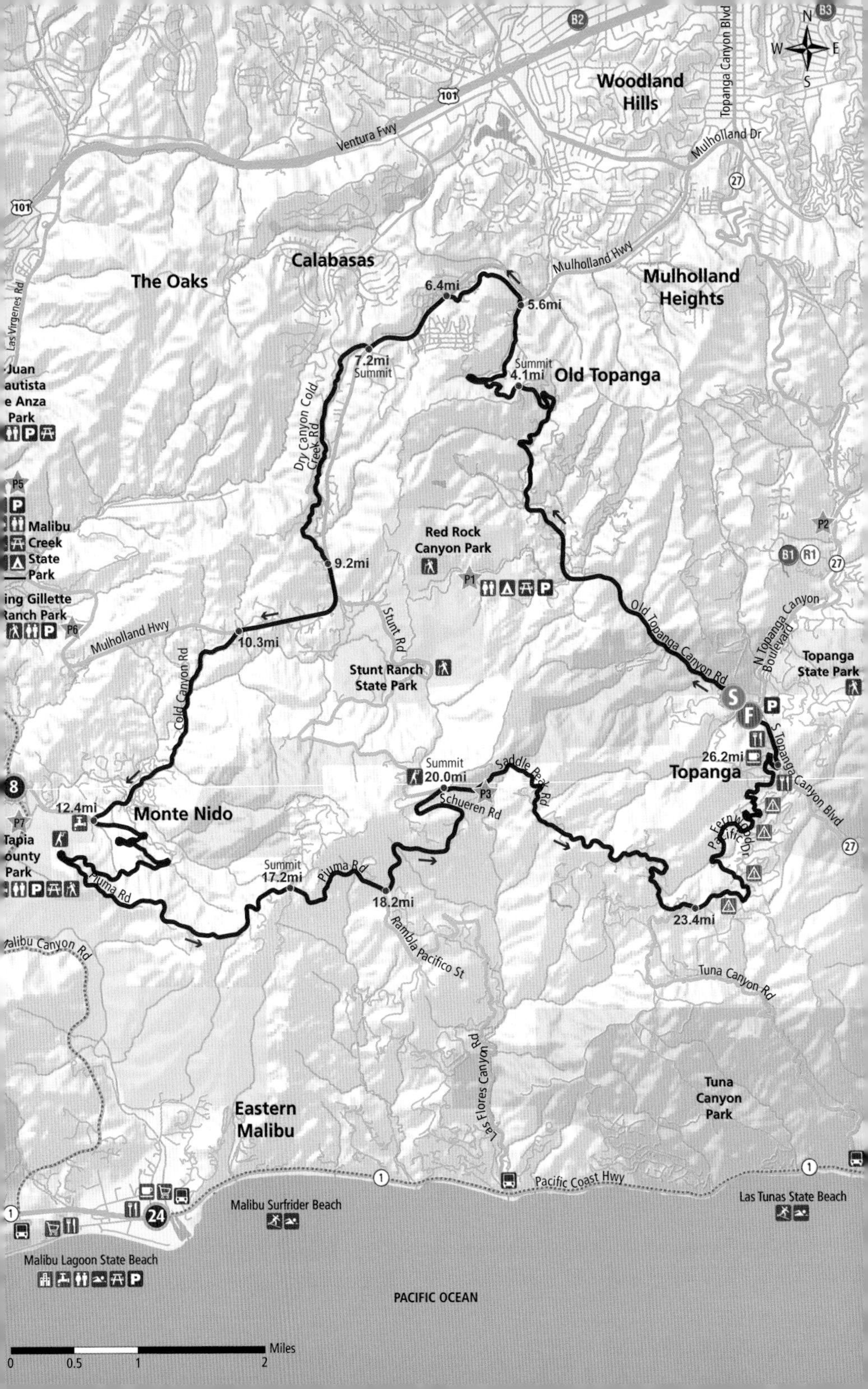
Woodland Hills
Topanga Canyon Blvd
Ventura Fwy
101
Mulholland Dr
27
Calabasas
The Oaks
Mulholland Hwy
Mulholland Heights
Las Virgenes Rd
6.4mi
5.6mi
7.2mi
Summit
Summit
4.1mi
Old Topanga
Juan
Bautista
de Anza
Park
Dry Canyon Cold Creek Rd
P5
Malibu
Creek
State
Park
Red Rock
Canyon Park
P1
P2
B1
R1
9.2mi
Stunt Rd
Gillette
Ranch Park
P6
Mulholland Hwy
10.3mi
Old Topanga Canyon Rd
N Topanga Canyon Boulevard
Topanga
State Park
Stunt Ranch
State Park
Cold Canyon Rd
S
F
P
S Topanga Canyon Blvd
26.2mi
Summit
20.0mi
Saddle Peak Rd
Topanga
8
P3
Schueren Rd
12.4mi
Monte Nido
P7
Tapia
County
Park
Fernwood Pacific Dr
Piuma Rd
Summit
17.2mi
Piuma Rd
18.2mi
23.4mi
Malibu Canyon Rd
Rambla Pacifico St
Tuna Canyon Rd
Las Flores Canyon Rd
Eastern
Malibu
Tuna
Canyon
Park
1
Pacific Coast Hwy
Malibu Surfrider Beach
Las Tunas State Beach
24
Malibu Lagoon State Beach
PACIFIC OCEAN
0
0.5
1
2
Miles
N
W
E
S
B2
B3

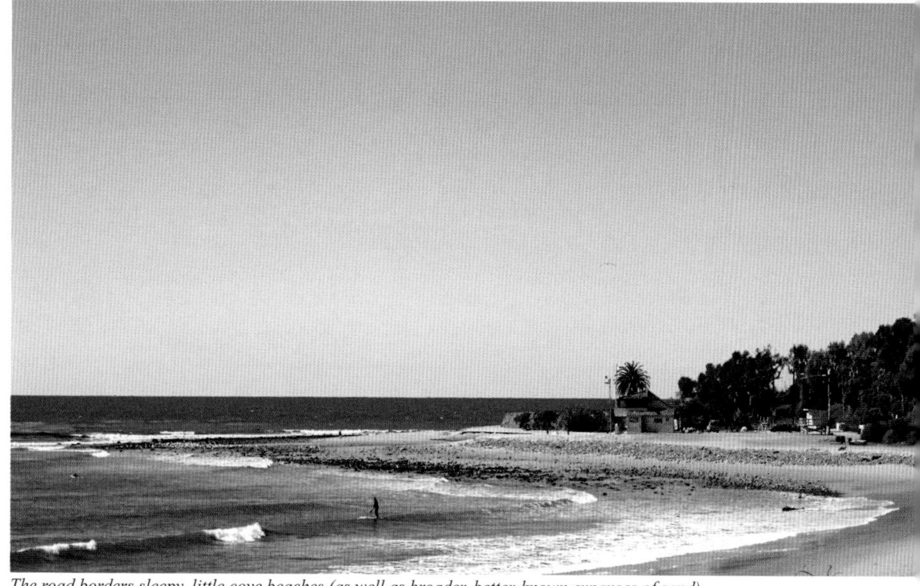

*The road borders sleepy, little cove beaches (as well as broader, better-known expanses of sand).*

## At a Glance

**Distance** 23.8 miles **Elevation Gain** 400 feet

### Terrain

Pacific Coast Highway, or PCH, is virtually flat for this entire coastal ride. Afternoon winds can sometimes make you feel you're riding up invisible hills toward Malibu and down them on the way home.

### Traffic

The route begins on a car-free bike path before transitioning to a wide shoulder that doubles as a bike lane along PCH. East of Topanga Canyon Boulevard on the trip home, be mindful of opening doors of parked cars. This ride is best on weekends or holidays, especially in the early morning.

### How to Get There

The route begins at the north end of the Santa Monica Pier parking lot. From the 10 Freeway, take the Fouth/Fifth Street exit and follow signs to the pier's paid parking area. Free parking is sometimes available on nearby streets.

### Food and Drink

You can fuel up numerous eateries along PCH or at the shopping centers across PCH from Malibu Lagoon State Park.

### Side Trip

Along PCH, stop by the Getty Villa to see oil baron J. Paul Getty's villa, gardens and outstanding collection of ancient Greek, Roman and Etruscan art. Or visit the 1930 Adamson House, a Spanish Colonial-style home-turned-museum integrating the most extensive holdings of Malibu Potteries ceramic tile.

**Links to** 8 25 26 27 k13

**Where to Bike Rating** 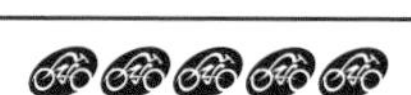

 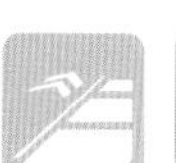 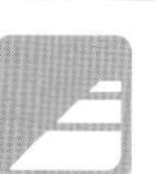 

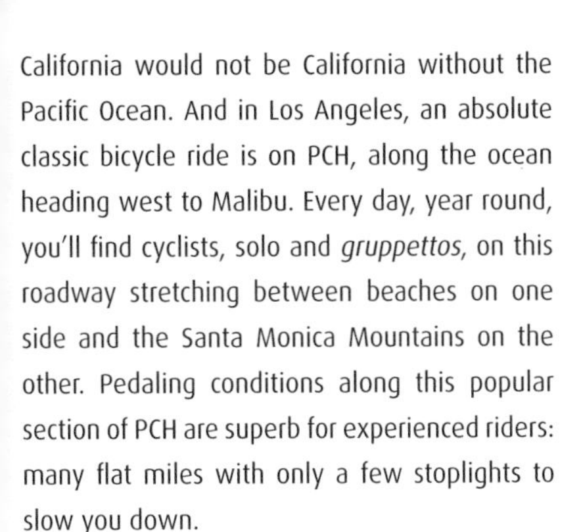

## About...

California would not be California without the Pacific Ocean. And in Los Angeles, an absolute classic bicycle ride is on PCH, along the ocean heading west to Malibu. Every day, year round, you'll find cyclists, solo and *gruppettos,* on this roadway stretching between beaches on one side and the Santa Monica Mountains on the other. Pedaling conditions along this popular section of PCH are superb for experienced riders: many flat miles with only a few stoplights to slow you down.



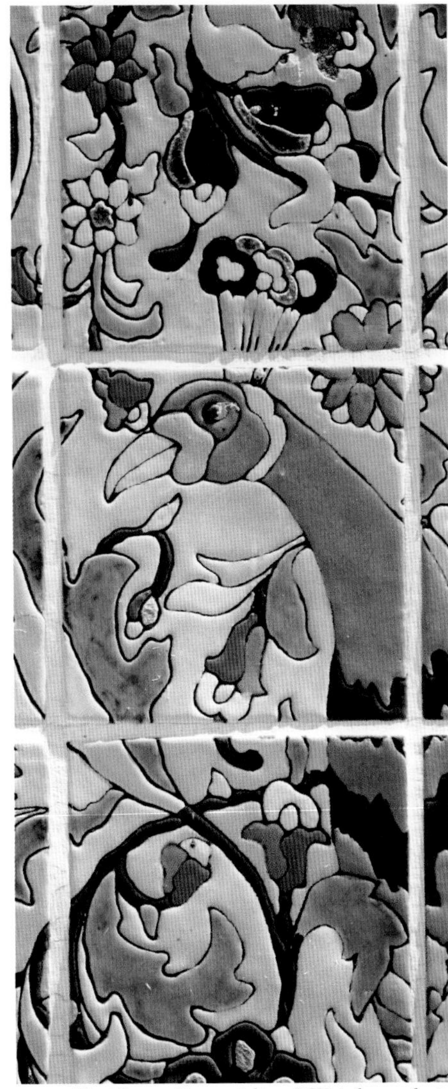

*The Adamson House, right on PCH, is famous for its Malibu Potteries ceramic tile.*

From the Santa Monica Pier, it's a three-mile warm-up along the car-free Marvin Braude Bike Trail—a time to gauge how comfortable the saddle's going to be today, feel the first pressure of the pedals and tentatively decide if it's a small- or big-chain ring day.

From Will Rogers State Beach, you'll cross Pacific Coast Highway and turn your handlebars west. Here, on PCH, the best part of the ride begins through an area once dubbed "the Riviera of America" for its striking places of sun, surf and sand against a backdrop of mountains.

The shoulder ahead is mostly blissfully flat. Maybe shift to a bigger cog or two for the bump between Sunset Boulevard and the Getty Villa. Another little rise just past the Charthouse restaurant leads up to Topanga Canyon Boulevard. After that, find the right gear, settle into a comfortable cadence and enjoy the ride.

As the turnaround at Cross Creek Road comes into view, it's time to decide on a rest stop. Will it be a quick espresso at one of the shopping centers on the right, or a few minutes of meditation along the vast wetlands of Malibu Lagoon State Park, or maybe a stroll through the Getty Villa or Adamson House grounds? From the Adamson, you can take in first-rate views of the aptly named Surfrider Beach.

Once you're back in the saddle, turn those handlebars toward Santa Monica. With any luck, the almost daily on-shore winds will whisk you home. As you pedal, South Bay panoramas will eventually come into view—coastal vistas all the way south to the Palos Verdes Peninsula.

# Ride Log

**0.0** From the north corner of the Santa Monica Pier parking lot, ride northwest on the Marvin Braude Bike Trail/ Santa Monica bike path.

**2.9** Arrive at Will Rogers State Beach. Turn right, and—taking care to watch for cross traffic—traverse the parking lot's exit and entrance lanes and Pacific Coast Hwy at Temescal Canyon Rd. At this busy intersection, be sure to use the cross walk or turn lane.

**4.1** Cross Sunset Blvd.

**4.9** Pass Getty Villa. There's bicycle parking near the entry kiosk. From there it's a short walk up to the villa. Admission is free, but timed tickets are required for any visit (tickets on-line at **www.getty.edu/visit**).

**5.6** Cross Topanga Canyon Blvd.

**8.9** Cross Los Flores Canyon Rd.

**11.9** Turn left into Malibu Lagoon State Beach at Cross Creek Dr. After a rest and/or a visit to the park, turn right onto Pacific Coast Hwy (towards Santa Monica and Los Angeles).

**12.2** Pass Adamson House and Malibu Lagoon Museum (tours Wed. to Sat. 10:00 a.m. to 2:00 p.m. Info at 310-456-8432).

**12.5** Pass the Malibu Pier.

**18.1** Pass Topanga State Beach.

**20.9** Turn into the Will Rogers State Beach parking lot at Temescal Canyon Rd. Cross the entry and exit lanes to the bike path. Watch for traffic. Turn left and continue south on the Marvin Braude Bike Trail/ Santa Monica bike path.

**23.8** Santa Monica Pier parking lot. End of ride.

*P1* Pacific Park on the Santa Monica Pier
*P2* The Getty Villa
*P3* Malibu Legacy Park
*P4* Adamson House & Malibu Lagoon Museum
*P5* Malibu Sport Fishing Pier
*P6* Paramount Ranch
*P7* King Gillette Ranch Park
*P8* Old M*A*S*H set
*P9* Saddle Peak
*P10* Temescal Gateway Park
*P11* Eames House

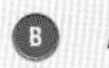

*B1* Blazing Saddles
320 Santa Monica Pier, Santa Monica
*B2* Spokes N'Stuff
1715 Ocean Front Walk, Santa Monica
*B3* Performance Bicycle Shop
501 Broadway, Santa Monica
*B4* Helen's Cycles
2501 Broadway, Santa Monica
*B5* Palisades Bicycles
871 Via de la Paz, Pacific Palisades
*B6* Topanga Creek Bicycles
1273 N. Topanga Canyon Blvd, Topanga

R

*R1* Perry's Café & Rentals, several locations on the Marvin Braude Bike Trail
*R2* Sea Mist Rentals
Santa Monica Pier
*R3* Helen's Cycles
2501 Broadway, Santa Monica

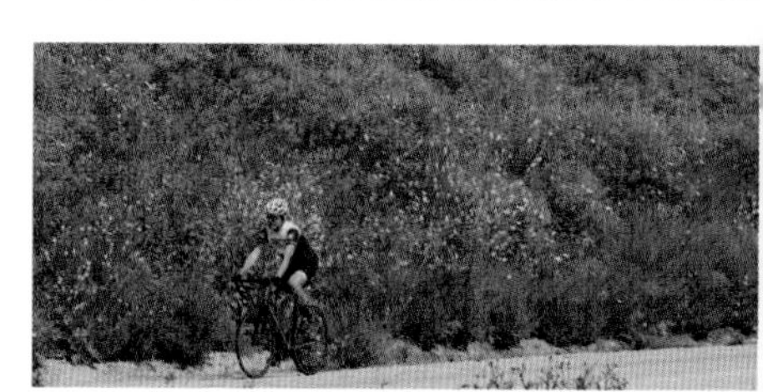

*In springtime, tiny, yellow wild mustard blossoms dot the hillsides.*

## Pacific Coast Highway

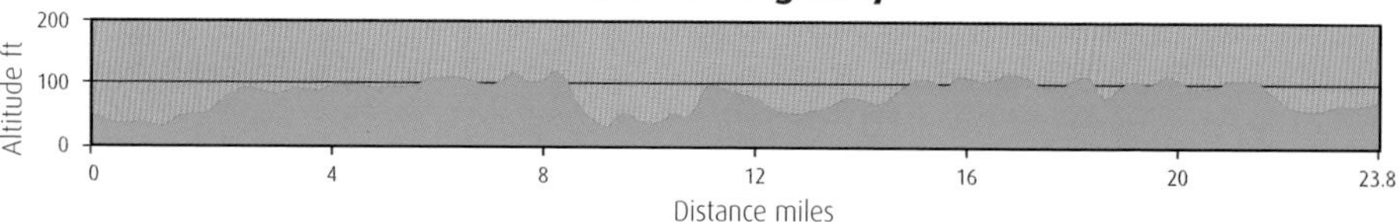

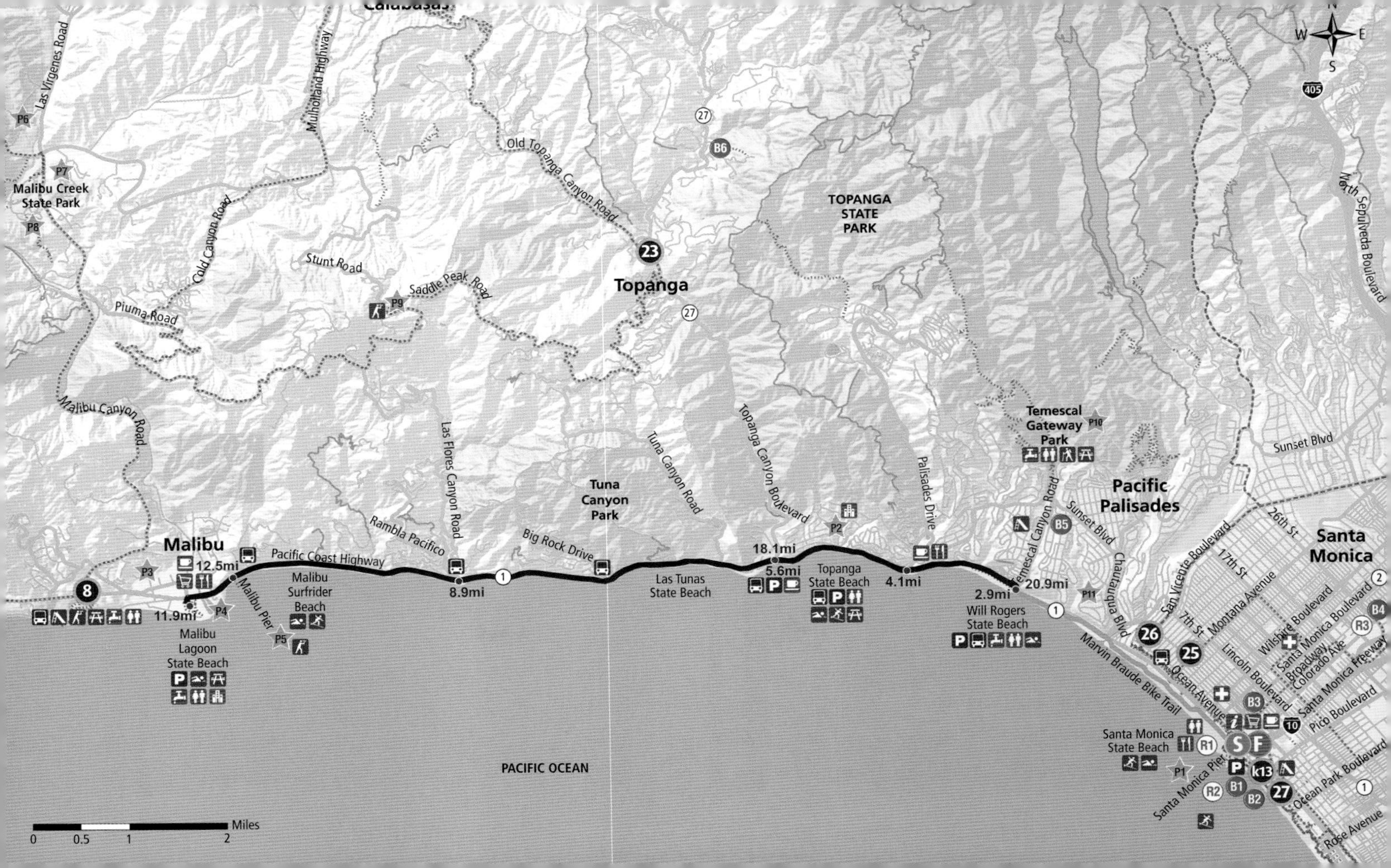

Las Virgenes Road
Mulholland Highway
Malibu Creek State Park
Old Topanga Canyon Road
Cold Canyon Road
Stunt Road
Saddle Peak Road
Piuma Road
Topanga
TOPANGA STATE PARK
North Sepulveda Boulevard
Malibu Canyon Road
Las Flores Canyon Road
Tuna Canyon Road
Topanga Canyon Boulevard
Palisades Drive
Temescal Gateway Park
Sunset Blvd
Tuna Canyon Park
Pacific Palisades
Rambla Pacifico
Big Rock Drive
Temescal Canyon Road
Malibu
Pacific Coast Highway
12.5mi
18.1mi
5.6mi
8.9mi
4.1mi
2.9mi
20.9mi
11.9mi
Malibu Pier
Malibu Surfrider Beach
Las Tunas State Beach
Topanga State Beach
Will Rogers State Beach
Chautauqua Blvd
San Vicente Boulevard
26th St
17th St
7th St
Montana Avenue
Wilshire Boulevard
Santa Monica Boulevard
Broadway
Colorado Ave
Santa Monica Freeway
Lincoln Boulevard
Pico Boulevard
Ocean Avenue
Ocean Park Boulevard
Rose Avenue
Santa Monica
Malibu Lagoon State Beach
Marvin Braude Bike Trail
Santa Monica State Beach
Santa Monica Pier
PACIFIC OCEAN
Miles
0
0.5
1
2

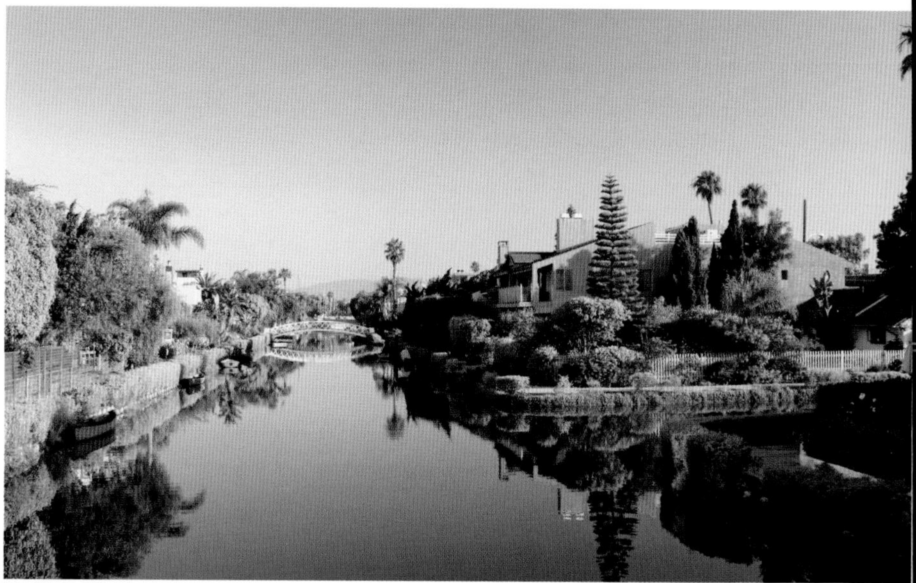

*The Venice Canals can be amazingly serene.*

## At a Glance

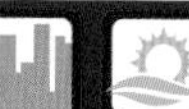

**Distance** 18.8 miles **Elevation Gain** 900 feet

### Terrain

On this essentially flat ride, you'll encounter one short downhill heading west on Ocean Park Boulevard.

### Traffic

This route through Santa Monica and Venice links bike lanes, bike routes and relatively quiet neighborhood streets. Car traffic tends to increase during peak times, such as rush hours.

### How to Get There

Exit the 10 Freeway at Fourth/Fifth Streets in Santa Monica, turn left on Fourth Street and then, right into Olympic Drive. There's metered parking along Main Street and paid parking in the many parking structures and lots near City Hall.

### Food and Drink

This *Tour* passes through several prime dining and snacking corridors, notably in its segments on Montana Avenue, Main Street and Abbot Kinney Boulevard and leading into the Third Street Promenade.

### Side Trip

The 1949 Eames House (Case Study House No. 8) is a landmark of Mid-century Modern architecture and well worth a visit. Continue north on Ocean Avenue, turn left on West Channel Road. At Pacific Coast Highway, make a sharp right onto Chautauqua Boulevard to the private drive marked 203/205. The house is at the end of the driveway. For a self-guided tour of the (very transparent) exterior, reservations are required (310-459-9663).

**Links to** 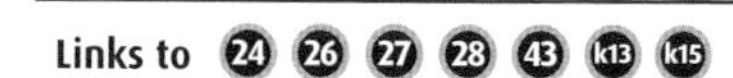


**Where to Bike Rating** 

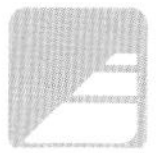

# About...

Santa Monica and Venice offer a veritable smorgasbord of fun and interesting things to experience. This versatile tour—which can be shortened as desired or readily extended to include the beachfronts (Ride 27)—gives you a taste of that varied fare, including farmers' markets, architectural milestones, hip and funky shopping streets, historic landmarks, restaurant rows, the great cluster of art galleries at Bergamot Station and the idyllic Venice Canals.

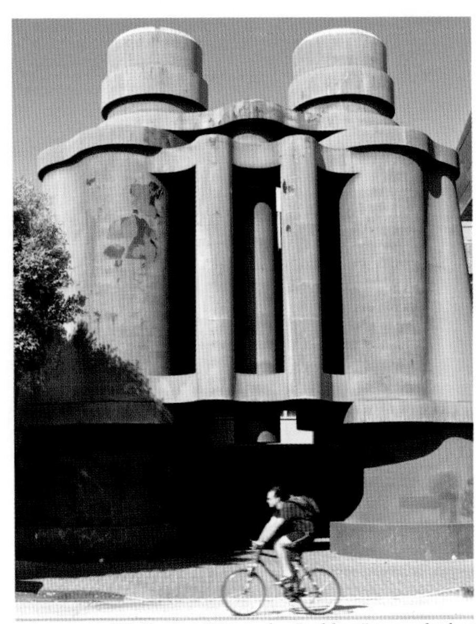

*The famous "Binocular Building" is perched on Main Street.*



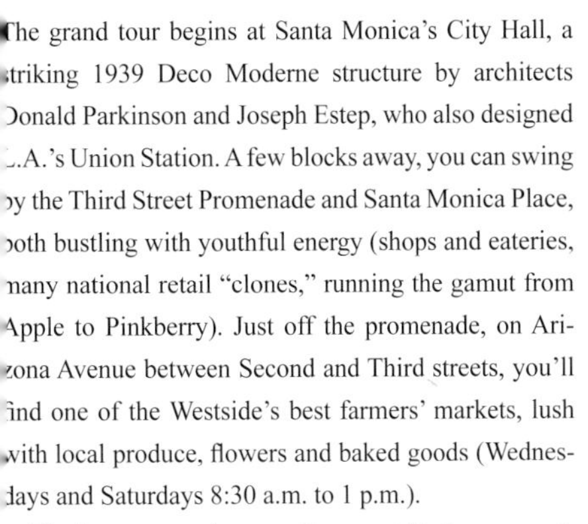

The grand tour begins at Santa Monica's City Hall, a striking 1939 Deco Moderne structure by architects Donald Parkinson and Joseph Estep, who also designed L.A.'s Union Station. A few blocks away, you can swing by the Third Street Promenade and Santa Monica Place, both bustling with youthful energy (shops and eateries, many national retail "clones," running the gamut from Apple to Pinkberry). Just off the promenade, on Arizona Avenue between Second and Third streets, you'll find one of the Westside's best farmers' markets, lush with local produce, flowers and baked goods (Wednesdays and Saturdays 8:30 a.m. to 1 p.m.).

The journey continues to Bergamot Station, a quasi-industrial, 8-acre complex with 30 contemporary art galleries, the Santa Monica Museum of Art and a café. Dating back to 1875, Bergamot was originally a depot for steam rail (later trolley) service from downtown L.A. to the Santa Monica Pier.

Next, pedal through industrial and residential areas, past the shops and food emporia on Montana Avenue, all the way west to Ocean Avenue, bordering Palisades Park. This esplanade—with abundant palm trees and a packed-dirt path for strolling and biking—overlooks a long stretch of beach.

After turning inland, you'll have another opportunity to visit a farmers' market, but this one, right on Main Street, can feel more like block fair. Beyond plentiful fresh produce, its stalls serve up everything from tamales, stir fries and crepes to fresh-squeezed juices; live bands play; vendors offer pony rides and more. The market's "bike valet" will mind your wheels free of charge, though tipping is welcome (2640 Main Street, Sundays 9:30 a.m. to 1:00 p.m.).

Along Main Street, watch for architect Frank Gehry's Binoculars Building (1985-91) with its entryway of giant binoculars by artist Claes Oldenburg. Hovering down the street against another building is sculptor Jonathan Borofsky's disquieting *Ballerina Clown* (1988).

Abbot Kinney Boulevard, with hip, one-of-a-kind stores and restaurants, angles off Main Street. Abbot Kinney was an early developer of Venice, California, and the canals he created there around 1904 highlight the end of our tour. This serene and picturesque historic district is what remains of a 16-mile network of man-made canals, romantically evoking Venice, Italy. Cottages line these waterways, originally plied by crooning gondoliers. You can ride on the streets and bridges, but must walk your bike on the waterside paths.

# Ride Log

**0.0** Starting from the ocean side of Santa Monica City Hall, turn right onto Main St.

**0.1** Turn left onto Colorado Ave. Go into the right turn lane.

**0.2** Turn right onto Second St.

**0.3** Turn right onto Broadway St. Join the bike lane at Seventh St.

**1.6** Turn right onto 20th St.

**1.9** Turn left onto Olympic Blvd.

**2.0** Turn right onto 21st St.

**2.1** 21st St bends to the left and becomes Michigan Ave.

**2.3** Cross Cloverfield Blvd.

**2.5** Arrive at Bergamot Station Arts Center. After exploring the galleries, the Santa Monica Museum of Art, or visiting the café, continue back along Michigan Ave to Cloverfield Blvd.

**2.7** Turn right onto Cloverfield Blvd then turn right onto 26th St.

**3.1** Turn right onto Colorado Ave.

**3.3** Turn right onto Stewart St (becomes 28th St south of Pico Blvd).

**4.5** Turn right onto Ocean Park Blvd. Join the bike lane at Cloverfield.

**5.8** Turn right onto 11th St.

**7.1** Turn right onto Arizona Ave.

**7.6** Turn left on 17th St.

**8.3** Turn left onto Montana Ave. Join the bike lane.

**9.5** Turn right onto Ocean Ave. Join the bike lane.

**10.0** Turn left, making a U-turn past San Vicente. Continue south on Ocean Ave.

**11.9** Angle slightly to the right at Pico Blvd. Ocean becomes Barnard Ave.

**12.8** Barnard Ave turns to the left and becomes Marine S

**13.0** Turn right onto Main St.

**13.9** Continue on Main St through the roundabou then turn left onto Venice Way.

**14.3** Cross both lanes of Venice Blvd, then turn lef onto Mildred Ave at Kim's Food Corner market.

**14.8** Turn right onto Washington Blvd. Join the bike lane

**15.4** Turn right onto Dell Ave at the signal (become Riviera Ave north of Mildred Ave).

**16.1** Turn right onto Grand Blvd.

**16.3**. Continue in the left lane when Grand meets Venice Blvd.

**16.4** Turn right onto Rialto Ave and then left onto Abbot Kinney Blvd.

**17.0** Turn right onto Main St. Join the bike lane at Marine

**18.8** Cross Pico Blvd, arrive back at City Hall.

B
*B1* Performance Bicycle Shop
501 Broadway, Santa Monica
*B2* Bike Effect
910 Broadway #100, Santa Monica
*B3* Cynergy Cycles
2300 Santa Monica Blvd, Santa Monica
*B4* Helen's Cycles Santa Monica
2501 Broadway, Santa Monica
*B5* The Bicycle Workshop
1638 Ocean Park Blvd, Santa Monica
*B6* Bike Attack
2400 Main St, Santa Monica
R
*R1* Helen's Cycles Santa Monica
2501 Broadway, Santa Monica
*R2* Perry's Café and Rentals, several locations on the Marvin Braude Bike Trail

## A Tour of Santa Monica

Altitude ft: 300, 200, 100, 0
Distance miles: 0, 3, 6, 9, 12, 15, 18.8

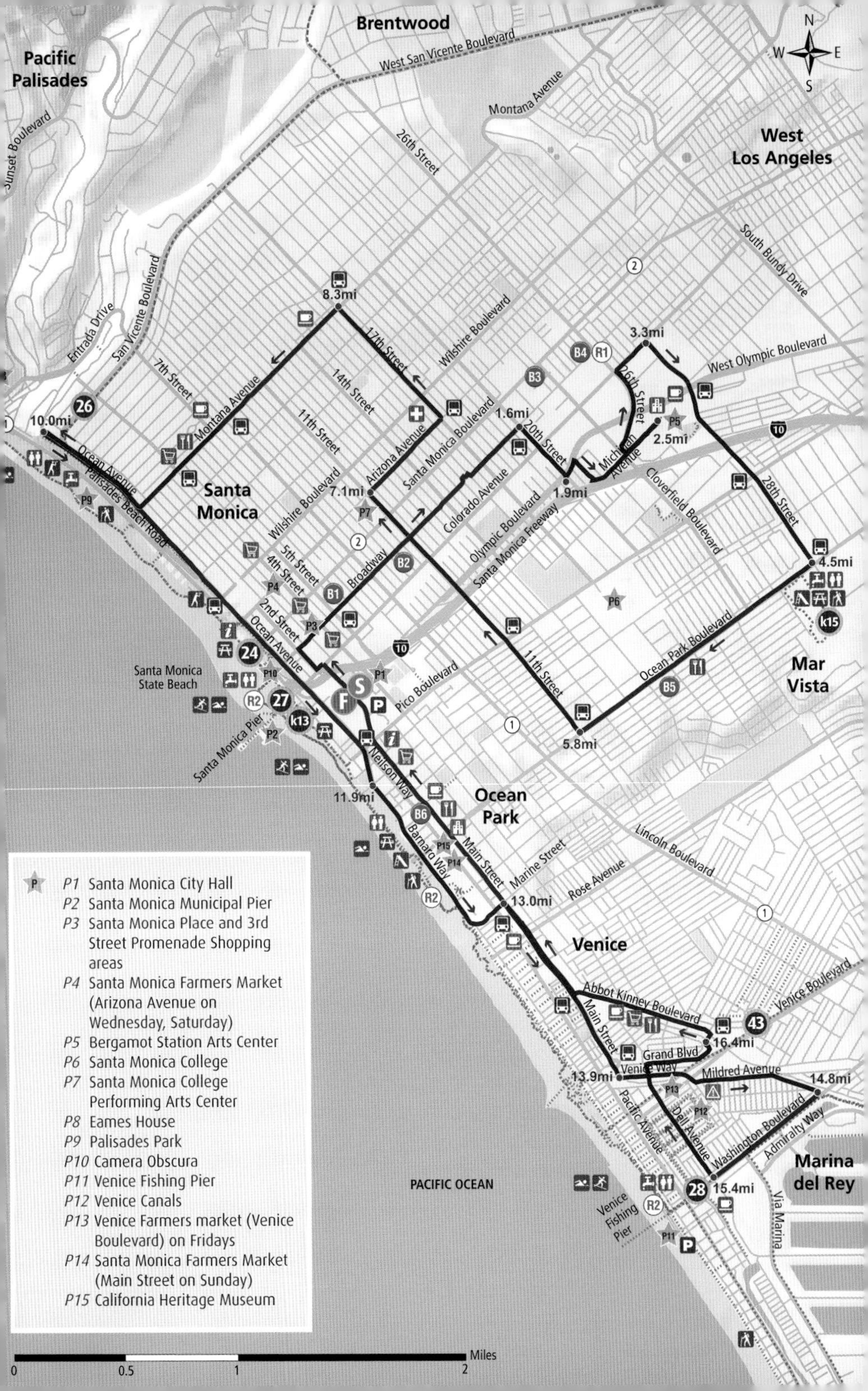

Brentwood
Pacific Palisades
West Los Angeles
Santa Monica
Ocean Park
Venice
Mar Vista
Marina del Rey
PACIFIC OCEAN
Santa Monica State Beach
Santa Monica Pier
Venice Fishing Pier
West San Vicente Boulevard
Montana Avenue
26th Street
Sunset Boulevard
South Bundy Drive
Wilshire Boulevard
Entrada Drive
San Vicente Boulevard
7th Street
14th Street
11th Street
17th Street
Arizona Avenue
Santa Monica Boulevard
20th Street
Colorado Avenue
Olympic Boulevard
Santa Monica Freeway
Michigan Avenue
Cloverfield Boulevard
West Olympic Boulevard
28th Street
Ocean Avenue
Palisades Beach Road
5th Street
4th Street
2nd Street
Broadway
Pico Boulevard
11th Street
Ocean Park Boulevard
Nelson Way
Barnard Way
Main Street
Marine Street
Rose Avenue
Lincoln Boulevard
Abbot Kinney Boulevard
Venice Boulevard
Grand Blvd
Venice Way
Mildred Avenue
Pacific Avenue
Dell Avenue
Washington Boulevard
Admiralty Way
Via Marina
10.0mi
8.3mi
7.1mi
1.6mi
1.9mi
2.5mi
3.3mi
4.5mi
5.8mi
11.9mi
13.0mi
13.9mi
14.8mi
15.4mi
16.4mi
P1 Santa Monica City Hall
P2 Santa Monica Municipal Pier
P3 Santa Monica Place and 3rd Street Promenade Shopping areas
P4 Santa Monica Farmers Market (Arizona Avenue on Wednesday, Saturday)
P5 Bergamot Station Arts Center
P6 Santa Monica College
P7 Santa Monica College Performing Arts Center
P8 Eames House
P9 Palisades Park
P10 Camera Obscura
P11 Venice Fishing Pier
P12 Venice Canals
P13 Venice Farmers market (Venice Boulevard) on Fridays
P14 Santa Monica Farmers Market (Main Street on Sunday)
P15 California Heritage Museum
Miles
0
0.5
1
2

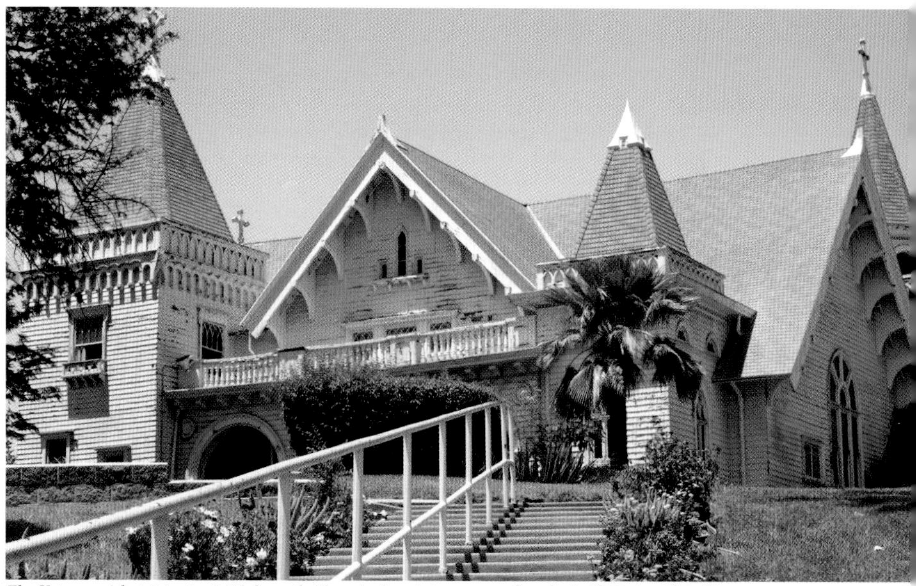

*The Veterans Administration's Wadsworth Chapel, closed since an earthquake in 1971, is still striking.*

## At a Glance

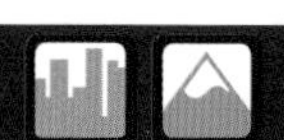

**Distance** 23.7 miles **Elevation Gain** 1,700 feet

### Terrain

This ride is entirely on paved roads with gradual climbs on San Vicente and a moderate, sustained ascent into Mandeville Canyon.

### Traffic

San Vicente has generous bike lanes. Traffic is relatively light in Mandeville Canyon.

### How to Get There

From the 405 Freeway, either exit at Wilshire Boulevard, take Wilshire east and then, Veteran Avenue south; or exit at Santa Monica Boulevard, head east on Santa Monica and north on Sepulveda Boulevard. On Westwood Recreation Center's north, south and west sides, you'll find free parking lots.

### Food and Drink

The well-to-do enclave of Brentwood has plentiful restaurants and cafés (Caffe Luxxe, Starbucks, Peets' and Coffee Bean), plus a Whole Foods. Toward the ride's coastal terminus, near the Santa Monica Pier or Third Street Promenade, other refreshment options abound.

### Side Trip

The ascent of Bundy Drive to Mount St. Mary's College offers the experience of another canyon. This ride is shorter and more manageable than Mandeville Canyon, but also a bit more suburban, less rustic. On the final climb, you can glimpse the ocean on a clear day—and on the descent, the Getty Center appears.

**Links to**

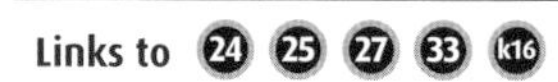


**Where to Bike Rating**

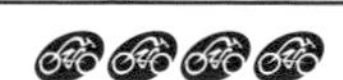

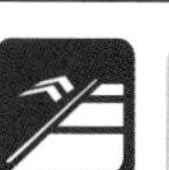

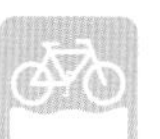

# About...

This ride takes advantage of San Vicente Boulevard's wide bike lanes through the calm, leafy, upscale residential neighborhoods of upper Santa Monica and Brentwood. The route offers the added option of a classic Los Angeles canyon ride: up the length of Mandeville Canyon and back. Mandeville's five-mile road—lined with abundant trees and high-end rustic homes—rises gradually through a cleft in the foothills of the Santa Monica Mountains.

The journey begins at the Westwood Community Center and soon wends its way across the Veterans Affairs Center grounds. On this 388-acre campus, you'll pass the white Wadsworth Chapel, ca. 1900, a confection of intricate and eclectic wood detailing, housing a Catholic and a Protestant chapel, separated by a heavy wall. Closed since the damaging Sylmar earthquake, of 1971, the deteriorating building remains striking.

Depending on your mood and energy level, you can simply ride San Vicente to the ocean (11.1 miles round trip), or you can make an excursion to Mandeville Canyon before continuing west to the coast (23.7 miles round trip).

Mandeville Canyon Road, five miles from end to end, is one of Los Angeles's longest paved dead-ends—and undeniably a mecca for cyclists. The canyons, at the interface of inhabited terrain and the wild Santa Monica Mountains, tend to be cooler and fresher than the rest of the city—and Mandeville is no exception. Quasi-rustic in character, the road is edged with lush trees and flowering front yards. Its slope is gradual but sustained, becoming slightly steeper toward the upper end. En route, you'll pass well-heeled but seemingly unpretentious homes against a backdrop of canyon walls. Quietly, such celebrities as actors Michael Douglas, Barbara Stanwyck and Eva Marie Saint and former California governor Arnold Schwarzenegger have lived along this road. After you reach the turnaround, you'll be rewarded with the joy of sailing all those miles downhill.

The route then winds back to San Vicente, another favorite among cyclists: a straight, broad, coral tree-lined avenue through the tony enclaves of upper Santa Monica and Brentwood. While nearby Sunset Boulevard (with direct connections to the 405 Freeway and Pacific Coast Highway) tends to attract fast vehicular traffic, San Vicente—blessed with a green, shady median and two lanes in either direction—is far more civilized and lightly traveled. Yet this boulevard extends all the way from the veterans center to the Santa Monica beach, some five miles, with only a handful of traffic signals—making it all the more pleasurable (and blessedly unencumbered) for riders. Coasting downhill, you'll finally arrive at the Palisades Park turnaround, with the ocean and horizon just beyond.



# Ride Log

## San Vicente

**0.0** From the Westwood Recreation Center, cross Sepulveda Blvd using the cross walk and ride south.
**0.2** Turn right onto Ohio Ave.
**0.4** Turn right onto Sawtelle Blvd, entering the VA Center. If the main gates are closed, use the pedestrian access-way on the right.
**0.5** Turn right onto Dowlen Dr.
**1.0** Turn right onto Bonsall Ave.
**1.2** Turn left onto Eisenhower Ave.
**1.6** Exit the VA Center and turn right onto Bringham Ave. If the main gates are closed, use the pedestrian access-way on the right.
**1.7** Turn left on Darlington Ave.
**1.8** Turn right onto San Vicente Blvd.
**2.4** Cross South Bundy Dr.
**3.5** Cross South 26th St.
**5.5** Cross Ocean Ave and arrive at Palisades Park in

## Ride Log continued...

Santa Monica. Return via San Vicente Blvd.

**9.3** Turn left on Darlington Ave, cross the westbound lane of San Vicente Blvd.

**9.4** Turn right onto Bringham Ave.

**9.5** Turn left into the VA Center and onto Eisenhower Ave.

**9.8** Turn right onto Bonsall Ave.

**10.0** Turn left onto Dowlen Dr.

**10.6** Turn left onto Bonsall Ave.

**10.7** Turn left onto Ohio Ave, leaving the VA Center.

**10.9** Turn left onto Sepulveda Blvd.

**11.1** Arrive at Westwood Recreation Center.

*P1* Los Angeles Veterans Center
*P2* Palisades Park
*P3* Eames House
*P4* University of California Los Angeles (UCLA)
*P5* Getty Center

### Mandeville Canyon

**0.0** Turn right onto 26th St—becomes Allenford Ave.

**0.7** Turn right onto Sunset Blvd (you can use the side-walk running parallel to Sunset).

**1.2** Turn left onto Mandeville Canyon Rd.

**6.3** Arrive at the "top" of the canyon at a security gate Rest, then turn around.

**11.4** Turn right onto Sunset Blvd (or cross and use th sidewalk parallel to Sunset).

**11.9** Turn left on Allenford Ave.

**12.6** Rejoin San Vicente Blvd.

### A Side Trip up Bundy to Mount St. Mary's

**0.0** Turn right onto Bundy Dr.

**0.3** Turn right, continuing on Bundy Dr.

**0.6** Cross Sunset Blvd.

**1.7** Stay to the left, do not turn onto Norman Pl (don' follow the sign indicating Mount St Mary's College).

**2.4** Turn right at the stop sign onto Chalon Rd.

**2.8** Arrive at the summit and entrance to Mount S Mary's College. Continue on Chalon Rd.

**3.0** Sharp right turn onto Norman Pl. Watch downhill speec

**3.8** Turn left, rejoining Bundy Dr.

**4.8** Cross Sunset Blvd.

**5.1** Turn left where Bundy Dr joins Kenter Ave.

**5.4** Rejoin San Vicente Blvd.

**San Vicente**

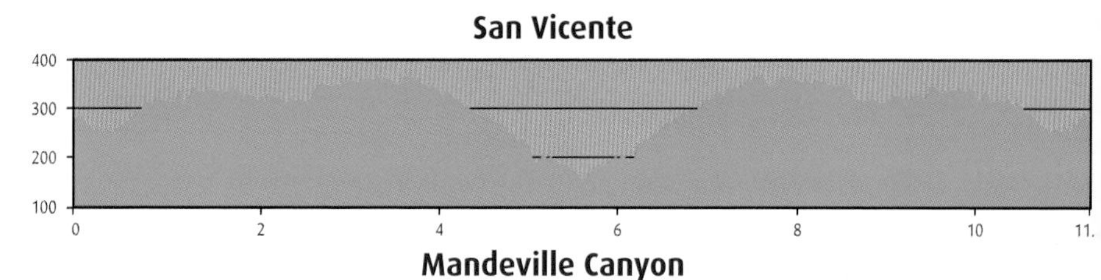


**Mandeville Canyon**

*Please note: the profile for Ride 26 (Mandeville) is depicted in 300ft vertical increments due to unusually high elevation.*

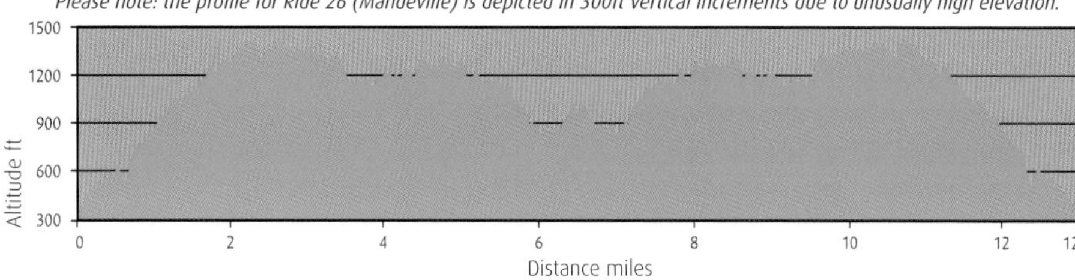

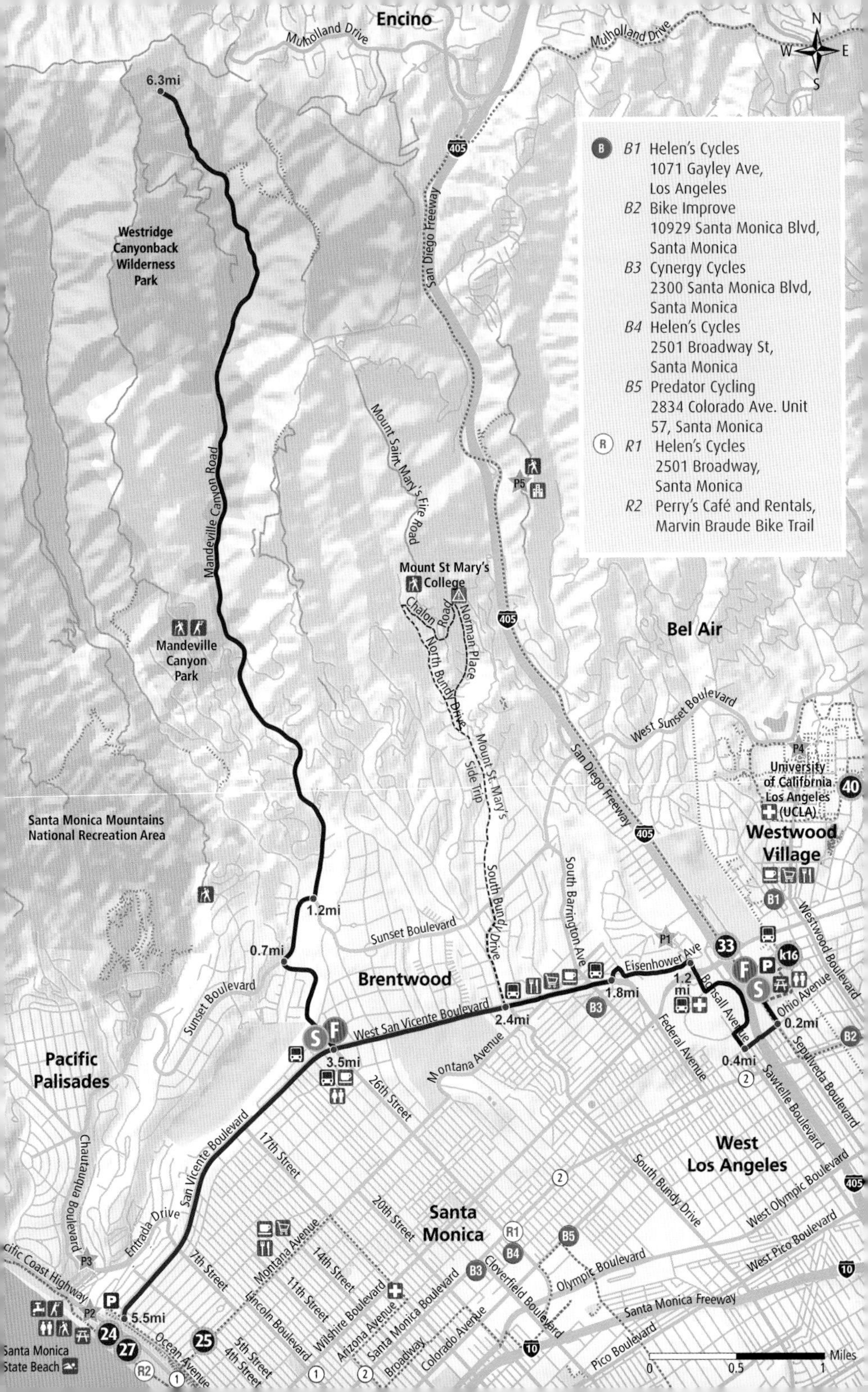

Encino
Mulholland Drive
Mulholland Drive
6.3mi
405
San Diego Freeway
B1 Helen's Cycles
1071 Gayley Ave,
Los Angeles
B2 Bike Improve
10929 Santa Monica Blvd,
Santa Monica
B3 Cynergy Cycles
2300 Santa Monica Blvd,
Santa Monica
B4 Helen's Cycles
2501 Broadway St,
Santa Monica
B5 Predator Cycling
2834 Colorado Ave. Unit
57, Santa Monica
R1 Helen's Cycles
2501 Broadway,
Santa Monica
R2 Perry's Café and Rentals,
Marvin Braude Bike Trail
Westridge
Canyonback
Wilderness
Park
Mount Saint Mary's Fire Road
Mandeville Canyon Road
P5
Mount St Mary's
College
Chalon Road
Norman Place
North Bundy Drive
Mount St Mary's
Side Trip
Bel Air
Mandeville
Canyon
Park
West Sunset Boulevard
San Diego Freeway
P4
University
of California
Los Angeles
(UCLA)
40
Westwood
Village
Santa Monica Mountains
National Recreation Area
South Barrington Ave
South Bundy Drive
B1
1.2mi
Sunset Boulevard
Westwood Boulevard
P1
33
k16
0.7mi
Eisenhower Ave
Brentwood
1.2
mi
1.8mi
Bonsall Avenue
Ohio Avenue
Sunset Boulevard
West San Vicente Boulevard
2.4mi
B3
0.2mi
B2
Federal Avenue
Sepulveda Boulevard
3.5mi
Montana Avenue
0.4mi
Pacific
Palisades
26th Street
Sawtelle Boulevard
San Vicente Boulevard
17th Street
West
Los Angeles
Chautauqua Boulevard
South Bundy Drive
West Olympic Boulevard
405
Entrada Drive
20th Street
Santa
Monica
Montana Avenue
R1
B5
West Pico Boulevard
P3
Pacific Coast Highway
7th Street
14th Street
B4
Olympic Boulevard
B3
Cloverfield Boulevard
10
P2
5.5mi
11th Street
Lincoln Boulevard
Wilshire Boulevard
Arizona Avenue
Santa Monica Boulevard
Santa Monica Freeway
24
27
25
Ocean Avenue
5th Street
4th Street
Broadway
Colorado Avenue
10
Pico Boulevard
Santa Monica
State Beach
R2
Miles
0
0.5
1
N
W
E
S

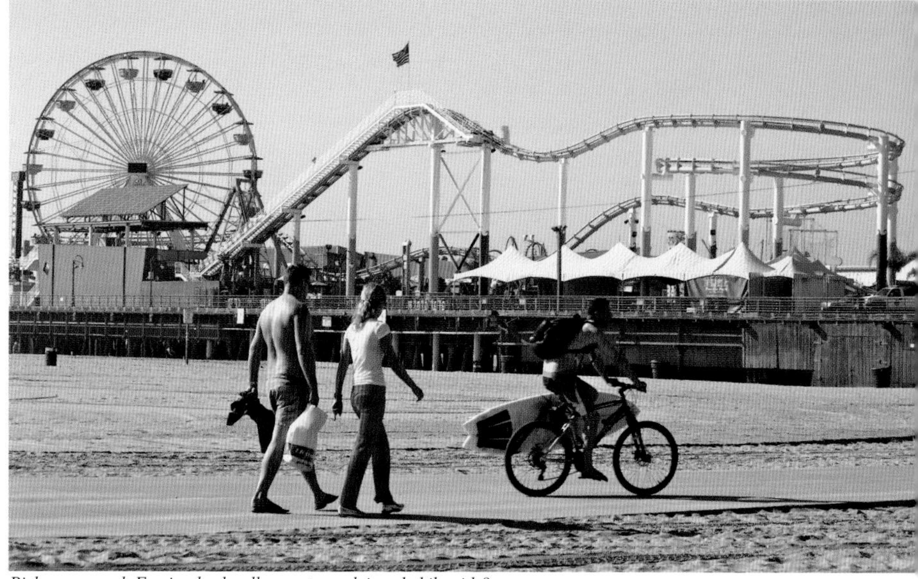

*Pick your speed: Ferris wheel, rollercoaster or leisurely bike ride?*

## At a Glance

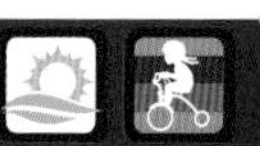

**Distance** 12.4 miles **Elevation Gain** 400 feet

### Terrain

This is a flat ride entirely on paved bike path. (Occasionally onshore winds blow sand onto the paving, producing slippery patches.)

### Traffic

The path is car-free. Though marked "bicycles only," it attracts some walkers, joggers and skaters. So be prepared to share. The most blissfully un-crowded times to bicycle here are weekday mornings and winter weekends.

### How to Get There

The ride begins at the Venice Fishing Pier, at the western end of Washington Boulevard in Marina del Rey. Take the 405 Freeway to the Venice/Washington exit. Follow Venice Boulevard west to Pacific Avenue, turn left onto Washington Boulevard, then right into the pier's parking lot. Or look for metered street parking along Washington.

### Food and Drink

You'll encounter an abundance of eateries and snack spots along Washington Boulevard near the Venice Fishing Pier, on the Venice Boardwalk, around the Santa Monica Pier and, during the summer, from concession stands at Will Rogers State Beach.

### Side Trip

Several fun excursions are within easy reach by bike. You can readily explore the scenic Venice Canals, Venice Fishing Pier, Venice Boardwalk and Santa Monica Pier, as well as the Third Street Promenade and Main Street shopping areas.

**Links to** 

**Where to Bike Rating** 

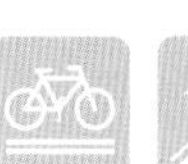 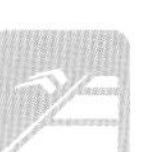  

# About...

This six-mile segment of the Marvin Braude Bike Trail, along Venice and Santa Monica beaches, is L.A. County's most famous leisurely bike "stroll," snaking past Venice's wild and colorful Boardwalk, with its lively potpourri of everyone and everything, from fortune tellers and skateboarders to organic juice bars and tattoo parlors. Next, you pass under Pacific Park, the last survivor of Santa Monica Bay's once plentiful amusement piers, before re-emerging along wide sandy beaches toward the turnaround at Will Rogers State Beach.

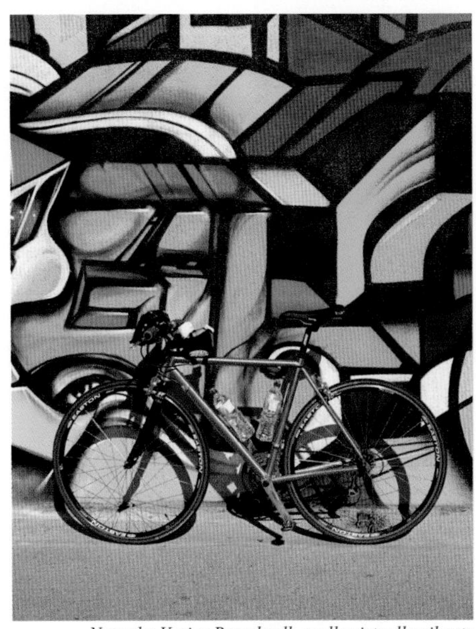

*Near the Venice Boardwalk, walls virtually vibrate with color.*



Venice, Ocean Park and Santa Monica—all bordering this route—date back more than 100 years as popular recreation magnets. In the 1890s, Abbot Kinney and his partners began developing the marshy beachfronts south of Santa Monica. Inspired by Kinney's exotic travels abroad, his creations here included "Venice of America," replete with picturesque canals and bridges. By 1905, the growing crowds descending on these sunny shores (thanks in part to train travel) prompted him to build the first of nearly a dozen amusement piers that would eventually perch over Santa Monica Bay. Much like Coney Island, these venues featured roller coasters, Ferris wheels and midways full of games and contests, casinos, bathhouses, restaurants, and music halls, where bands played into the night.

Fraser's Million Dollar Pier, the Sunset, Lick, Pickering, Venice Amusement and Pacific Ocean Park piers have all gone the way of the high-wheeled penny-farthing, but not their spirit of popular entertainment—still very much alive at Pacific Park on the Santa Monica Pier.

Less than a mile from the start, you'll be pedaling near the curiously board-free Venice Boardwalk, that two-and-a-half-mile-long, quirky, artsy circus of a promenade, packed with every ilk of street performer or artist and trinket-and-sarong vendor. Here, shops hawk offerings from body piercing and tattoos to funky sunglasses and t-shirts, from junk snacks to health food, Botox and medicinal herbs. Nearby, ripped bodybuilders at the Venice Weight Pen carry on the area's Muscle Beach tradition. Also a short stretch away is the Venice Skate Park, a hangout for skateboarders you might catch performing grabs, inverts, ollies and other tricks. Continuing north, the ride ducks briefly under Pacific Park at the Santa Monica Pier, the only remaining amusement pier, with its historic carousel, Ferris wheel, roller coaster and game arcade.

From there, you'll ride along a much less crowded part of Santa Monica State Beach, with deep sandy shores, past concession stands, and several beach clubs (including the Annenberg Community Beach House, with a swimming pool, yoga classes and other amenities—open to the public for a modest admission fee). The turnaround is at Will Rogers State Beach, named for the humorist, who counseled us: "You've got to go out on a limb sometimes because that's where the fruit is." And this ride offers quite a bounty.

# Ride Log

**0.0** Start at parking lot for the Venice Fishing Pier and pedal north on the Marvin Braude Bike Trail. The access point to the path is near the parking lot entry kiosk.

**0.6** Pass the Venice Beach Weight Pen, successor to the famous Muscle Beach.

**0.8** Pass the south end of the Venice Beach Boardwalk.

**3.0** Pass under the Santa Monica Pier and Pacific Park.

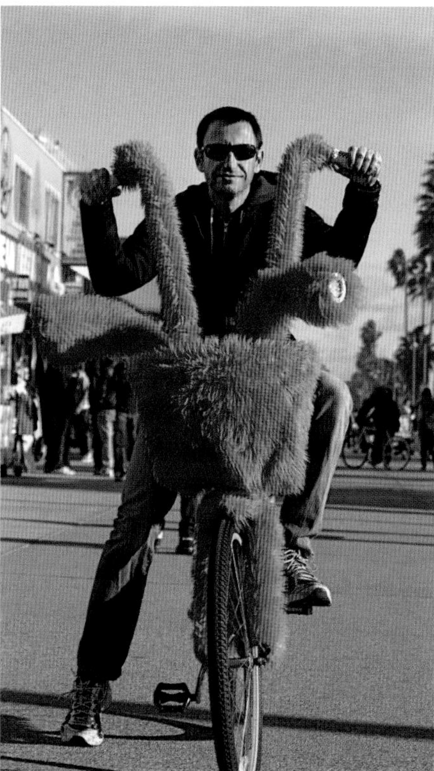

*A flamingo-pink fuzzy bike heads down the Venice Boardwalk.*

**4.6** Pass the Annenberg Community Beach House.

**6.2** Arrive at Will Rogers State Beach where the bike path ends at Temescal Canyon Rd. Take a moment—or more—to enjoy this typically less crowded stretch of beach. Make a U-turn and then follow the breadcrumbs back south.

**7.8** Pass the Annenberg Community Beach House.

**9.4** Pass under the Santa Monica Pier and Pacific Park.

**10.8** Pass the north end of the Venice Beach Boardwalk.

**12.4** Arrive back at the Venice Fishing Pier parking lot.

B *B1* Helen's Cycles
2472 Lincoln Blvd, Marina del Rey

*B2* MDR Bike Company
4051 Lincoln Blvd, Marina del Rey

*B3* Bike Attack
2400 Main St, Santa Monica

*B4* Veloworx
3106 Lincoln Blvd, Santa Monica

*B5* Performance Bicycle Shop
501 Broadway, Santa Monica

*B6* Helen's Cycles
2501 Broadway, Santa Monica

*B7* Bike Effect
910 Broadway, Santa Monica

R *R1* Perry's Café & Rentals
several locations on the Marvin Braude Bike Trail

*R2* Sea Mist Rentals
Santa Monica Pier

*R3* Blazing Saddles
320 Santa Monica Pier, Santa Monica

*R4* Spokes N'Stuff
1715 Ocean Front Walk, Santa Monica

*R5* Helen's Cycles
2501 Broadway, Santa Monica

**Santa Monica Bike Path**

Altitude ft
100
0
0 2 4 6 8 10 12.4
Distance miles

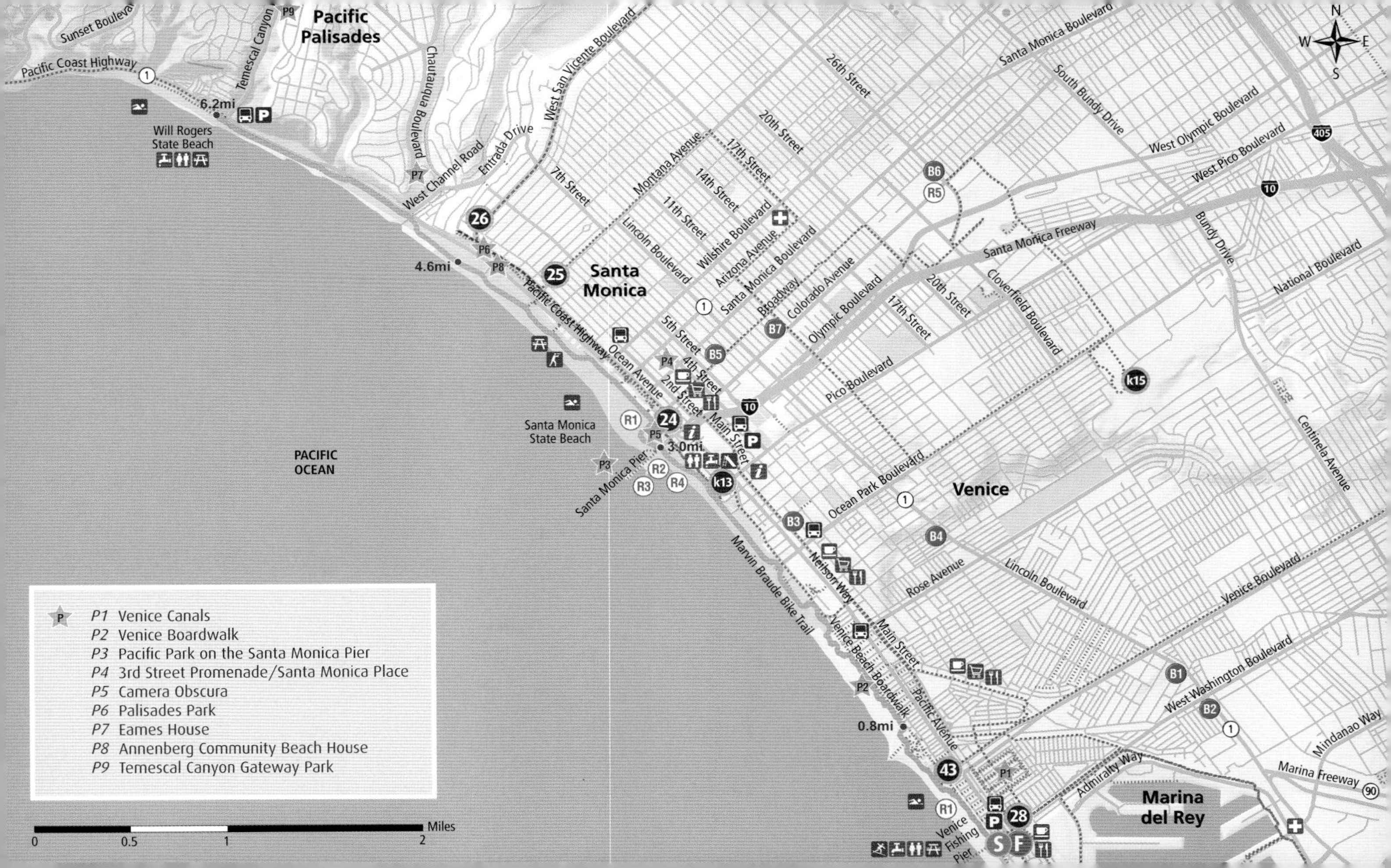
Pacific Palisades
Santa Monica
Venice
Marina del Rey
PACIFIC OCEAN
Will Rogers State Beach
Santa Monica State Beach
Santa Monica Pier
Venice Fishing Pier
Sunset Boulevard
Pacific Coast Highway
Temescal Canyon
Chautauqua Boulevard
West Channel Road
Entrada Drive
West San Vicente Boulevard
7th Street
Montana Avenue
17th Street
14th Street
11th Street
Lincoln Boulevard
Wilshire Boulevard
Arizona Avenue
Santa Monica Boulevard
Broadway
Colorado Avenue
Olympic Boulevard
5th Street
4th Street
2nd Street
Ocean Avenue
Main Street
26th Street
20th Street
South Bundy Drive
West Olympic Boulevard
West Pico Boulevard
Santa Monica Freeway
Bundy Drive
National Boulevard
Cloverfield Boulevard
Pico Boulevard
Centinela Avenue
Ocean Park Boulevard
Rose Avenue
Nielson Way
Marvin Braude Bike Trail
Venice Beach Boardwalk
Pacific Avenue
Venice Boulevard
West Washington Boulevard
Mindanao Way
Marina Freeway
Admiralty Way
6.2mi
4.6mi
3.0mi
0.8mi
P1 Venice Canals
P2 Venice Boardwalk
P3 Pacific Park on the Santa Monica Pier
P4 3rd Street Promenade/Santa Monica Place
P5 Camera Obscura
P6 Palisades Park
P7 Eames House
P8 Annenberg Community Beach House
P9 Temescal Canyon Gateway Park
0
0.5
1
2
Miles

# Marina del Rey Loop

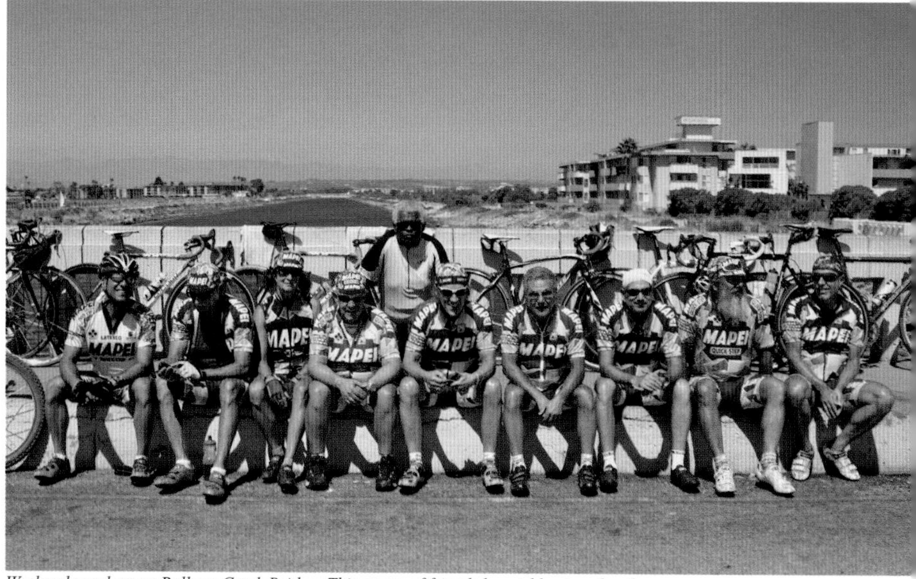


*Weekend regulars on Ballona Creek Bridge: This group of friends has ridden together for years.*

## At a Glance

**Distance** 11.0 miles **Elevation Gain** 100 feet

### Terrain

The roads and bike paths around the marina are flat and in good condition.

### Traffic

The bike path is car-free, and traffic on the ride's street sections tends to be light. Be attentive around the Venice Fishing Pier and crossing Washington Boulevard, as well as at Admiralty, Bali and Mindanao ways.

### How to Get There

To reach the ride start—the Venice Fishing Pier, at the foot of Washington Boulevard, in Marina del Rey—exit the 405 Freeway at Venice/Washington. Follow Venice west to Pacific Avenue, turn left to Washington and then, right into the pier's parking lot. Alternatively, you can look for metered or free street parking spots along Washington Boulevard.

### Food and Drink

Restaurants, ice cream parlors and coffee bars abound near the pier, in the shopping center at Admiralty and Mindanao, and in Playa del Rey just east of Del Rey Lagoon Park.

### Side Trip

For an entirely different experience of the marina, rent a kayak (Boat Rentals of America, Fisherman's Village: 310-574-2822; **www.boats4rent.com**) and paddle the calm waters of the basins and main channel. Watch for sea lions and harbor seals.

**Links to** 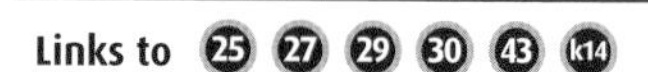


**Where to Bike Rating** 

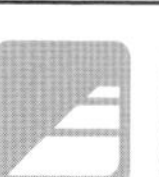

# About...

Marina del Rey's picturesque harbor cuts a rift into L.A.'s otherwise continuous stretch of coastal beaches and bike path. So, unless you can bicycle over water, you must go around this small-craft marina, built at the natural intersection of estuarial marshlands and ocean. Fortunately, this interlude from the beach is a pleasing change of scene—nautical, rather than surfside, in spirit. In summer, the temptation to linger here is heightened by such offerings as Burton Chase Park's free concerts and outdoor movies.

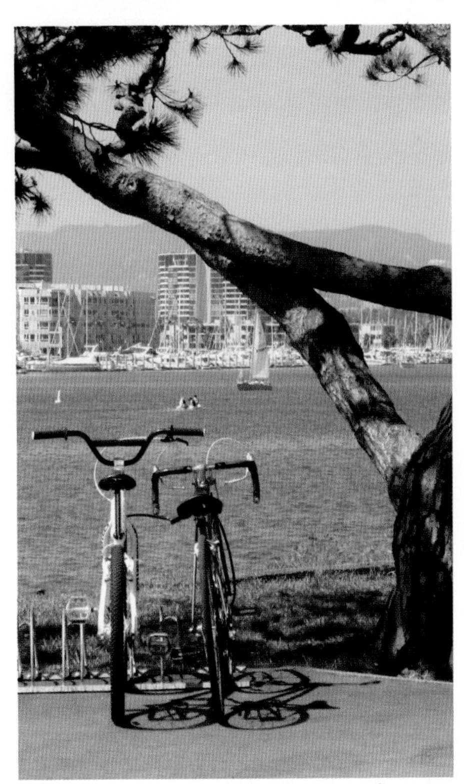

*Boats and bikes abound near the marina.*



A little more than a half century ago, the area now called Marina del Rey was a marshy ocean outlet for Ballona Creek, a wetlands estuary then known for duck hunting. In the early 1960s, after years of controversy, Los Angeles County and the United States Congress launched construction of the Marina, one of the nation's largest recreational boat harbors. In the wake of sailboats and yachts came condos, harbor-side restaurants, shops and parks. Leisurely cycling also drifted into this maritime scene.

Our ride begins from the Venice Fishing Pier, at the southern end of the Santa Monica Bike Path (Ride 27). After a short cruise through a residential area, houses to the north give way to wetlands. Here, and again on the south side of the main channel at Del Rey Lagoon Park, you'll glimpse the native character of this area: narrow tidal channels and saltwater marshes fringed in pickleweed and inhabited by many shorebird species.

After crossing a series of lanes with nautical names like Quarterdeck and Spinnaker, you'll follow the route's sweeping U-turn past Aubrey E. Austin Jr. Park, breezing past dockside streets with names alluding to Tahiti, Bora Bora and other exotic islands. Views of the main channel and harbor area unfold as you make your way around the marina, along this stretch, near Marina Mother's Beach and Burton Chase Park and, later, on the spit of land extending out toward the Ballona Creek Bridge. En route, you're likely to spot all sorts of small craft, as well as collegiate rowing teams plying the waters of the main channel and Ballona Creek.

As you continue around the marina, you'll transition onto bike lane, then the Marvin Braude Bike Trail, bisecting the grassy, tree-lined Yvonne B. Burke Park and then, back onto bike lane along Fiji Way. You'll pass dry docks, ship chandleries and the brightly multicolored "Fisherman's Village," a Hollywood take on a New England fishing hamlet. The village, accented by a faux lighthouse, has some tourist-oriented restaurants and a short harbor-side promenade. Finally following the route back onto car-free bike path, you'll reach the Ballona Creek Bridge, a crossroads with the South Bay Bike Path (Ride 29), back on the beach.

# Ride Log

**0.0** From the Venice Fishing Pier, ride east on Washington Blvd and then right onto Pacific Ave.

**1.2** Where Pacific dead-ends, make a left onto Via Marina.

**1.4** Via Marina turns to the left.

**2.5** Continue past Admiralty Way.

**2.6** Turn right onto Washington Blvd, joining the bike lane.

**3.0** Turn right onto the bike path at the stop light just before Mildred Ave.

**3.7** Cross Admiralty Way at the signal, then turn left, following the bike path around the library.

**3.9** Cross Bali Way (watch for cross traffic).

**4.1** Turn right on Mindanao Way.

**4.3** Burton W. Chace Park. For excellent views of all action in the marina, ride through the parking lot and follow the paved promenade that circles the park. Return to Mindanao Way.

**4.5** Turn right on the bike path.

**4.8** Turn right on Fiji Way, joining the bike lane.

**5.5** Follow the roundabout counterclockwise to the entry of the Marvin Braude Bike Trail.

**5.6** Turn right at the junction with the Ballona Creek Bike Path.

**6.3** Turn left and cross the Ballona Creek Bridge.

**6.4** Turn right at the end of the bridge, continuing on the South Bay Bike Path.

**6.8** Turn left off the bike path onto Trolley Place just past the restroom building (the first left after the Ballona Creek Bridge).

**6.9** Turn left at Pacific Ave.

**7.3** Continue straight onto the Ballona Creek Bridge.

**7.4** Turn right onto the Ballona Creek Bike path at the end of the bridge.

**8.0** Turn left just before the gate leading to Ballona Creek.

**8.1** Turn right onto Fiji Way, joining the bike lane.

**8.8** Turn left onto the bike path (use the left turn lane)

**9.1** Cross Mindanao Way (watch the cross traffic).

**9.3** Cross Bali Way (watch the cross traffic).

**9.4** Follow the bike path around the library, turn right and cross Admiralty Way using the crosswalk.

**10.1** Cross Washington Blvd at Mildred Ave, then turn left, joining the bike lane.

**11.0** Cross Pacific Ave and end the ride at the Venice Fishing Pier.

P

*P1* Venice Fishing Pier
*P2* Aubrey E. Austin, Jr. Park
*P3* Marina Mother's Beach
*P4* Yvonne B. Burke Park
*P5* Burton Chase Park
*P6* Fisherman's Village
*P7* Ballona Saltwater Marsh and Dunes
*P8* Del Rey Lagoon Park
*P9* Venice Canals

B

*B1* MDR Bike Company
4051 Lincoln Blvd, Marina del Rey
*B2* Helen's Cycles
2472 Lincoln Blvd, Marina del Rey

R

*R1* Perry's Café & Rentals, several locations on the Marvin Braude Bike Trail
*R2* Venice Beach Rentals
3100 Ocean Front Walk, Marina del Rey
*R3* Venice Bike & Skates
21 Washington Blvd, Marina del Rey
*R4* Daniel's Bicycle Rentals
13737 Fiji Way, Marina del Rey
*R5* Spokes N'Stuff
4200 Admiralty Way, Marina del Rey

**Marina del Rey Loop**

Altitude ft: 100, 0
Distance miles: 0, 2, 4, 6, 8, 10, 11.0

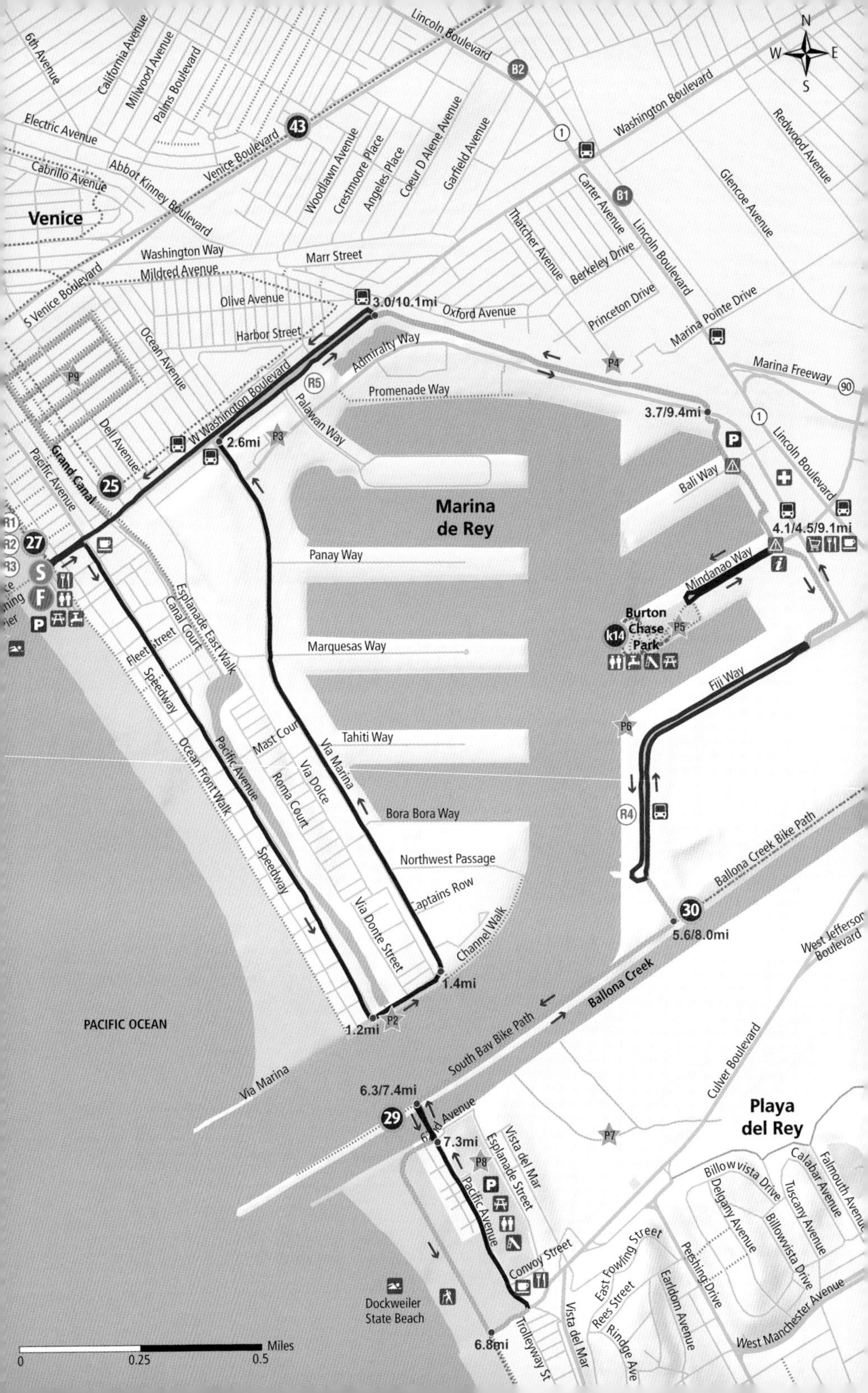

Venice
Marina de Rey
Playa del Rey
PACIFIC OCEAN
Lincoln Boulevard
Washington Boulevard
Venice Boulevard
Abbot Kinney Boulevard
Washington Way
Mildred Avenue
Marr Street
Olive Avenue
Harbor Street
Oxford Avenue
Admiralty Way
Promenade Way
Palawan Way
W Washington Boulevard
Grand Canal
Pacific Avenue
Ocean Avenue
Dell Avenue
Panay Way
Marquesas Way
Tahiti Way
Bora Bora Way
Northwest Passage
Captains Row
Channel Walk
Via Marina
Via Dolce
Mast Court
Roma Court
Via Donte Street
Esplanade East Walk
Canal Court
Fleet Street
Speedway
Ocean Front Walk
Bali Way
Mindanao Way
Burton Chase Park
Fiji Way
Ballona Creek Bike Path
Ballona Creek
South Bay Bike Path
West Jefferson Boulevard
Culver Boulevard
Marina Freeway
Marina Pointe Drive
Princeton Drive
Berkeley Drive
Thatcher Avenue
Carter Avenue
Glencoe Avenue
Redwood Avenue
Garfield Avenue
Coeur D Alene Avenue
Angeles Place
Crestmoore Place
Woodlawn Avenue
6th Avenue
California Avenue
Milwood Avenue
Palms Boulevard
Electric Avenue
Cabrillo Avenue
S Venice Boulevard
62nd Avenue
Esplanade Street
Vista del Mar
Convoy Street
Trolleyway St
East Fowling Street
Rees Street
Rindge Ave
Earldom Avenue
Pershing Drive
Delgany Avenue
Billowvista Drive
Calabar Avenue
Tuscany Avenue
Falmouth Avenue
West Manchester Avenue
Dockweiler State Beach
3.0/10.1mi
2.6mi
3.7/9.4mi
4.1/4.5/9.1mi
5.6/8.0mi
1.4mi
1.2mi
6.3/7.4mi
7.3mi
6.8mi
Miles
0
0.25
0.5
N
S
E
W

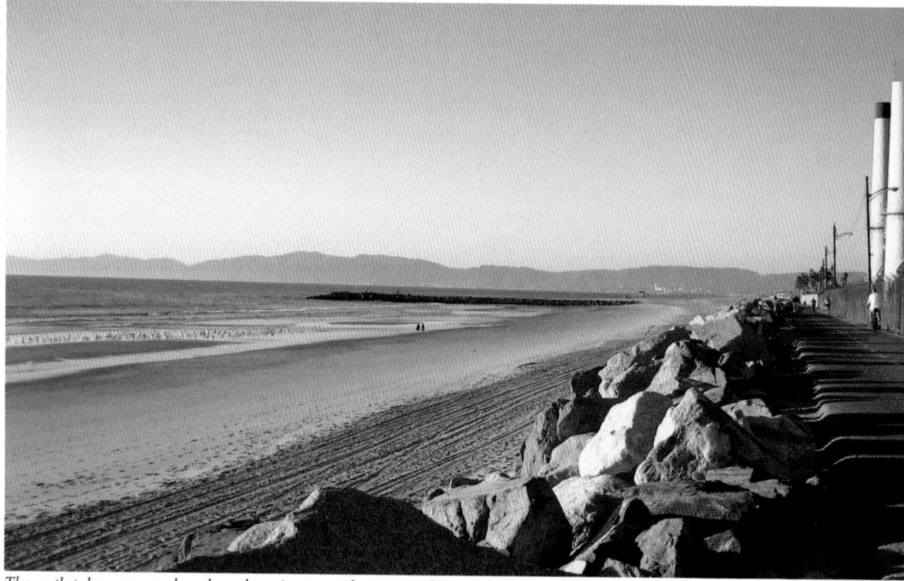

*The path takes on a rocky edge where it passes the power plant.*

## At a Glance

**Distance** 23.5 miles **Elevation Gain** 500 feet

### Terrain

This ride is flat bike path and lanes with two small climbs.

### Traffic

Following 6.9 miles of car-free bike path, the ride transitions onto a city street through Hermosa Beach. Here "sharrows"—chevrons with a bicycle symbol—indicate continuous right of way for cyclists. In Redondo Beach, the route shifts onto bike lanes, then two miles of dedicated cycling path. In these beach communities, vehicular traffic tends to be light to moderate.

### How to Get There

From the 405 Freeway, take the 90 Freeway west to Marina del Rey's Culver Boulevard exit. Turn left through Playa del Rey. Make a right on Pacific. Park on either side of this street or at the lot at its north end or at Del Rey Lagoon Park.

### Food and Drink

From ice cream parlors to restaurants, refreshment options abound, especially near the piers. Tanner's Coffee Company, on Culver Boulevard in Playa del Rey, is great for post-ride lattes, coffees and muffins.

### Side Trip

Sand Dune Park has a 100-foot-high dune you can hike up and slide down on cardboard mats. Reservations required (**www.ci.manhattan-beach.ca.us**); admission $1. (From the bike path, take Marine Avenue about 0.4 of a mile, then left on Bell Avenue to 33rd Street.)

**Links to** 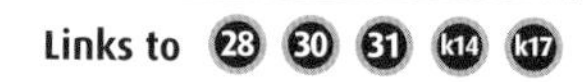


**Where to Bike Rating** 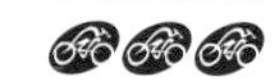

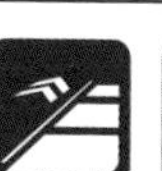
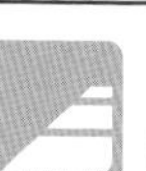
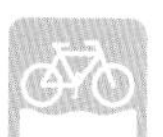

# About...

Often called the South Bay Bike Path, this is the southern leg of the Marvin Braude Bike Trail, linking Marina del Rey to the South Bay communities of Manhattan, Hermosa, Redondo and Torrance Beach. With some of the best seaside bicycling around, this route also connects three piers—at Manhattan, Hermosa and Redondo Beach, respectively—each near a hub of activity.

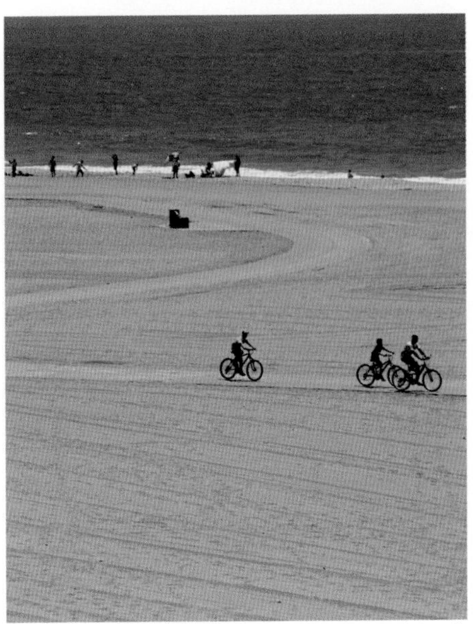

*The bike trail snakes across a wide sandy beach.*



From Ballona Creek to the Manhattan Beach Pier, this paved path snakes over the shore like a ribbon of concrete with acres of sand to either side. A quintessential Southern California beach, it's miraculously wide, fine-grained and mostly flat, accented by bright umbrellas, wet-suited surfers, sun-worshipping volleyball players and bicycles of every stripe: from candy-colored cruisers and slick racing wheels to rusty beaters. Though crowds flock here on sunny weekends, during mid-week you sometimes have the path almost to yourself. And for much of this South Bay leg of the Marvin BraudeTrail, barely a commercial venue is in sight—yet you're never far from plenty of refreshment and diversion options. Three piers punctuate the route: at Hermosa, Manhattan and Redondo Beach, respectively. (While you can't ride on them, you can walk your bicycle or lock it to a rack.)

All along the bike path, adjacent communities and piers gradually reveal their distinctive character. Beyond Playa del Rey's low-rise homes, you'll coast beneath planes taking off from LAX and then past other "big birds," at Dockweiler Beach's hang-gliding park (where you can learn to fly). Around the bend, alongside El Segundo's power-plant chimneys, the beach narrows, the bike path gains a picturesque rugged edge of boulders, and surfers or dolphins may appear in the waves. The trail continues along the Manhattan Beach Strand, lined with small, cheek-by-jowl dwellings—from faux-palazzos to glass silos and wooden beach shacks. Here, the open-air pier ends with a 1922 octagonal building, housing a café and modest aquarium (admission free).

At Hermosa Beach, the ride shifts inland a block, onto a street marked with sharrows, yielding right-of-way to cyclists. Alternatively, you could continue along the oceanfront on the popular and frequently jam-packed Hermosa Beach Strand—at posted speed of eight miles per hour. Pier Avenue, a wide pedestrian way extending inland from the pier, also offers plenty of eateries.

While Manhattan and Hermosa Beach have simple linear piers, Redondo's is multi-limbed and encrusted with restaurants, music clubs and snack stands. Just before it, the bike path passes through a parking garage. There, you must dismount and walk a few yards before breezing down the rest of the beach to mile zero of the Marvin Braude Trail—with the Palos Verdes hills rising just ahead.

*While Ride 29 has not been deemed kid-friendly in its entirety, it does include substantial sections which are entirely safe for family use.*

# Ride Log

**0.0** Start at the south end of the Ballona Creek Bridge at 62nd Ave. Turn onto the South Bay Bike Path.

**3.6** Pass the Dockweiler State Beach Hang Glider Training Park.

**6.3** Pass by Manhattan Beach Pier.

**6.9** The route changes from bike path to bike route (marked with sharrows after 26th St). Or you could continue along the beachfront on the popular and frequently jam-packed Hermosa Beach Strand, edged with restaurants, motels and beach houses by turning a right at 24th St. Rejoin the main route at Herondo St.

**8.0** Pass by Hermosa Beach Pier.

**9.4** The route transitions from bike lane to bike path where North Harbor Dr turns to the left. Continue straight on the path beginning in front of Captain Kidd's Fish Market and Restaurant.

**9.6** The bike path enters a parking garage—watch for pedestrian and automobile traffic.

**9.7** Dismount and walk past the Redondo Beach Pier.

**9.8** Remount and resume riding.

**11.7** Bike path ends at Torrance Beach. Enjoy a few minutes at the concession stand, Lifeguard Operations building, and the beach, then make a U-turn—you can't miss the 0.00 mile marker painted on the pavement—and begin the return trip north.

**13.5** Dismount and walk your bike past Redondo Beach Pier.

**14.1** Bike path ends. Cross North Harbor Dr using the crosswalk and resume the ride using the northbound bike lane.

**15.4** Pass the Hermosa Beach Pier.

**16.2** Continue straight on Hermosa Ave at 26th St. Pass the North End Bar & Grill on the right.

**16.6** Turn left on 35th St and then right onto the South Bay Bike Path at the end of Hermosa Ave.

**17.2** Pass the Manhattan Beach Pier.

**19.9** Pass Hang Glider International Airport.

**23.5** Arrive back at the Ballona Creek Bridge. End of the ride.

**Note:** For a detour from weekend crowds, turn inland at mile 6.0, onto South Marine Ave and follow this service road that roughly parallels the bike path, but closer to the bluffs. At the southern end of this 2.3-mile bypass, cut across the parking lot and re-enter the bike path.

B
*B1* Helen's Cycles
1570 Rosecrans Ave, Manhattan Beach
*B2* REI Co-Op
1800 Rosecrans Ave, Manhattan Beach
*B3* Hermosa Cyclery
20 13th St, Hermosa Beach
*B4* Ted's Manhattan Cycles
110 N. Sepulveda Blvd, Manhattan Beach
*B5* Triathlon Lab
600 N. Catalina Ave, Redondo Beach
*B6* The Old Bike Shop
430 Pier Ave, Hermosa Beach

R
*R1* Hermosa Cyclery
20 13th St., Hermosa Beach
*R2* Marina Bike Rentals
500 N. Harbor Dr., Redondo Beach

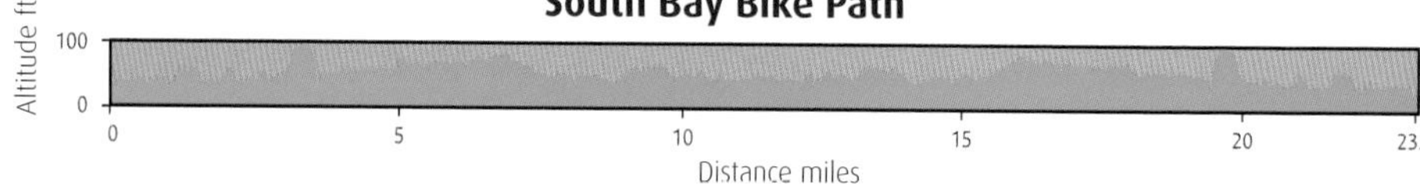

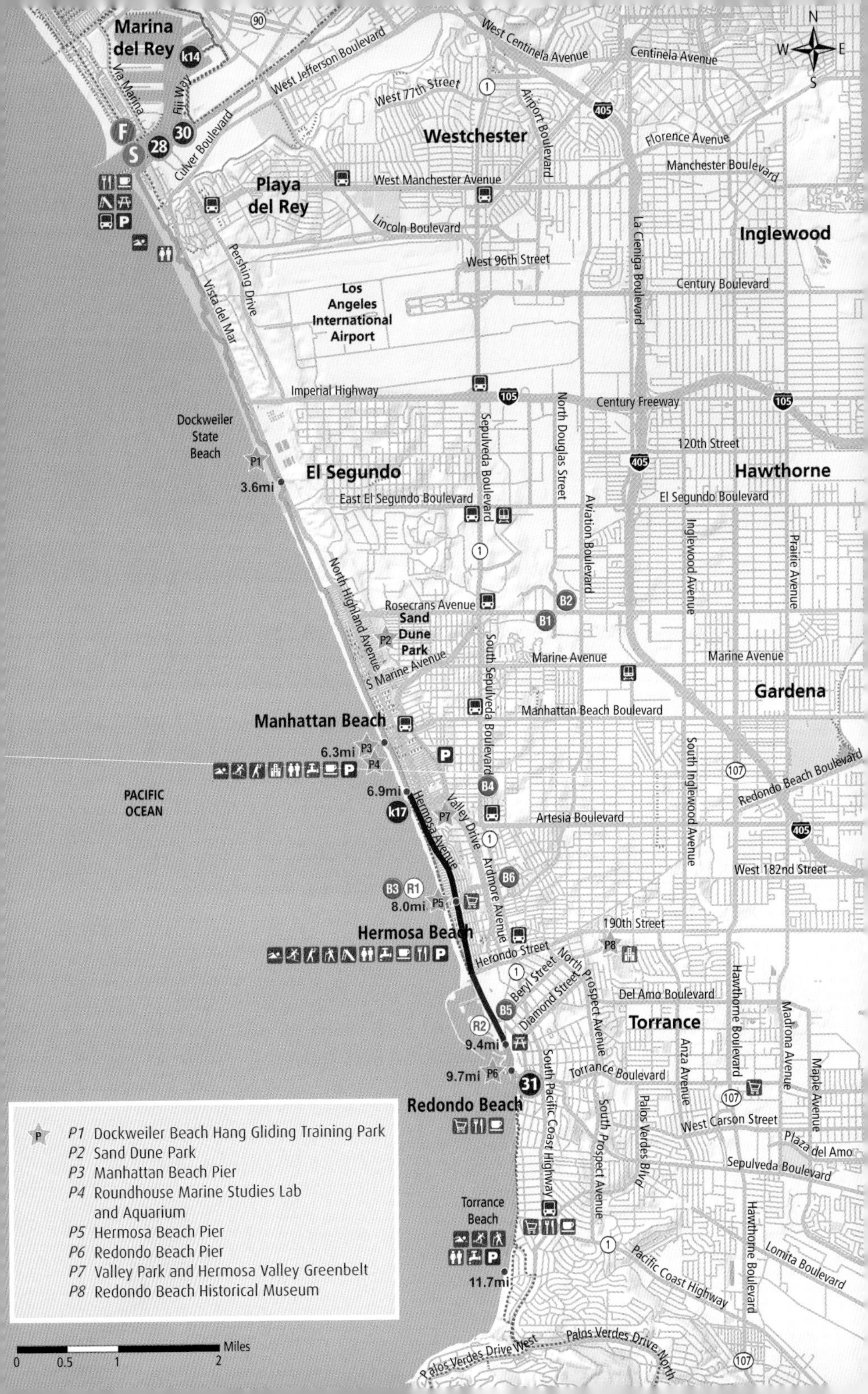

Marina del Rey
Via Marina
Fiji Way
West Jefferson Boulevard
West Centinela Avenue
Centinela Avenue
West 77th Street
Airport Boulevard
Westchester
Culver Boulevard
Florence Avenue
Manchester Boulevard
West Manchester Avenue
Playa del Rey
Lincoln Boulevard
La Cienega Boulevard
Inglewood
West 96th Street
Pershing Drive
Vista del Mar
Los Angeles International Airport
Century Boulevard
Imperial Highway
Century Freeway
North Douglas Street
Sepulveda Boulevard
Dockweiler State Beach
120th Street
El Segundo
Hawthorne
3.6mi
East El Segundo Boulevard
El Segundo Boulevard
Aviation Boulevard
Inglewood Avenue
Prairie Avenue
North Highland Avenue
Rosecrans Avenue
Sand Dune Park
S Marine Avenue
South Sepulveda Boulevard
Marine Avenue
Gardena
Manhattan Beach Boulevard
Manhattan Beach
6.3mi
South Inglewood Avenue
Redondo Beach Boulevard
PACIFIC OCEAN
6.9mi
Hermosa Avenue
Valley Drive
Artesia Boulevard
Ardmore Avenue
West 182nd Street
8.0mi
Hermosa Beach
190th Street
Herondo Street
North Prospect Avenue
Beryl Street
Diamond Street
Del Amo Boulevard
Torrance
Hawthorne Boulevard
Madrona Avenue
Anza Avenue
Maple Avenue
9.4mi
9.7mi
South Pacific Coast Highway
Torrance Boulevard
Redondo Beach
South Prospect Avenue
Palos Verdes Blvd
West Carson Street
Plaza del Amo
Sepulveda Boulevard
Torrance Beach
Lomita Boulevard
Pacific Coast Highway
11.7mi
Palos Verdes Drive West
Palos Verdes Drive North
P1 Dockweiler Beach Hang Gliding Training Park
P2 Sand Dune Park
P3 Manhattan Beach Pier
P4 Roundhouse Marine Studies Lab and Aquarium
P5 Hermosa Beach Pier
P6 Redondo Beach Pier
P7 Valley Park and Hermosa Valley Greenbelt
P8 Redondo Beach Historical Museum
Miles
0 0.5 1 2

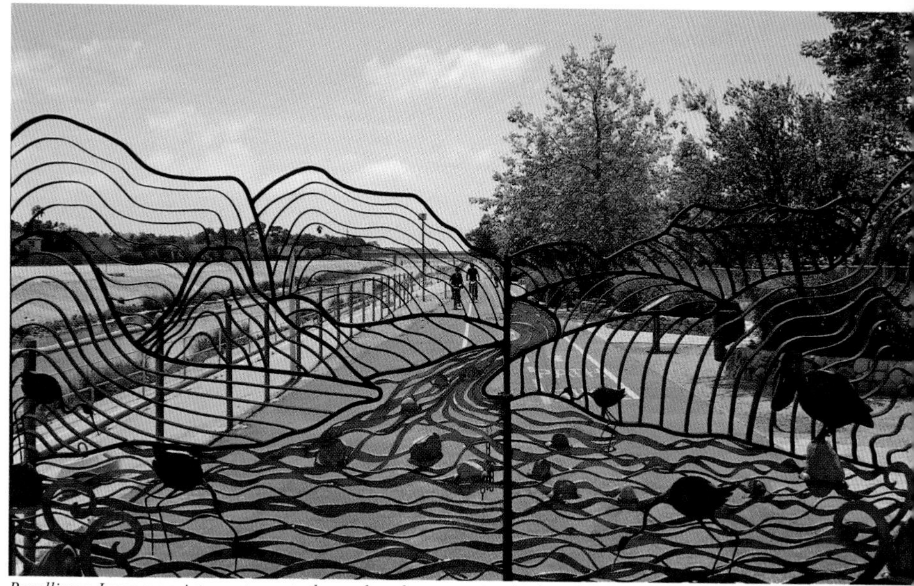
*Recalling a Japanese print, a gateway to the creek evokes mountains, birds and flowing water.*

## At a Glance

**Distance** 13.2 miles **Elevation Gain** 300 feet

### Terrain

This smooth concrete path is composed of long flat stretches, punctuated by deep dips where the bike path swoops down to cross under surface streets.

### Traffic

The creek is free of automobile traffic and street crossings.

### How to Get There

Exit the 10 Freeway at Washington/Fairfax (westbound) or Fairfax (eastbound), turn west on Washington Boulevard, then left onto Reid Avenue. Go two blocks to Syd Kronenthal Park, the ride's trailhead. Or, from Metro's Expo Line Cienega/Jefferson station, ride the bike path west about one block to Ballona Creek.

### Food and Drink

Playa del Rey refreshment choices include The Shack (famous burgers) and Tanners (coffee, lattes, muffins, cookies). In Downtown Culver City, (via Duquesne Avenue to Culver Boulevard), Tender Greens is exceptional for salads and sandwiches, with a Starbucks, Coldstone Creamery and many other options nearby.

### Side Trip

The Baldwin Hills Overlook offers panoramas of the L.A. Basin, Pacific Ocean and surrounding mountains. Hiking trails meander across the hills. Exit Ballona Creek at Duquesne Avenue and pedal south one block, then east on Jefferson to the entrance. The road up is an arduous climb, so you might lock your wheels to a bike rack at the hill's base and scale the stairs to the summit.

**Links to** 28 29 40 43 k14

**Where to Bike Rating** 

 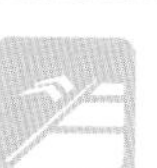 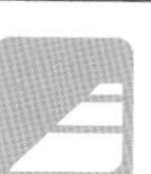 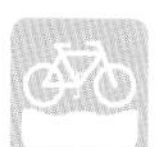

# About...

Bordering a wide storm channel, this bike path performs as a key connector within L.A., allowing cyclists to ride from inland areas to the beach communities, traversing entire neighborhoods without a single street crossing. The route—accented by occasional murals, tilework, gates and sculptures by local artists—also provides access to the re-emerging Ballona wetlands, the natural habitat of many bird and plant species. (Note: This unlit path is *not* recommended for riding after dusk.)

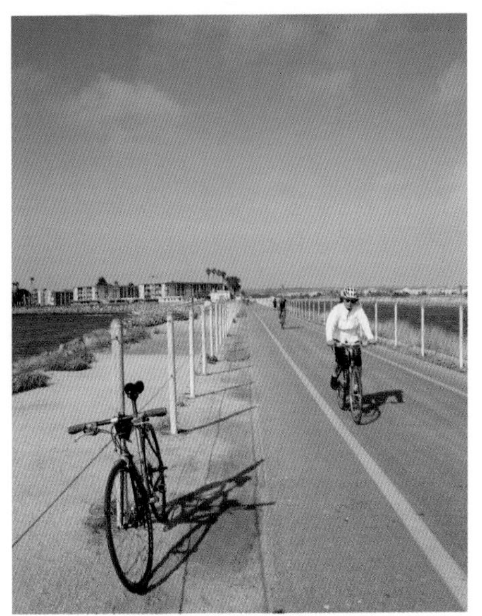

*The bikeway extends onto a spit of land between the creek and Marina del Rey's harbor.*



Ballona Creek was once a picturesque waterway with plentiful fish, birdlife and fertile banks with sycamores, willows, tules and even wild watercress. But its tendency to flood during storms ultimately prompted the Army Corps of Engineers to muscle it into submission in the 1930s, transforming its silt-rich streambed into a broad concrete channel, much the way the Corps changed the Los Angeles and San Gabriel rivers in the same era. The creek—sometimes flowing abundantly; sometimes virtually dry for long stretches—is still part of an essential watershed, directing rain flow from the Hollywood Hills to the ocean.

Though only seven miles long, the Ballona path provides a crucial bicycling conduit between inland and the coast. Without encountering any cars, you can ride this path from Culver City to Playa del Rey, before turning onto the Marvin Braude Bike Trail to Marina del Rey, Venice and Santa Monica to the north (Ride 26), or Manhattan, Hermosa and Redondo beaches to the south (Ride 28). Bike lanes on Venice Boulevard are a short distance away. The network will expand dramatically when the Metro's Expo Line and its bordering bike route open in 2012. You'll be able to pedal a continuous route from the downtown area—or hop the train from there—to this ride's Culver City trailhead.

The future also looks brighter for the creek's native landscapes and habitats. After years of contention between developers and environmentalists, hundreds of acres of Ballona Creek wetlands and open space are gradually being reclaimed. While the waterway's eastern end skirts industrial and residential areas, the western end, nearing the ocean, will offer access to the wetlands, its fresh and saltwater ecosystems. Some 300 bird species have been sighted here in recent times, including the Great Blue Heron, California Killifish, Snowy Egret and Belding's Savannah Sparrow. Ballona Qallflowers, Southern Tarplants, Lewis' Primroses and Orcutt's Yellow Pincushions are among the native plant species making their return. As you pedal along, you may also pass UCLA's crew teams, plying the waters where native Tongva tribes once fished and paddled. On approach to the Ballona Creek Bridge, the path extends onto a narrow a spit of land between the billowing sailboats in Marina del Rey's harbor and the creek itself, flowing into the ocean.

# Ride Log

P *P1* Hayden Tract
*P2* Kenneth Hahn State Recreation Area
*P3* Baldwin Hills Scenic Overlook
*P4* Bill Botts Field
*P5* Museum of Jurassic Technology
*P6* Sony Pictures Studios
*P7* The Culver Studios
*P8* Culver Ice Rink
*P9* Ballona Wetlands Freshwater Marsh
*P10* Ballona Saltwater Marsh and Dunes

B *B1* Palms Cycle
3770 Motor Ave, Culver City
*B2* Chubby's Cruisers
5431 Sepulveda Blvd, Culver City
*B3* Wheel World Cycles
4051 Sepulveda Blvd, Culver City
*B4* Abba Padre Bikes and Books
4219 Sepulveda Blvd, Culver City
*B5* MDR Bike Company
4051 Lincoln Blvd, Marina del Rey
R *R1* Daniel's Bicycle Rentals
13737 Fiji Way, Marina del Rey

*Springtime wildflowers bloom along the creek.*

**0.0** This ride begins at the southeastern corner of Sy Kronenthal Park, past the baseball diamonds, under th Expo light rail line. If you are coming from an Exp Line station, you'll enter the park from National Blvd Make a U-turn at the bottom of the ramp where th path starts in earnest.

**1.1** Cross under Duquesne Ave (alternate entrance/exi point).

**2.0** Cross under Overland Ave (alternate entrance/exi point).

**2.6** Cross under Sepulveda Blvd (alternate entrance exit point).

**2.9** Cross under Sawtelle Blvd (alternate entrance/exi point).

**3.6** Cross under Inglewood Blvd (alternate entrance exit point).

**3.9** Cross under Centinela Ave (alternate entrance/exi point).

**5.1** Cross under Lincoln and Culver boulevards (alternate entrance/exit point).

**6.0** Join the Marvin Braude/South Bay Bike Trail Continue straight.

**6.6** Turn left onto the Ballona Creek Bridge. From her you can join the South Bay bike path (cross the bridg and then turn left, following the signs). Turn arounc and ride the same route back to the park or Metro.

**13.2** End of ride.

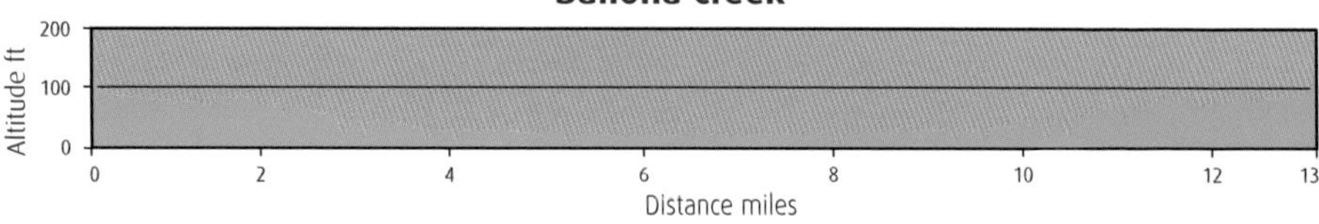

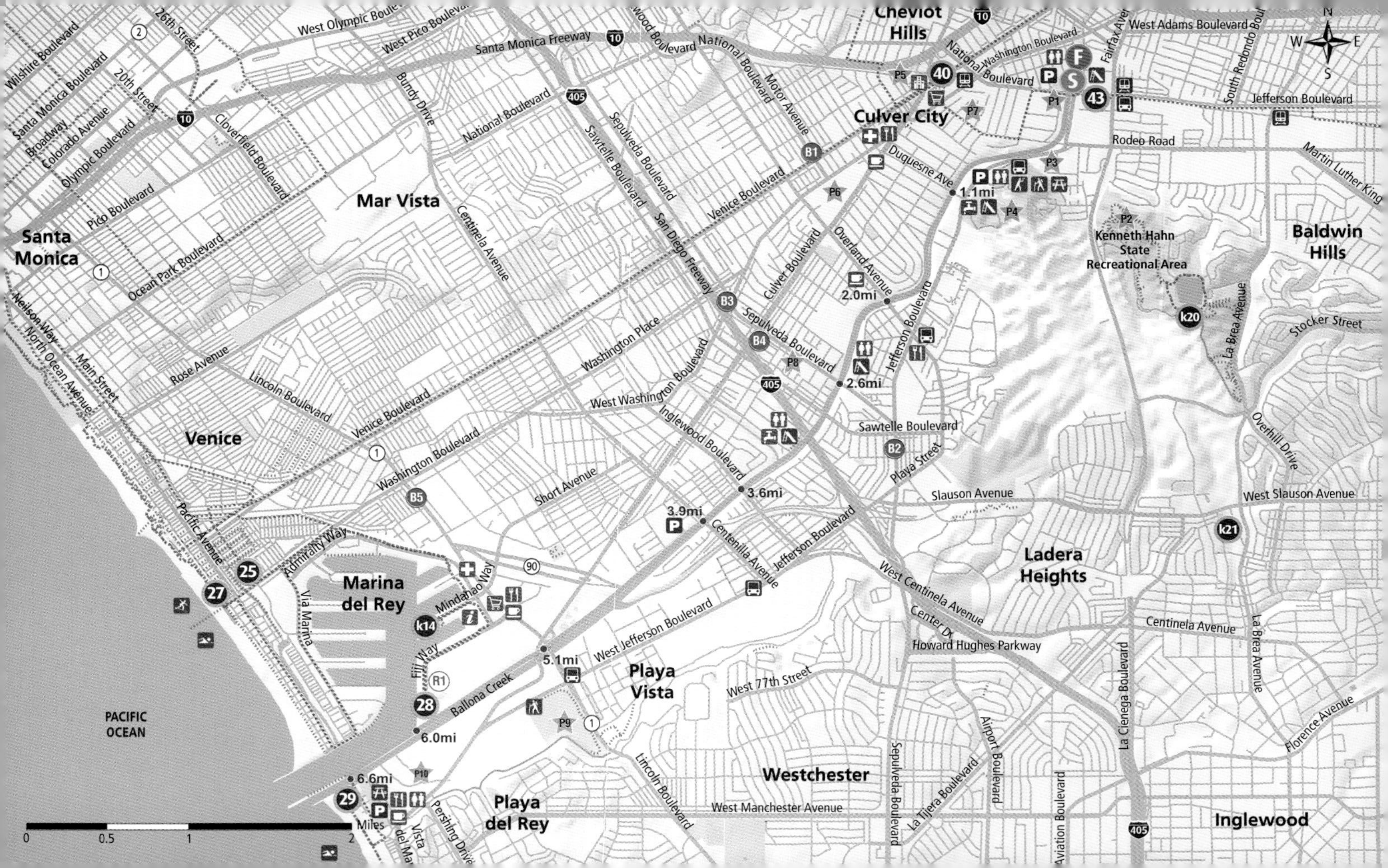
Cheviot Hills
Culver City
Baldwin Hills
Kenneth Hahn State Recreational Area
Santa Monica
Mar Vista
Venice
Marina del Rey
Playa Vista
Ladera Heights
Westchester
Playa del Rey
Inglewood
PACIFIC OCEAN
Wilshire Boulevard
Santa Monica Boulevard
Broadway
Colorado Avenue
Olympic Boulevard
Pico Boulevard
26th Street
20th Street
West Olympic Boulevard
West Pico Boulevard
Santa Monica Freeway
Cloverfield Boulevard
Bundy Drive
National Boulevard
Ocean Park Boulevard
Centinela Avenue
Sawtelle Boulevard
Sepulveda Boulevard
San Diego Freeway
Venice Boulevard
Motor Avenue
Washington Boulevard
Fairfax Ave
West Adams Boulevard
South Redondo Boulevard
Jefferson Boulevard
Rodeo Road
Martin Luther King
Duquesne Ave
Overland Avenue
Culver Boulevard
Stocker Street
La Brea Avenue
Overhill Drive
Slauson Avenue
West Slauson Avenue
Neilson Way
North Ocean Avenue
Main Street
Rose Avenue
Lincoln Boulevard
Washington Place
West Washington Boulevard
Inglewood Boulevard
Short Avenue
Playa Street
Centenilla Avenue
Pacific Avenue
Admiralty Way
Via Marina
Mindanao Way
Fiji Way
West Jefferson Boulevard
Ballona Creek
West Centinela Avenue
Center Dr
Howard Hughes Parkway
West 77th Street
Airport Boulevard
La Tijera Boulevard
La Cienega Boulevard
Aviation Boulevard
Florence Avenue
West Manchester Avenue
Pershing Drive
Vista del Mar
1.1mi
2.0mi
2.6mi
3.6mi
3.9mi
5.1mi
6.0mi
6.6mi
0
0.5
1
2
Miles
N
S
E
W

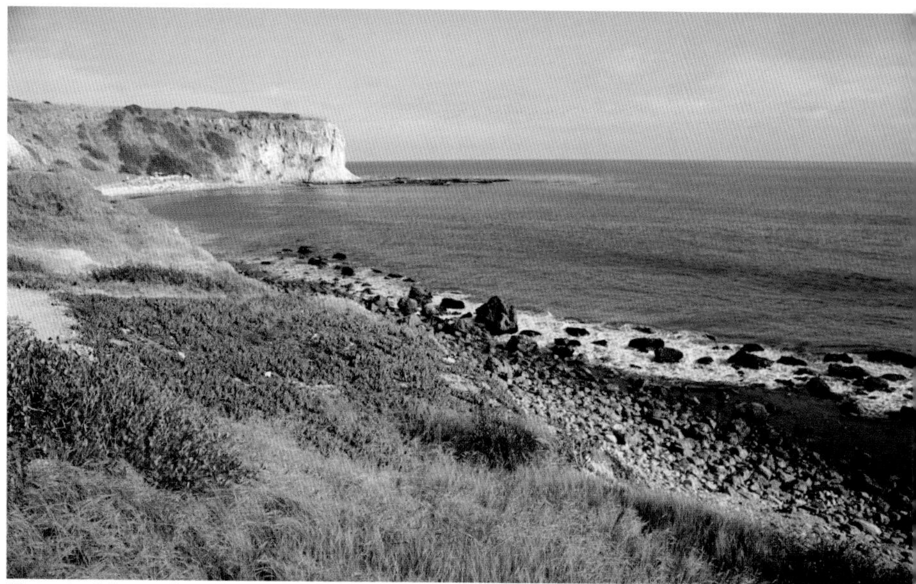

*The peninsula's rugged coastline curves at Abalone Cove.*

## At a Glance

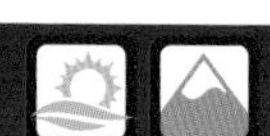

**Distance** 27.1 miles **Elevation Gain** 2,300 feet

### Terrain

The Donut combines rolling hills with a single sustained ascent. Road surfaces are average, although constant tectonic activity periodically roughens Palos Verdes Drive South at Portuguese Bend.

### Traffic

Bike lanes and routes form most of the loop, except on Palos Verdes Drive East, which has a paved shoulder nearly as wide as a traditional bike lane.

### How to Get There

From Pacific Coast Highway, turn on Pearl Street toward the ocean. Cross South Catalina Avenue to Veterans Park. The parking lot has coin meters, so bring enough quarters for at least three hours. More parking is at the Redondo Beach Pier.

### Food and Drink

Food stops are sprinkled across The Donut, at Malaga Cove Plaza, Golden Cove, Miraleste Plaza and Kelly's Korner. The unofficial après-ride hangout for locals is Catalina Coffee Company (four blocks north of Veterans Park on South Catalina Avenue) with excellent sandwiches, aromatic coffee drinks, fresh-baked muffins and brownies.

### Side Trip

For a refreshing breather, consider hiking one of the coastal trails between Malaga and Abalone coves, meandering through diverse ecosystems, among seasonal wildflowers or tidal pools with sea urchins and starfish.

**Links to** 

**Where to Bike Rating** 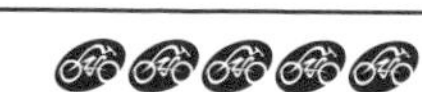

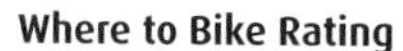

# About...

The Donut is an outstanding ride, a virtual institution among L.A. cyclists. It encircles the Palos Verdes Peninsula—on a clear day unfolding panoramic coastal views from Santa Monica to Orange County, taking in Catalina Island, the ports of Los Angeles and Long Beach and Downtown's skyline. Beyond this feast of amazing scenery, the ride is a great work-out with rolling, semi-rural terrain linking its five featured climbs and breezy downhill runs.

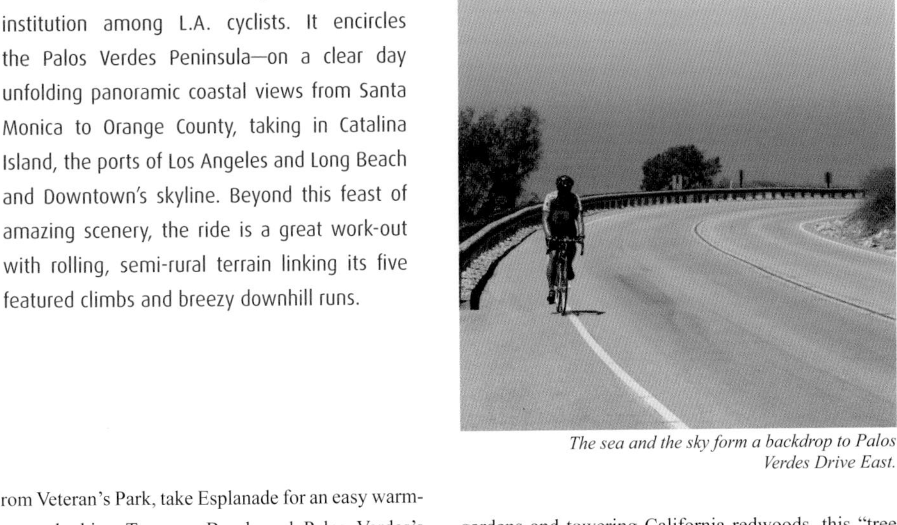

*The sea and the sky form a backdrop to Palos Verdes Drive East.*



From Veteran's Park, take Esplanade for an easy warm-up overlooking Torrance Beach and Palos Verdes's northern tip. Dolphins often share the ocean with swimmers and surfers, so keep watch. After a short, fairly steep climb to the first summit, turn right onto Palos Verdes Boulevard. Then veer right, descending through the traffic Y, past Malaga Cove Plaza (with its Market & Deli, a favorite cyclist rendez-vous spot).

Continue south along the coast, cresting the second summit. Take a right onto Paso Del Mar with its stunning views of Bluff Cove and, later, Lunada Bay. In 1961, the Greek freighter *Dominator* ran aground in this bay, leaving rusted skeletal remains, visible on the rocks at low tide. Where Paso Lunado intersects Palos Verdes Drive West, turn right and continue south. The classic white 1926 Point Vicente Lighthouse appears on the road's seaward side. The adjacent Point Vicente Interpretive Center focuses on the peninsula's natural and cultural history. Along this entire coastline, the bluffs provide excellent observation perches during the Pacific gray whales' December and April migration.

About two miles further along, on the hill opposite Abalone Cove, you'll see the Wayfarers Chapel, designed by Frank Lloyd Wright's son, Lloyd. Amid gardens and towering California redwoods, this "tree chapel" is a light-filtering arbor rendered in glass and redwood. Sometimes a wedding site for movies and Hollywood celebrities, it also offers a tranquil meditative spot within the spectacular coastal landscape.

The course turns inland at Palos Verdes Drive East and begins the famed switchbacks, yielding superb coastline and Peninsula views at the turns.

From the third summit, at Marymount College, the route snakes generally downhill, except for one short climb. As you take in the vistas along this winding descent, be prepared for a couple of sharp U-turns en route. At the bottom, turn left onto Palos Verdes Drive North, a lush tree-lined street through residential neighborhoods on the way back to the coast at Malaga Cove. A short ride through upper Redondo to Torrance Beach, a brief warm-down along Esplanade, and The Donut is done.

*Note: The Donut is best ridden counter-clockwise—a direction blessed with superior bike lanes and coastal vantage points.*

# Ride Log

**0.0** The Donut begins at Veteran's Park near the corner of Esplanade and South Catalina Ave. Turn right onto Esplanade.

**1.5** Turn right on Paseo De La Playa. Start the first climb.

**2.2** First summit.

**2.3** Turn right on Palos Verdes Blvd (Becomes Palos Verdes Dr North/Granvia La Costa).

**2.6** Stay to the right at the Y, where Palos Verdes Blvd joins Palos Verdes Dr West. Be especially attentive to southbound automobile traffic through this intersection.

**2.8** Malaga Cove Plaza is on the left.

**2.9** Start the second climb.

**4.0** Second summit.

**4.5** Turn right on Paseo Del Mar.

**6.5** Paseo Del Mar becomes Paseo Lunado.

**6.6** Turn right on Palos Verdes Dr West.

**8.0** Hawthorne Blvd and Golden Cove Shopping Center.

**8.5** Point Vicente Lighthouse and Interpretive Center.

**8.6** Palos Verdes Dr West becomes Palos Verdes Dr South.

**8.9** Observation point.

**10.3** Abalone Cove Shoreline Park.

**10.4** Wayfarers Chapel.

**10.6** Historic Tuscan-style gatehouse to the old Vanderlip estate and start of Portuguese Bend. Be extra attentive to rough road conditions for the next mile.

**12.4** Marilyn Ryan Sunset Point Park.

**13.2** Turn left onto Palos Verdes Dr East. Watch the cross-traffic when making this turn. Start the third climb up the famous switchbacks.

B *B1* Bill Ron's Bicycles
807 Torrance Blvd, Redondo Beach
*B2* Corbins Redondo Bicycle
607 South Pacific Hwy, Redondo Beach
*B3* Sprocket Cycles
1408 South Pacific Hwy, Redondo Beach
*B4* Triathlon Lab
600 N. Catalina Ave, Redondo Beach
*B5* Palos Verdes Bicycle Center,
Corner Hawthorne & Silver Spur Rd,
Rolling Hills Estates

R *R1* Palos Verdes Bicycle Center
Corner Hawthorne & Silver Spur Rd,
Rolling Hills Estates

**14.4** Scenic overlook. You may want to stop here and take in the view of the Pacific Ocean, the coast as far as you can see and Catalina Island. Take extra care when crossing to the overlook.

**15.1** Third summit and Marymount College.

**16.6** Miraleste Plaza. Begin the fourth climb.

**17.4** Fourth summit.

**19.7** Turn left on Palos Verdes Dr North and start the fifth climb.

**20.8** Kelly's Korner at Palos Verdes Dr North and Rolling Hills Rd.

**22.1** Fifth summit.

**24.3** Stay to the right at the Y where Palos Verdes Dr North/Granvia La Costa joins Palos Verdes Blvd.

**25.2** Turn left at Calle Miramar (second signal—use crosswalk if traffic is too crazy).

**25.6** Follow the right side of the roundabout to Esplanade.

**27.1** Left at Harbor Dr into the Veterans Park.

## The Donut: Palos Verdes Peninsula

*Please note: the profile for Ride 31 is depicted in 250ft vertical increments due to unusually high elevation.*

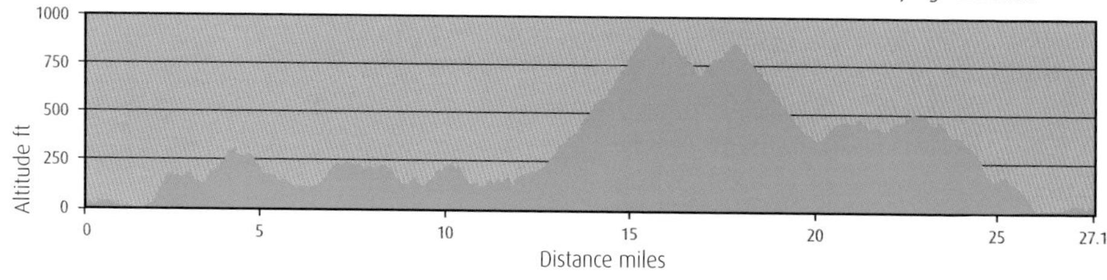

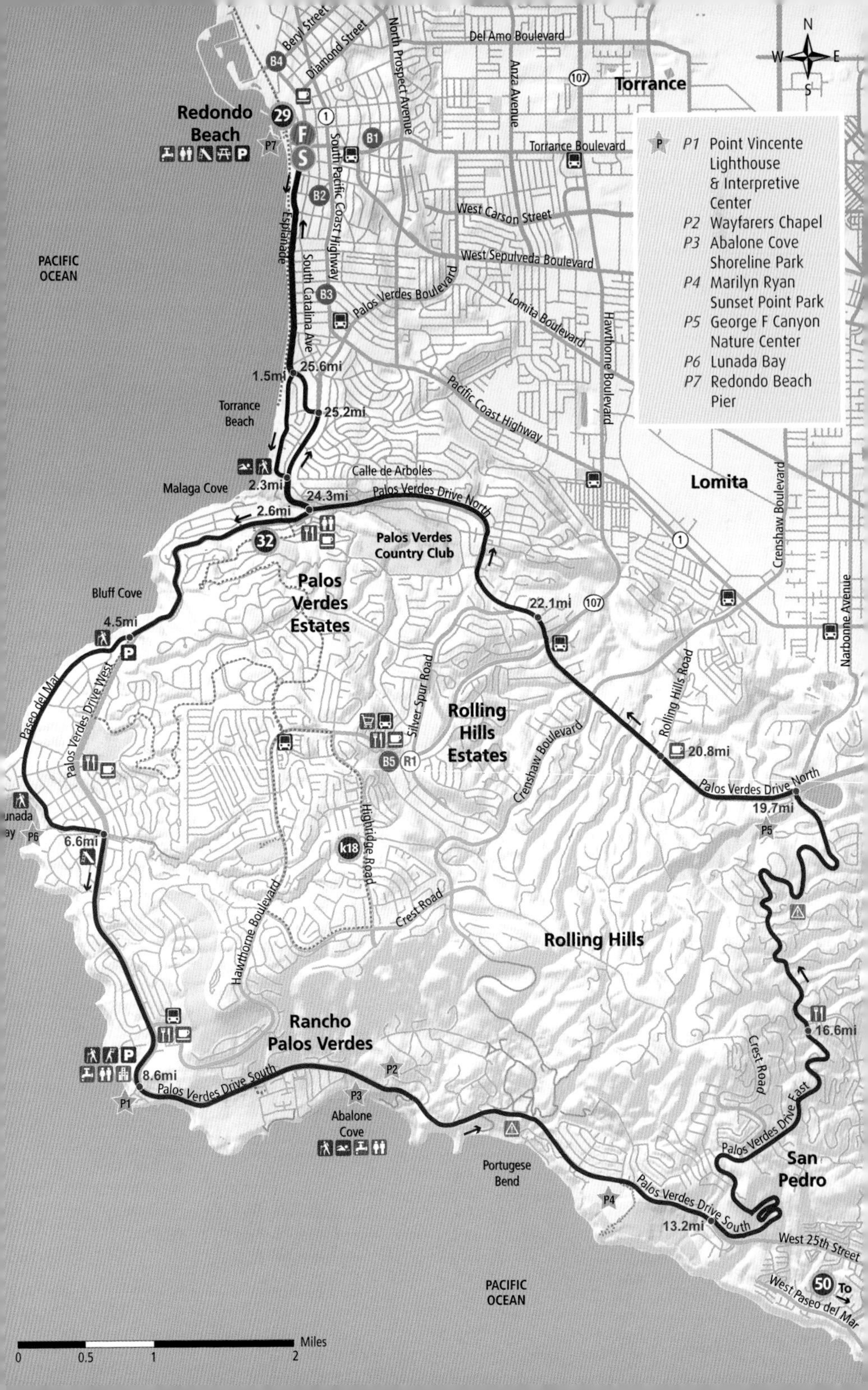

Beryl Street
Diamond Street
North Prospect Avenue
Del Amo Boulevard
Anza Avenue
107
Torrance
N
W
E
S
Redondo Beach
29
F
S
1
B4
B1
B2
B3
P7
South Pacific Coast Highway
Torrance Boulevard
P1 Point Vincente Lighthouse & Interpretive Center
P2 Wayfarers Chapel
P3 Abalone Cove Shoreline Park
P4 Marilyn Ryan Sunset Point Park
P5 George F Canyon Nature Center
P6 Lunada Bay
P7 Redondo Beach Pier
West Carson Street
Esplanade
South Catalina Ave
West Sepulveda Boulevard
PACIFIC OCEAN
Palos Verdes Boulevard
Lomita Boulevard
Hawthorne Boulevard
Pacific Coast Highway
1.5mi
25.6mi
25.2mi
Torrance Beach
Malaga Cove
2.3mi
Calle de Arboles
24.3mi
Palos Verdes Drive North
Lomita
Crenshaw Boulevard
2.6mi
32
Palos Verdes Country Club
Palos Verdes Estates
Bluff Cove
4.5mi
22.1mi
107
Narbonne Avenue
Paseo del Mar
Palos Verdes Drive West
Silver Spur Road
Rolling Hills Estates
Rolling Hills Road
Crenshaw Boulevard
20.8mi
B5
R1
Palos Verdes Drive North
19.7mi
P5
Lunada Bay
P6
6.6mi
Hightide Road
k18
Crest Road
Rolling Hills
Hawthorne Boulevard
16.6mi
Rancho Palos Verdes
P2
Crest Road
8.6mi
Palos Verdes Drive South
P1
P3
Abalone Cove
Palos Verdes Drive East
Portugese Bend
San Pedro
P4
Palos Verdes Drive South
13.2mi
West 25th Street
PACIFIC OCEAN
50
To
West Paseo del Mar
Miles
0
0.5
1
2

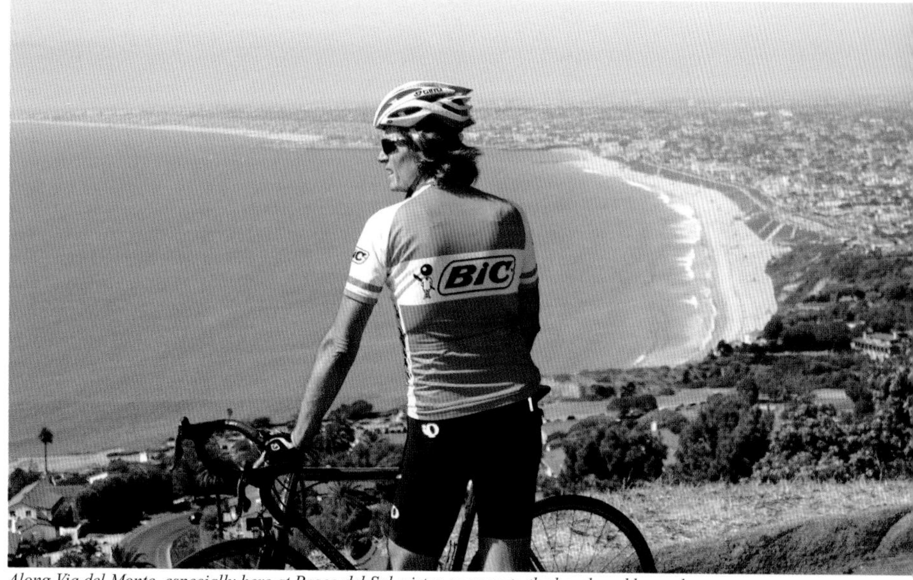


*Along Via del Monte, especially here at Paseo del Sol, vistas open up to the beach and beyond.*

## At a Glance

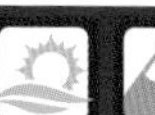
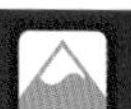

**Distance** 13.0 miles **Elevation Gain** 1,400 feet

### Terrain

The road quality is good, with typical Palos Verdes (P.V.) topography: rolling coastal bluffs, gradual sustained climbs and fast downhills.

### Traffic

Palos Verdes Drive West and Hawthorne Boulevard have generous bike lanes and typically moderate traffic. Higher up, the residential neighborhoods have wide streets and light traffic.

### How to Get There

Exit the 405 Freeway onto Artesia Boulevard and drive west. Turn left onto Pacific Coast Highway, then right onto Palos Verdes Boulevard. At the Y, merge right onto Palos Verdes Drive West. Continue south about two miles to Paseo Del Mar, where you'll find free parking.

### Food and Drink

Malaga Cove Ranch Market and the Yellow Vase, both in Malaga Cove Plaza, serve coffee, pastries and more. Higher up, where Hawthorne meets Granvia Altamira, is a Valero gas-station convenience store.

### Side Trip

Point Vicente Interpretive Center, on Palos Verdes Drive West, three and one-half miles south of Paseo Del Mar, features exhibitions on the Peninsula's natural and cultural history. Set on coastal bluffs beside an iconic lighthouse, the center is also an excellent whale-watching site (December to April). Open daily.

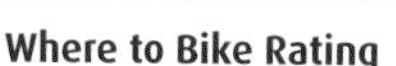
**Links to** 31 k18

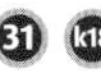

**Where to Bike Rating** 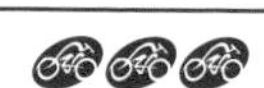

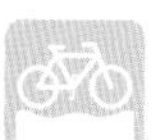

# About...

The ride we've named The Double Donut Holes is the little brother of The Donut (Ride 31). The "holes" nests within that classic, longer, more climb-intensive loop—hence the names. Yielding spectacular views, this journey ascends from Malaga Cove, winding through upscale residential neighborhoods to a high point on the Palos Verdes Peninsula. As short rides go, it offers plenty of opportunity for variation: two possible routes up, two ways back down and the option to continue on to a second loop.

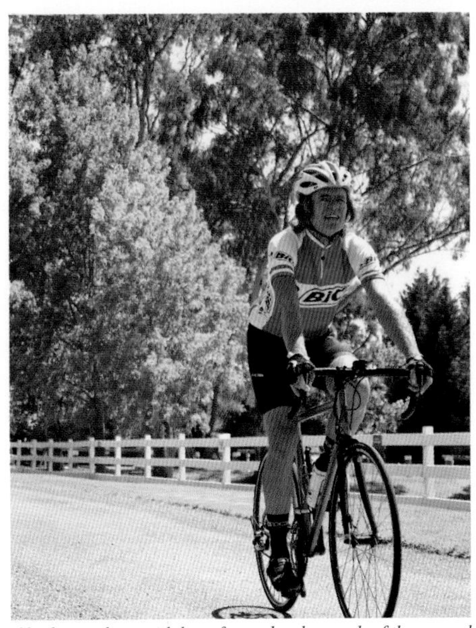

*Shady meadows with long fences border much of the second loop, or donut hole.*



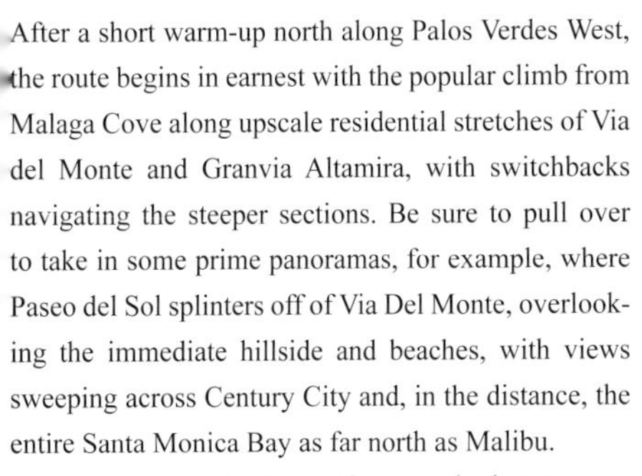

After a short warm-up north along Palos Verdes West, the route begins in earnest with the popular climb from Malaga Cove along upscale residential stretches of Via del Monte and Granvia Altamira, with switchbacks navigating the steeper sections. Be sure to pull over to take in some prime panoramas, for example, where Paseo del Sol splinters off of Via Del Monte, overlooking the immediate hillside and beaches, with views sweeping across Century City and, in the distance, the entire Santa Monica Bay as far north as Malibu.

The elegance of a loop, of course, is that you can attack it from either direction. So, too, with The Holes. If you choose, instead, to ride the first "hole" counterclockwise, here's the progression: After a short warm-up southward on Palos Verdes Drive West, your climb will be slightly longer yet more gradual, rising from the coast along Via Coronel and snaking up through lightly trafficked suburbs on P.V.'s Pacific Ocean side. Though not as spectacular as the steeper Granvia Altamira ascent, the route in this direction offers some unexpected vistas (for instance, from the first switchback, you'll see the entire length of Catalina Island).

Whichever way you reach it, the highest point of this loop is the intersection of Granvia Altamira and Hawthorne Boulevard. From here, you can continue on to the second "hole," which, despite its decidedly more inland feel and moderate climbs, actually reaches the highest traversable part of the peninsula. The payoff: occasional stunning glimpses of the distant San Gabriel Mountains and Downtown L.A. From Hawthorne, as you turn onto Highridge, make sure you pull into the Day Adventist church's parking area for spectacular vistas. A little further along, take a quick detour (a couple hundred feet) to the left on Crestridge Road, just before Highridge Park, for views of Downtown. After arriving back at Hawthorne and Granvia Altamira, you can return along Via Coronel or down the Granvia Altamira-Via Del Monte route.

The Double Donut Holes gives you a good taste of the Palos Verdes Peninsula, even if you're not quite in the mood to wolf down the entire Donut, that more demanding classic P.V. classic. At the end, you can wash it all down with a real cup o' java or a steaming latte back at Malaga Cove.

# Ride Log

## The First Donut Hole

**0.0** Exit the parking lot, and turn onto Paseo Del Mar for a very short distance, cross the south-bound lane of Palos Verdes Dr West and turn left joining the bike lane. Watch the cross traffic through both turns.

**1.7** Turn right onto Via Corta at the stop sign. Malaga Cove Plaza is on the left.

**1.8** Turn right onto Via Del Monte.

**3.0** Pass Paseo Del Sol for spectacular vistas of Santa Monica Bay.

**3.7** Turn right onto Granvia Altamira at the stop sign.

**5.0** Arrive at the top of the first donut hole. The Valero gas station and 7-Eleven convenience store have cold drinks, plus snacks. The gas station also has a few utilitarian outdoor tables and chairs.

## The Second Donut Hole

**5.0** Turn left onto Hawthorne Blvd, joining the bike lane.

**5.3** Turn right onto Highridge Rd, joining the bike lane.

**6.3** Pass Highridge Park where you'll find restrooms and a drinking fountain.

**6.8** Turn right onto Crest Rd.

**7.8** Turn right onto Hawthorne Blvd, joining the bike lane.

## Return on Granvia Altamira and Via Del Monte

**9.1** Turn left onto Granvia Altamira. Use the crosswalk if traffic conditions warrant.

**10.3** Turn right onto Via Fernandez/Montemalaga Dr at the stop sign.

**10.4** Turn left onto Via Del Monte at the stop sign.

**12.3** Turn left onto Via Corta at the stop sign. Malaga Cove Plaza is on the right.

**12.4** Turn left onto Palos Verdes Dr West.

**14.0** Arrive back at the parking area on Paseo Del Mar.

## Return on Via Coronel

**9.1** Turn left onto Granvia Altamira. Use the crosswalk if traffic conditions warrant.

**9.4** Turn left onto Via Coronel at Coronel Plaza.

**9.5** Turn right onto Via Vargarita for a short distance, then left onto Via Coronel.

**10.0** Cross Paseo La Cresta.

**12.3** Turn right onto Palos Verdes Dr West, joining the bike lane.

**13.0** Arrive back at the parking area on Paseo Del Mar.

*P1* Malaga Cove Plaza Shopping Center
*P2* Highridge Park
*P3* Fred Hesse Jr. Community Park
*P4* Point Vicente Interpretive Center & Lighthouse
*P5* Lunada Bay Plaza

**Double Donut Holes: Palos Verdes Peninsula** - Returning on Via Coronel

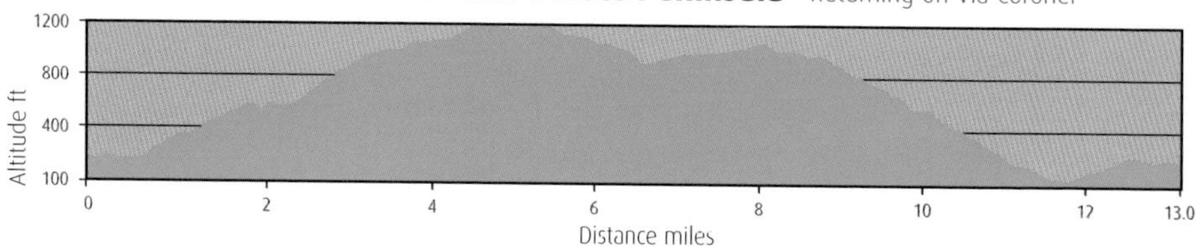

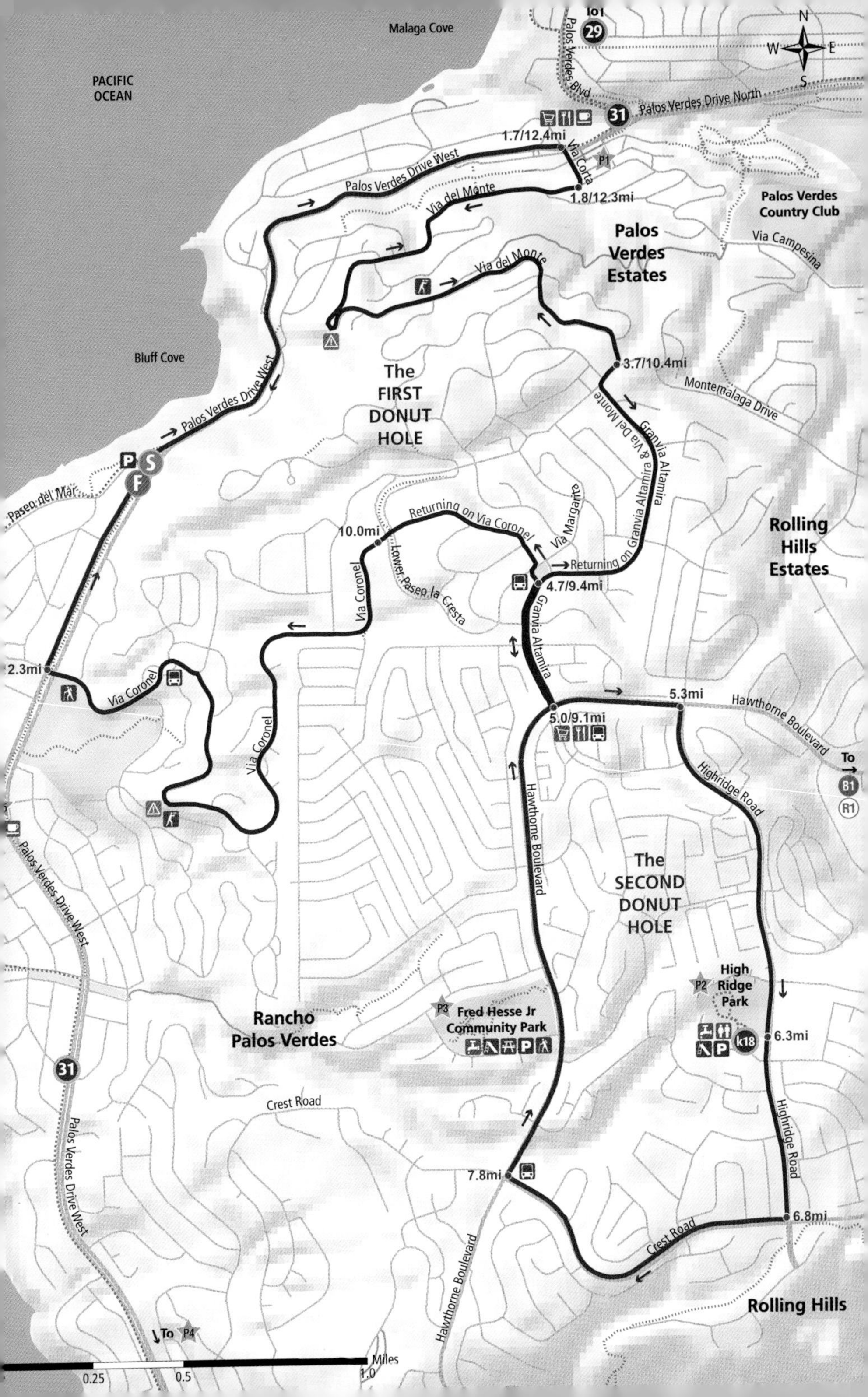

Malaga Cove
PACIFIC OCEAN
Palos Verdes Blvd
Palos Verdes Drive North
1.7/12.4mi
Via Corta
P1
Palos Verdes Drive West
Via del Monte
1.8/12.3mi
Palos Verdes Country Club
Palos Verdes Estates
Via Campesina
Via del Monte
Bluff Cove
3.7/10.4mi
The FIRST DONUT HOLE
Montemalaga Drive
Palos Verdes Drive West
Granvia Altamira & Via Del Monte
Paseo del Mar
Via Margarita
Returning on Via Coronel
10.0mi
Returning on Granvia Altamira
Rolling Hills Estates
Lower Paseo la Cresta
4.7/9.4mi
Via Coronel
Granvia Altamira
2.3mi
Via Coronel
5.3mi
Hawthorne Boulevard
5.0/9.1mi
Via Coronel
To B1 R1
Highridge Road
Hawthorne Boulevard
Palos Verdes Drive West
The SECOND DONUT HOLE
High Ridge Park
P2
P3
Fred Hesse Jr Community Park
Rancho Palos Verdes
6.3mi
k18
31
Crest Road
Highridge Road
Palos Verdes Drive West
7.8mi
6.8mi
Crest Road
Hawthorne Boulevard
Rolling Hills
To P4
Miles
0.25
0.5
1.0

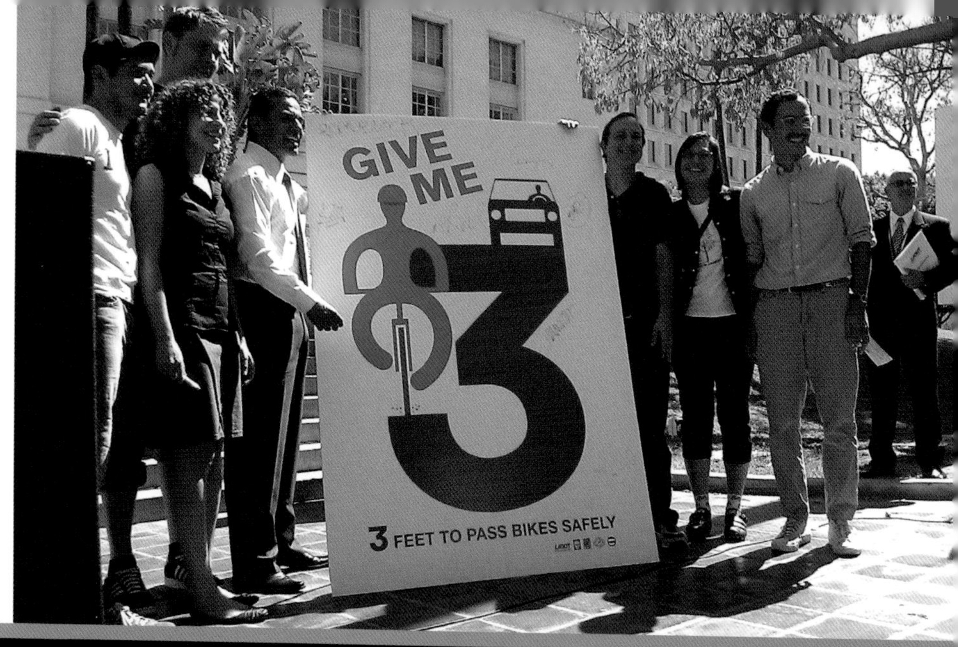


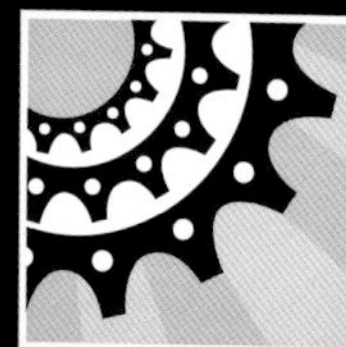

LOS ANGELES COUNTY
BICYCLE
COALITION
WWW.LA-BIKE.ORG

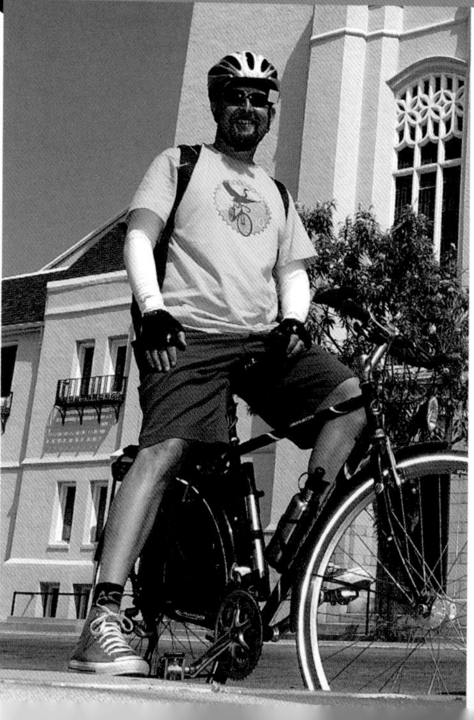

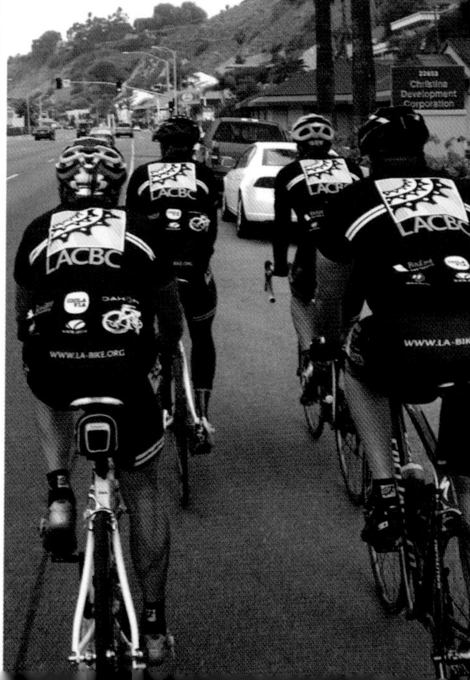

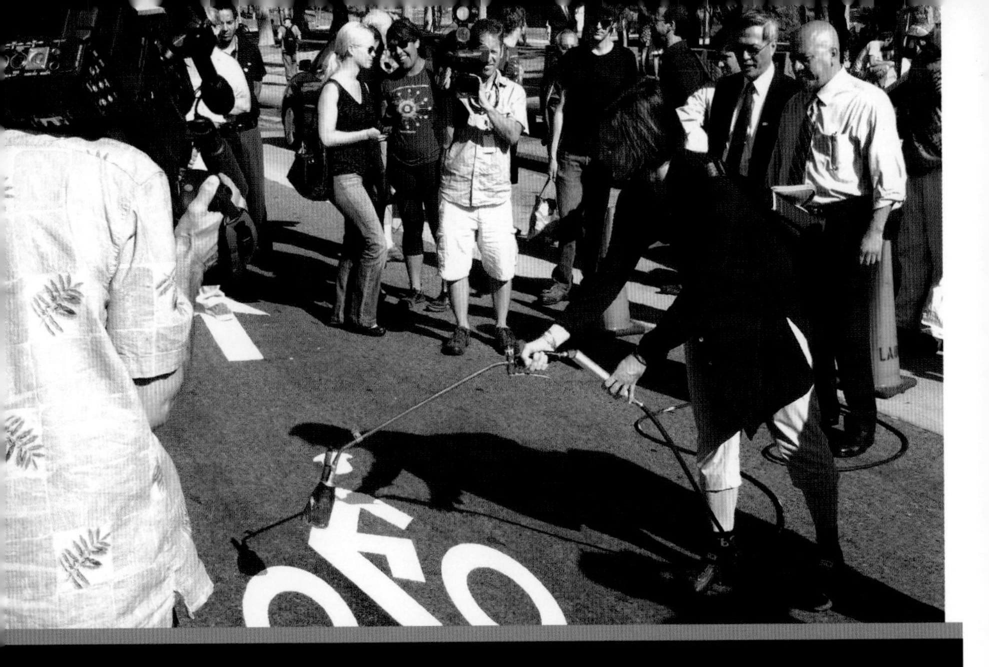

Founded in 1998, Los Angeles County Bicycle Coalition (LACBC) works to build a better, more bike-able Los Angeles County. LACBC is the only nonprofit, membership-based organization working exclusively for the millions of bicyclists in Los Angeles County. Through advocacy, education and outreach, Los Angeles County Bicycle Coalition brings together the diverse bicycling community in a united mission to make the entire L.A. region a safe and enjoyable place to ride.

Despite Los Angeles' reputation as a car-centric region, LACBC has emerged as one of the most innovative and wide-reaching bicycle advocacy non-profits in the country, playing a major role in the growing cycling movement here in LA. Our vision is to improve the built environment in Los Angeles, so that all cyclists--low-income, commuter, recreational, families, and women--can safely navigate LA County streets. Through the help of our strong volunteer network, we accomplish this in our campaigns to increase bicycle infrastructure throughout the 88 cities in the County. Our mission is to build a better, bike-able Los Angeles by improving the bicycle environment and quality of life in Los Angeles County through the following strategic goals:

- Increase bikes as a mode of transportation in Los Angeles County
- Advocate for improved bicycle and pedestrian infrastructure
- Serve as an umbrella organization for all bicyclists in LA County by fostering local chapters and regionally coordinated campaigns.
- Provide better education to both motorists and cyclists through our many educational, multi-lingual programs and resources.

Do you ride a bicycle in Los Angeles County? You can make a difference! Help make L.A. County a safe and enjoyable place to ride by joining, and/or donating to, the Los Angeles County Bicycle Coalition. Whether you ride for fun, transportation or both, LACBC works for you! There are a couple of ways you can help:

- **Membership**. By becoming a member, you join us in the fight for cyclists' rights. Join, renew or give the gift of LACBC membership and continue to build a better LA County.
- **Donate**. Make a donation to support our advocacy. As a grassroots organization, all tax-deductible monetary donations to our work are extremely crucial to improving the quality of life for LA County cyclists.
- **Volunteer** for LACBC and be part of the action as it happens: sign up to volunteer at upcoming events, in-office help, attend public meetings, bike valet, membership drives and more.

Your membership and donations are crucial to helping LACBC sustain its work to be the leading countywide bicycle advocacy non-profit and allow us to focus on issues most important to you!

**Find out more at www.la-bike.org**

# Downtown to Beverly Hills

Tinsel, glamour, grit and the great outdoors: Hollywood, Chinatown, Downtown, Beverly Hills and unexpected pockets of wilderness coexist in this region of Los Angeles, extending roughly from the Santa Monica Mountains-Hollywood Hills ridgeline south to Exposition Park and from the 405 Freeway east to the L.A. River. Diverse as the county itself, this area has multiple "centers of gravity." The old tag line "there's no there there" has often been affixed to L.A. – but, in truth, it's a place with both diffuse focus and an awesome abundance of "theres."

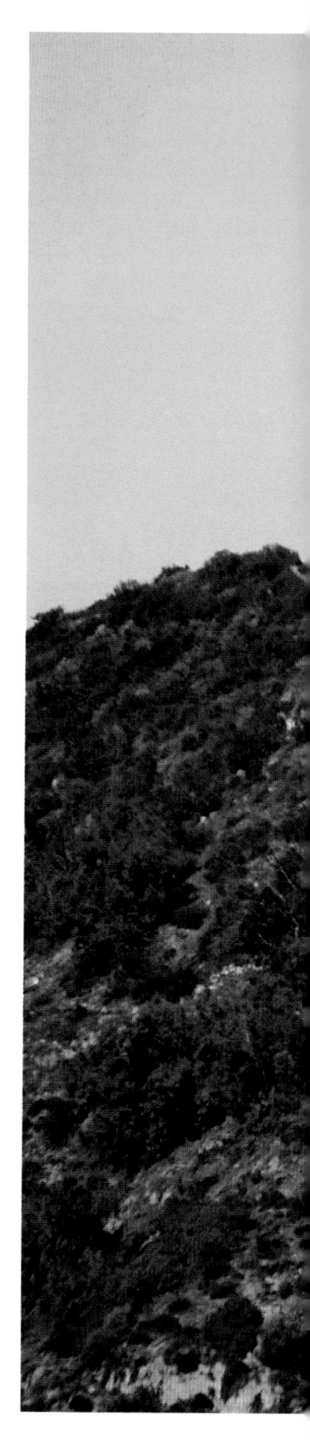

You'll find the highest concentration of "theres" in our Tour of Downtown L.A., an area so packed with landmarks and hot venues that we've provided a rolling list, a veritable smorgasbord, of top picks in the order you'll encounter them en route. Disney Concert Hall, Olvera Street and the Cathedral of Our Lady of the Angels are all part of the grand mix. Also at the urban end of the spectrum is this chapter's southernmost ride: the Crosstown Shuffle, a skyscrapers-to-surf route, taking in Miracle Mile's Museum Row, Exposition Park, the Coliseum and USC campus.

In a more rustic realm, the Mount Hollywood Drive ride ascends into "high country," along Griffith Park's rugged back roads, while the lush, tranquil Lake Hollywood Reservoir loop offers rare close-ups of the world-famous Hollywood sign. Another surprisingly idyllic spot is Elysian Park, juxtaposed with Downtown skyline views. And from our Mulholland Drive route, high along the city's spine, you'll get cross-county panoramas.

Hip, emerging parts of town, such as artsy Silver Lake, are the low-key stars of other rides. But for more glamour-seeking stargazing, our Beverly Hills jaunt sweeps by mansions and glitzy Rodeo Drive boutiques.

The Crosstown Shuffle and Downtown-to-Long Beach rides lead all the way to the Pacific Ocean, much the way Downtown's tangle of freeways extends into other regions. More literally evoking a bike freeway, our California Cycleway ride parallels one man's dream route: an elevated bicycle "highway," planked in wood, from Downtown L.A. to Pasadena (only partly realized and long ago demolished).

In the spirit of a bicycle freeway, we encourage you to experience the city center in its car-free glory during CicLAvia, a semiannual event that temporarily takes over Downtown streets. CicLAvia's current route coincides with parts of our Crosstown Shuffle and Tour of Downtown. Imagine over 100,000 cyclists, roller bladers and pedestrians flowing through the streets, with bands playing at intersections (for info: **www.ciclavia.org**).

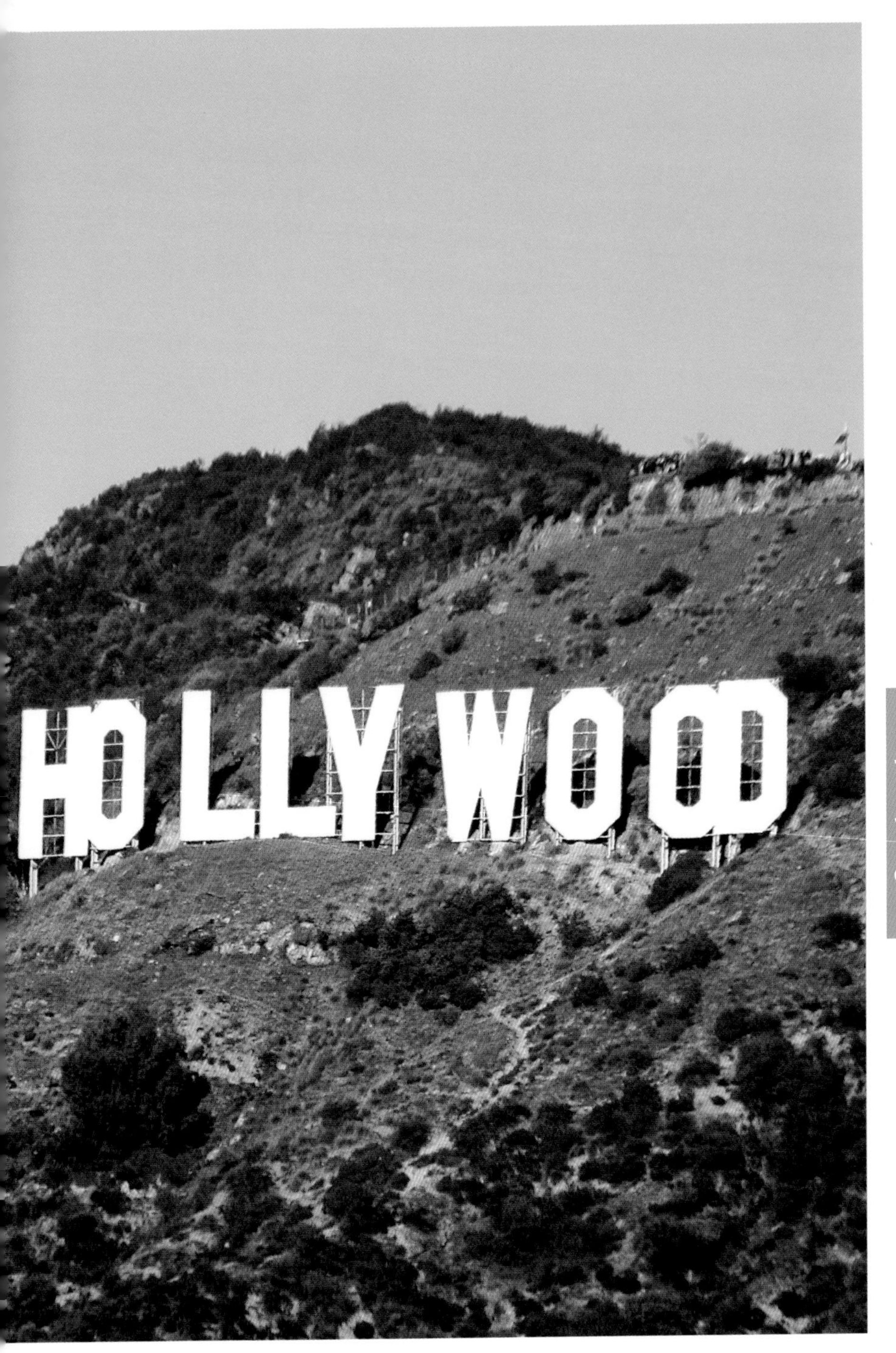
HOLLYWOOD

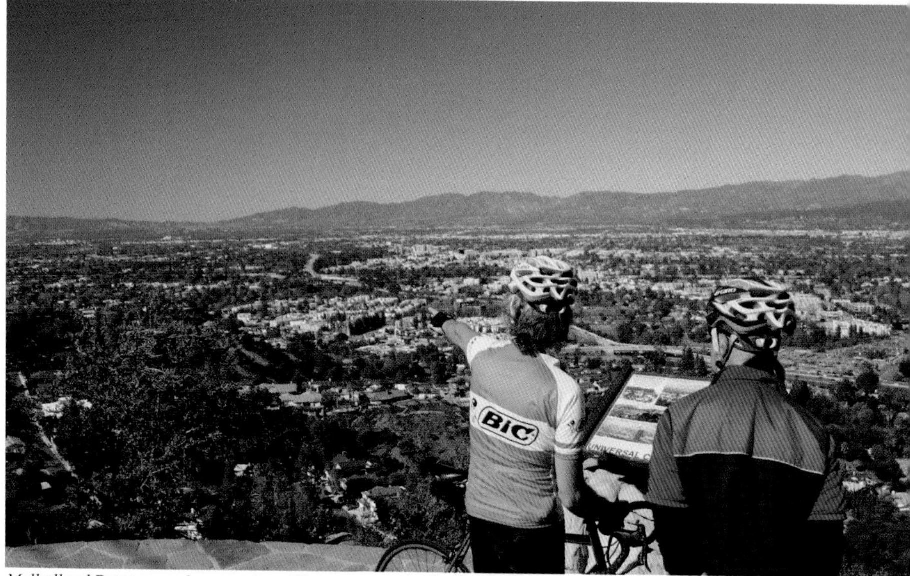


*Mulholland Drive runs along a ridge with panoramas opening beneath it.*

## At a Glance

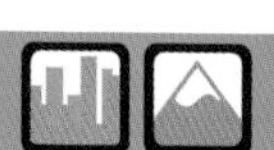

**Distance** 26.1 miles **Elevation Gain** 2,300 feet

### Terrain

Relatively flat city streets lead to a steep climb through Nichols Canyon, followed by rolling terrain along Mulholland Drive, a skyline ridge road. The loop finishes with a long descent back into the city. On Mulholland, watch for potholes and patches of rough pavement.

### Traffic

City traffic here is busiest on weekdays from late morning until early evening—though Nichols Canyon and stretches of Mulholland often remain uncrowded. This loop is not recommended for riders inexperienced with city traffic. The ride is at its tranquil best on weekend mornings.

### How to Get There

We begin from West Hollywood Park, near the corner of San Vicente and Santa Monica boulevards. To reach it from the 10 Freeway, take Robertson Boulevard north. (Parking is $1.00 per hour or $7.00 all day.)

### Food and Drink

Santa Monica Boulevard offers many choices. Best bets mid-ride are at Glen Centre, with the Beverly Glen Deli, Starbucks and more. To reach them, turn left from Mulholland onto Beverly Glen Boulevard, ride down to the signal and turn right.

### Side Trip

Off Sepulveda Boulevard, visit the famed Getty Center, with its collection of Western art from the Middle Ages to the present, prominent architecture, gardens and spectacular hilltop site. Free admission—and ample bicycle parking.

**Links to** 26 39 40 k16

**Where to Bike Rating** 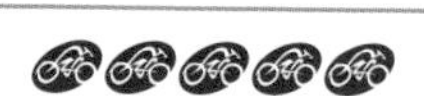

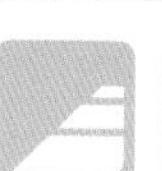

## About...

This route may seem daunting on paper—after all, we've awarded it a rating of five. Truly, it's easier than that, with most of the "suffering" in the three-mile Nichols Canyon climb. Otherwise, the ride isn't strenuous, with at least one-quarter of it pitched downhill through Sepulveda Pass! The pedaling is amply rewarded with unparalleled scenery—rural and urban—notably stunning panoramas that unfold to either side of Mulholland, combining some of the best bicycling in Westwood, Beverly Hills, West Hollywood, the Hollywood Hills and the Santa Monica Mountains.

This ride is a treat served in three courses. First, after a few blocks of city streets, you'll arrive at the appetizer: Nichols Canyon. Long favored by cyclists, this winding, narrow and (for that reason) little-used road provides a refreshing conduit between the city and Mulholland Drive. The lower reaches feature a moderate grade upward along a tree-lined, mossy streambed. You may hear gurgling water, especially after winter or spring rains. Nestled amid abundant trees and lush underbrush, the houses along the canyon walls tend to be small and old, lending the road a rustic aura. Further up, a series of switchbacks yield exceptional down-canyon views toward WeHo, or West Hollywood. For some riders, this section evokes a mountain stage of the Tour de France.

The main course, and centerpiece, is the scenic and legendary Mulholland Drive, winding along the spine of the Santa Monica Mountains. Begun in 1924, this skyline parkway was envisioned as a prime connector between the city, valleys, mountains and beaches (a link long ago supplanted by faster, wider, more streamlined routes). Several noteworthy scenic overlooks punctuate this nine-mile stretch, enticing riders with periodic rest stops and spectacular panoramas of the San Fernando and San Gabriel valleys, the Santa Monica Mountains, the ocean in the distance and the metropolis of Los Angeles.

Finally, dessert: a long, enjoyable, low-key downhill on wide shoulders through Sepluveda Pass, practically grazing the gateway to the Getty Center before continuing on flats through Westwood, near UCLA, then chic Beverly Hills, and finally hip WeHo. A mix of tall buildings, storefronts, galleries and upscale homes animates this all-purpose cross-town leg (almost making up for the unfortunate absence of cycling infrastructure in Beverly Hills, where Santa Monica Boulevard's bike lanes end abruptly, only to spring back to life in WeHo).

## Ride Log

**0.0** From West Hollywood Park, ride north on San Vicente Blvd then turn right, or east, onto the bike lane on Santa Monica Blvd.

**0.9** Turn left on North Kings Rd.

**1.1** Turn right on Fountain Ave.

**1.9** Turn left on Genesee Ave (the third street past Fairfax Ave).

**2.4** Genesee becomes Nichols Canyon Rd.

**3.5** At the stop sign, Nichols Canyon continues to the right. (Note: There are several intersections like this one along Nichols Canyon, where a wrong turn leads to a dead end, so follow the street signs and the yellow centerline.)

**5.2** Turn right on Woodrow Wilson Dr. Be prepared for a steep climb.

**5.4** Left on Mulholland Dr.

**5.9** Universal City overlook.

**7.2** Cross Laurel Canyon Blvd.

**8.0** Nancy Hoover Pohl overlook.

**9.3** Barbara A. Fine Summit overlook.

**9.8** Continue straight (actually, the right-hand branch of a Y) following the arrows indicating Mulholland Dr West and Coldwater Canyon Rd.

**10.1** Continue on Mulholland Dr (slightly uphill to the left) at Franklin Canyon Dr (don't ride downhill on

## Ride Log continued...

Coldwater Canyon Ave).

12.1 Charles and Lotte Melhorn overlook.

12.3 Pass through the intersection with Benedict Canyon Dr. For a shorter ride, turn right and descend Benedict Canyon. At Sunset, turn left onto Rodeo Dr. At Carmelita Ave, turn left and rejoin the long route.

12.6 Pass through the intersection at Beverly Glen Blvd.

13.1 Stone Canyon overlook.

14.8 Turn left on Skirball Center Dr just before the 405 Freeway (follow the arrows to Sepulveda Blvd). Do not continue straight on Mulholland Dr.

15.3 Turn left on Sepulveda Blvd.

17.9 The Getty Center.

21.3 Turn left on Santa Monica Blvd, joining the bike lane.

23.3 Continue straight on the "Local Access Only" (right) lane of Santa Monica Blvd at Century Park East.

24.0 Cross Wilshire Blvd, then turn left on Roxbury Dr.

24.2 Turn right on Carmelita Ave.

25.6 Turn left at the stop sign, continuing on Carmelita Ave.

25.7 Turn right on Doheny Dr, then left on Santa Monica, joining the bike lane.

26.1 Turn left on San Vicente and, then into West Hollywood Park.

P1 Skirball Cultural Center
P2 The Getty Center
P3 University of California Los Angeles (UCLA)
P4 Century City
P5 Rodeo Drive
P6 Melrose Avenue shopping district
P7 Schindler House
P8 The Los Angeles County Museum of Art
P9 Page Museum at La Brea Tar Pits

B1 I. Martin Imports
8330 Beverly Blvd, Los Angeles
B2 Spokes 'n Stuff
7777 Melrose Ave, Los Angeles
B3 Helen's Cycles Westwood Village
1071 Gayley Ave, Los Angeles
B4 Bike Improve
10929 Santa Monica Blvd, Los Angeles
B5 Bikecology
9006 West Pico Blvd, Los Angeles
B6 Beverly Hills Bike Shop
854 South Robertson Blvd, Los Angeles

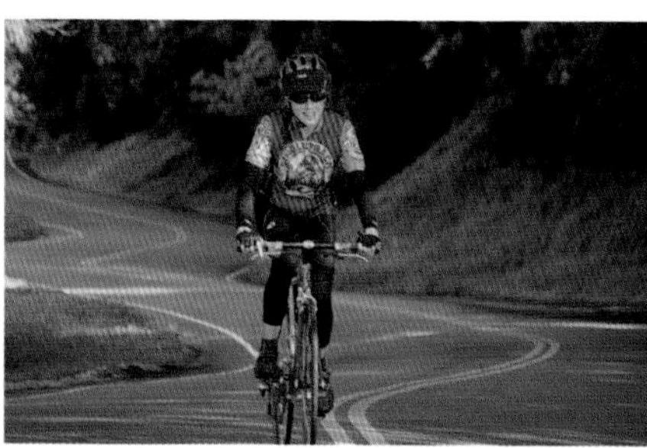

*Another serpentine little climb*

### Mulholland Drive

*Please note: the profile for Ride 33 is depicted in 300ft vertical increments due to unusually high elevation.*

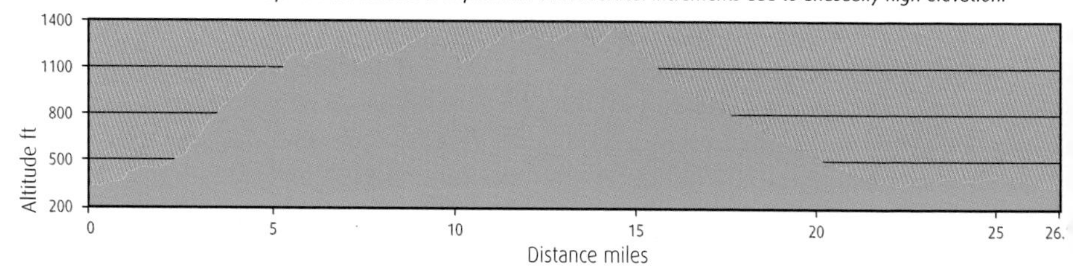

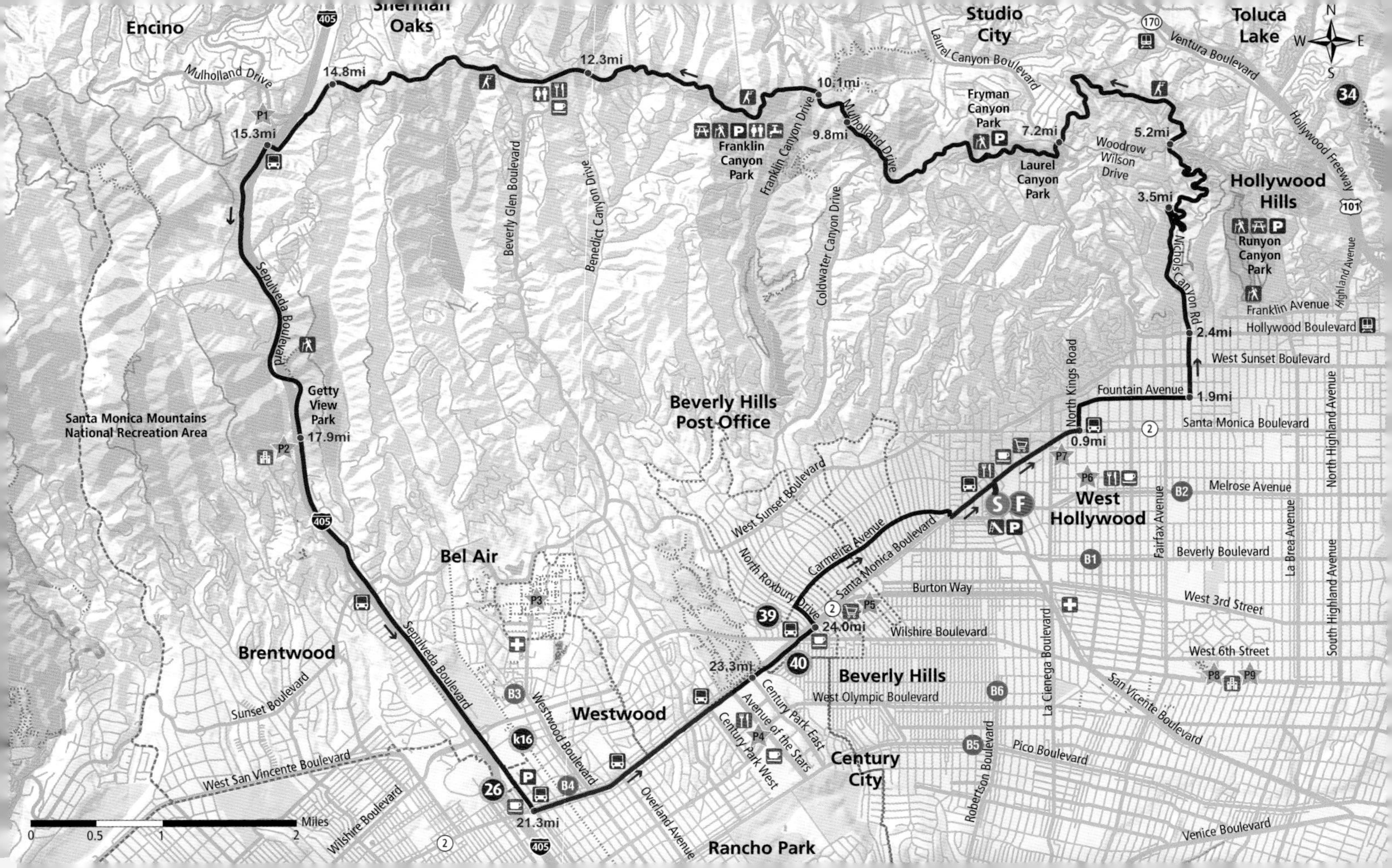
Encino
Oaks
Studio City
Toluca Lake
Mulholland Drive
14.8mi
12.3mi
10.1mi
9.8mi
7.2mi
5.2mi
3.5mi
2.4mi
1.9mi
0.9mi
15.3mi
17.9mi
21.3mi
23.3mi
24.0mi
Laurel Canyon Boulevard
Ventura Boulevard
Hollywood Freeway
Fryman Canyon Park
Laurel Canyon Park
Woodrow Wilson Drive
Hollywood Hills
Runyon Canyon Park
Franklin Canyon Park
Franklin Canyon Drive
Mulholland Drive
Coldwater Canyon Drive
Benedict Canyon Drive
Beverly Glen Boulevard
Nichols Canyon Rd
Franklin Avenue
Highland Avenue
Hollywood Boulevard
West Sunset Boulevard
Fountain Avenue
Santa Monica Boulevard
North Kings Road
North Highland Avenue
Melrose Avenue
Fairfax Avenue
La Brea Avenue
Beverly Boulevard
West Hollywood
West 3rd Street
West 6th Street
South Highland Avenue
San Vicente Boulevard
Burton Way
Wilshire Boulevard
La Cienega Boulevard
Beverly Hills
West Olympic Boulevard
Robertson Boulevard
Pico Boulevard
Venice Boulevard
Century City
Century Park East
Avenue of the Stars
Century Park West
Rancho Park
Overland Avenue
Westwood
Westwood Boulevard
Bel Air
Beverly Hills Post Office
West Sunset Boulevard
North Roxbury Drive
Carmelita Avenue
Santa Monica Mountains National Recreation Area
Getty View Park
Sepulveda Boulevard
Brentwood
Sunset Boulevard
West San Vincente Boulevard
Wilshire Boulevard
Miles
0
0.5
1
2

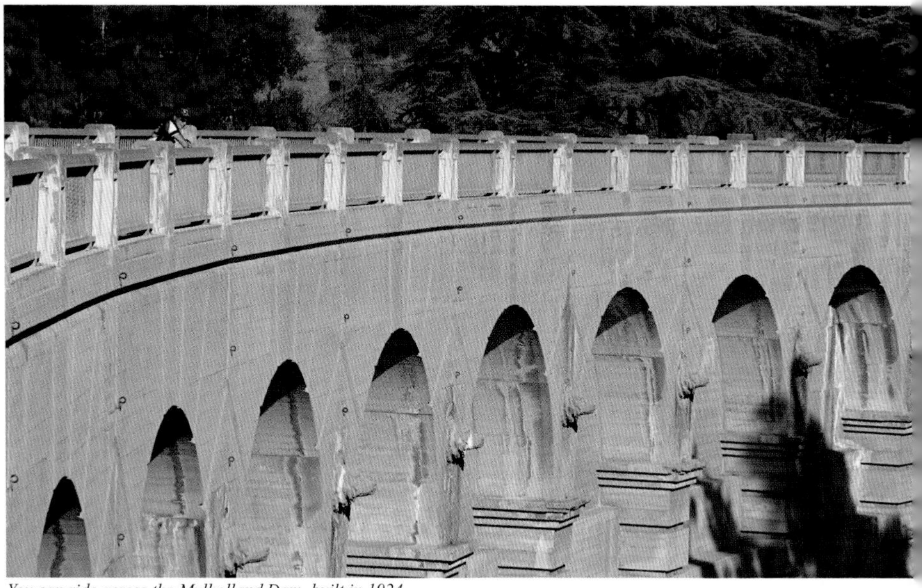

*You can ride across the Mulholland Dam, built in 1924.*

## At a Glance

**Distance** 4.8 miles **Elevation Gain** 150 feet

### Terrain

This out-and-back ride is flat, except for a modest climb on the outbound leg. Pavement surfaces are generally good—the few rough spots are easily avoided.

### Traffic

From the start to Tahoe Drive, the ride uses the shoulder of a lightly traveled neighborhood street. The rest of the route follows a wide, paved bike-and-pedestrian path, entirely free from vehicular traffic.

### How to Get There

Exit the 101 Freeway at Barham Boulevard and proceed northeast to Lake Hollywood Drive. Turn right and meander up through a residential neighborhood for about 0.5 mile. Turn right at the stop sign and park at the bottom of the hill.

### Food and Drink

The Hollywood Reservoir is secluded with no nearby snack options—so best to stock up on refreshments before starting the ride. You'll find convenience stores and sandwich shops on Barham Boulevard.

### Side Trip

For other views of the Hollywood Sign, the reservoir and Downtown, head north on Tahoe Drive, turn left on Canyon Lake Drive to its end—or, alternatively, turn right on Canyon Lake Drive and up a short distance to the overlook—on foot or by bike. (The climbs are murderous.)

**Where to Bike Rating** 

 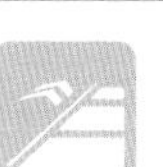  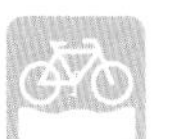

# About...

This is literally a hidden ride. Lake Hollywood Reservoir, with its encircling bike path, nestles into the Hollywood Hills, becoming almost invisible from the lower neighborhoods. (Only tiny bits of the dam show through the foliage.) This ride, especially on its long, lakeside stretch offers easy, tranquil cycling conditions with scenic glimpses of the iconic Hollywood Sign and Lake Hollywood. Aromas of pine and eucalyptus, plus the soft carpet of pine needles occasionally under your wheels, enhance the "far-from-civilization" character of this short spin.

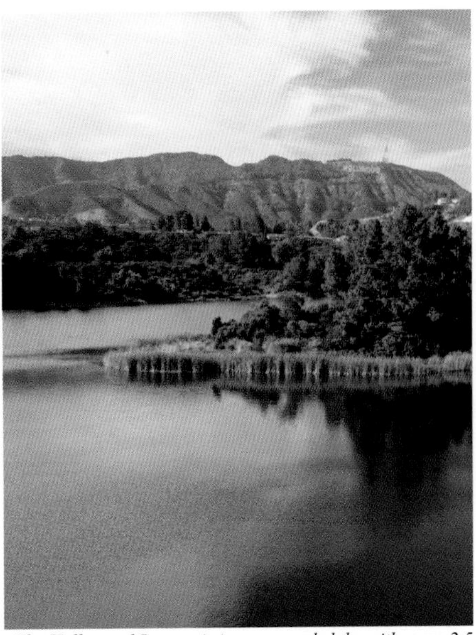

*The Hollywood Reservoir is a manmade lake with some 2.5 billion gallons of water.*

This mini-escapade from the gritty streets and car culture of Los Angeles immerses you in a setting so rustic it seems hard to believe it's only a short distance from intense urban areas. All along the way, you get fleeting glimpses, through towering shade trees, of the Hollywood Sign to one side and the sparkling green-blue waters of Lake Hollywood to the other.

The chain-link security fence surrounding the reservoir is initially off-putting, but the beauty of the scenery soon transcends it. Incidentally, this fence is a cinematic celebrity in its own right. In *Chinatown,* the famed noir classic set in pre-war Los Angeles, Jake Gittes, played by Jack Nicholson, has a run-in with bad guys who shove him against this fence as he tries to investigate falsified water levels in the reservoir. Fortunately, he escapes with only a bloody nick on his nose (administered by director Roman Polanski in cameo role as a hired thug).

Further on, views of the Hollywood Hills give way to panoramas of the castle-like architecture of the Mulholland Dam. This 1925 structure was named for the reservoir's designer, William Mulholland, the famed but highly controversial engineer of L.A.'s water system in the '20s—and the inspiration for Gittes's chief antagonists in *Chinatown*. Southern California is naturally arid and water-starved, despite the apparent abundance of moisture in lush lawns and landscaping across Greater Los Angeles, especially in posh neighborhoods. At one time, the 2.5-billion-gallon, manmade reservoir (still in use as a water supply), provided most of the city's drinking water.

Fittingly, a drinking fountain at the western end of the dam marks the turnaround point.

A footnote: The bicycling/pedestrian path actually encircles the entire lake, making a 3.4-mile loop. Unfortunately, the path between the north end (this ride's trailhead) and the west side of the dam has been closed indefinitely, due to landslide damage. In an ideal world, the Department of Water and Power will finish the repairs in the foreseeable future, allowing cyclists, runners and walkers to complete the full loop around the lake. That said, the currently accessible section is still well worth the trip, a refreshing out-and-back through a beautiful landscape, unlike any other in Los Angeles.

*While Ride 34 has not been deemed kid-friendly in its entirety, it does include substantial sections which are entirely safe for family use.*

# Ride Log

0.0 Park along Lake Hollywood Dr near the reservoir's north gate, then head southeast on Lake Hollywood Dr.
0.7 At Tahoe Dr, ride around either end of the "Hollywood" gate (if closed) and walk through the maze-like gate leading to the path dedicated to bicyclists and pedestrians.
2.2 Turn right and pedal across the top of the Mulholland Dam.
2.4 Make a U-turn at the end of the dam.
2.6 Turn left at the end of the dam and continue around the reservoir.
4.1 Walk through the gate and ride around the "Hollywood" gate.
4.8 End of ride.

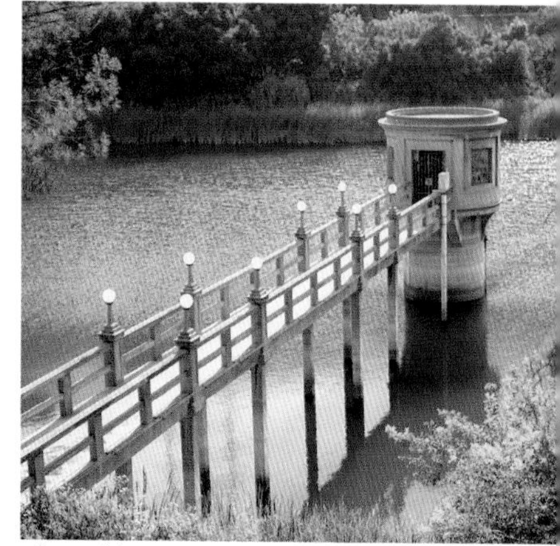

*Some of the most picturesque structures are only accessible to official personnel!*

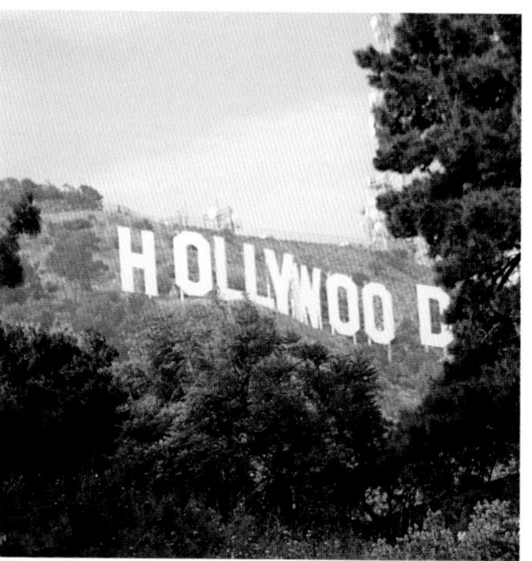


*The Hollywood Reservoir is directly below the famous Hollywood sign.*

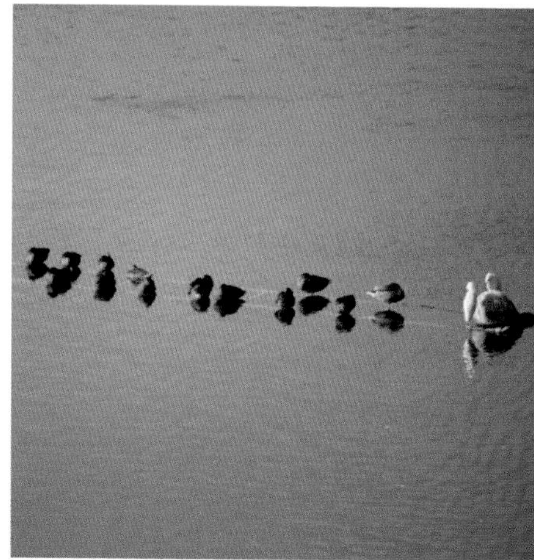

*Though swimming in this source of drinking water is verboten, birds make themselves at home.*

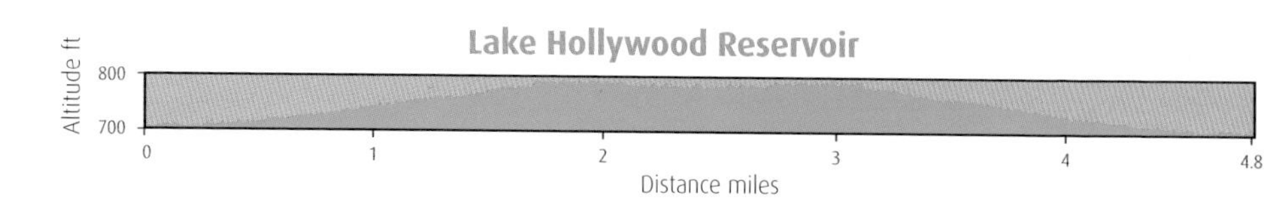

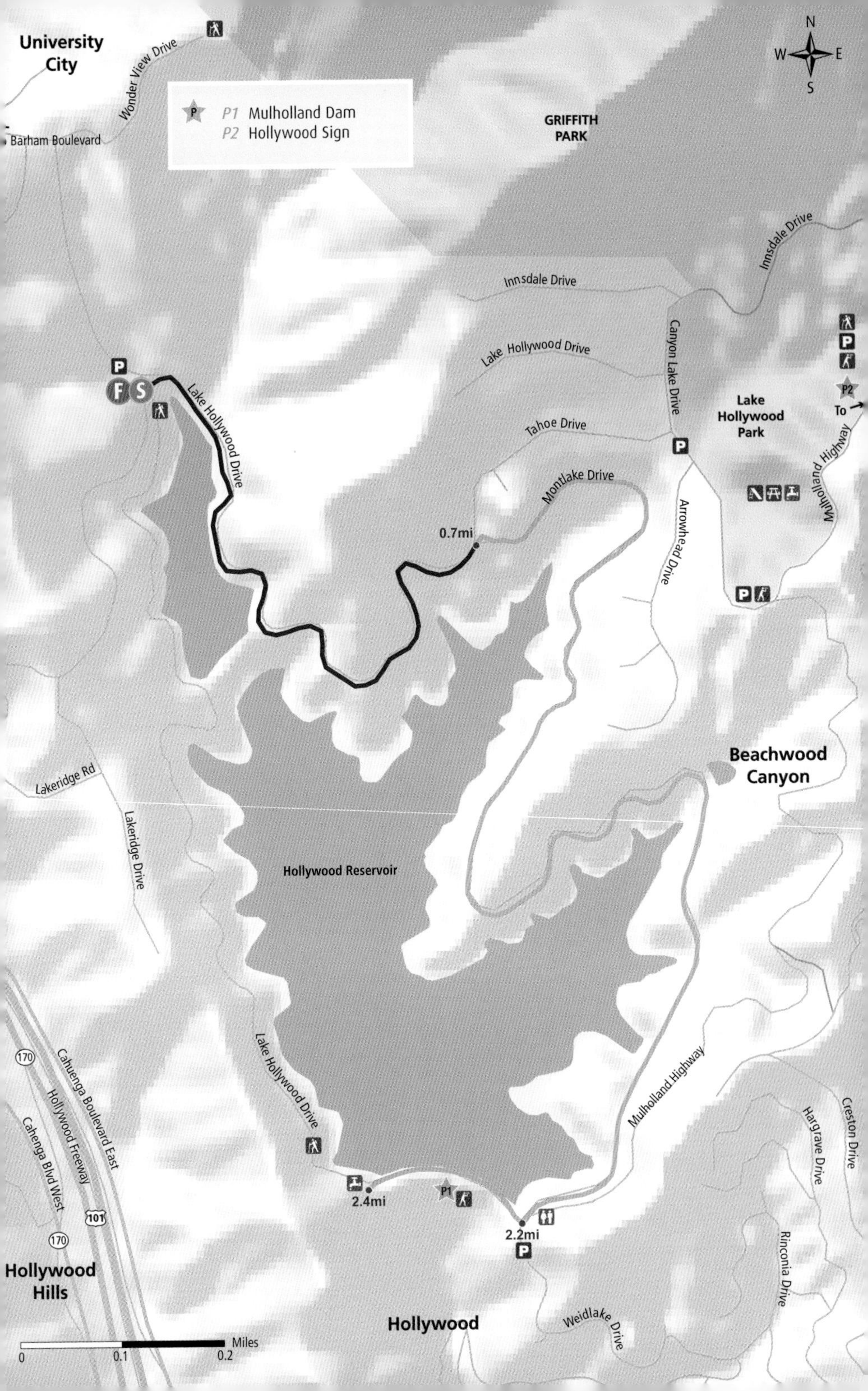

University City
Wonder View Drive
Barham Boulevard
P1 Mulholland Dam
P2 Hollywood Sign
GRIFFITH PARK
N
W
E
S
Innsdale Drive
Innsdale Drive
Lake Hollywood Drive
Canyon Lake Drive
Lake Hollywood Park
P2
To
Tahoe Drive
Montlake Drive
Lake Hollywood Drive
0.7mi
Arrowhead Drive
Mulholland Highway
Beachwood Canyon
Lakeridge Rd
Lakeridge Drive
Hollywood Reservoir
Lake Hollywood Drive
Mulholland Highway
170
Cahuenga Boulevard East
Hollywood Freeway
Cahenga Blvd West
101
170
Hollywood Hills
2.4mi
P1
2.2mi
Hargrave Drive
Creston Drive
Rinconia Drive
Hollywood
Weidlake Drive
Miles
0
0.1
0.2

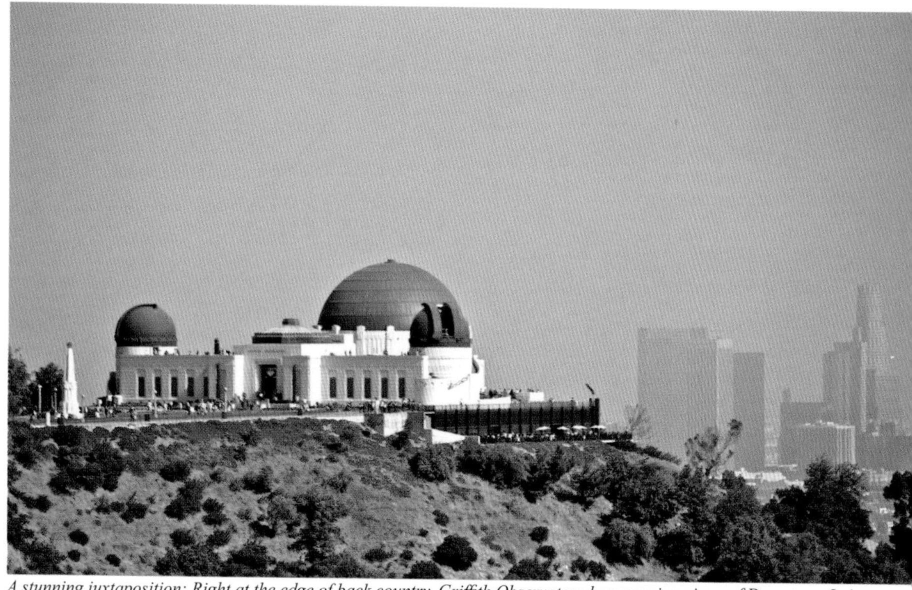
*A stunning juxtaposition: Right at the edge of back country, Griffith Observatory has amazing views of Downtown L.A.*

## At a Glance

**Distance** 19.3 miles **Elevation Gain** 2,100 feet

### Terrain

This route transverses Griffith Park, climbing Mount Hollywood twice—you ascend and descend, coast over a few easy flat miles, and then ascend and descend again. The roads are mainly good, except for a few rough patches on Mount Hollywood Drive (so watch for sand, gravel and potholes there).

### Traffic

Expect light traffic on Fern Dell Drive, Western Canyon Road, Observatory Avenue, and on the segment through the north side of Griffith Park. Mount Hollywood Drive is closed to motorized traffic.

### How to Get There

Drive west on Los Feliz from the 5 Freeway to Fern Dell. From the 101 Freeway, take Franklin Avenue east to Western Avenue, which becomes Los Feliz, then turn left onto Fern Dell. Park on Fern Dell, near Black Oak Drive.

### Food and Drink

For refreshments, try Griffith Observatory's Café at the End of the Universe, operated by Wolfgang Puck, the Autry National Center's Golden Spur Café, or fresh-baked goods at The Trails Café, on Fern Dell.

### Side Trip

Lock your bikes on racks at the observatory and make the easy trail hike to the top of Mount Hollywood for panoramic vistas of the Los Angeles Basin.

**Links to**  

**Where to Bike Rating** 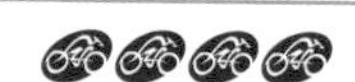

 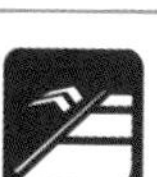 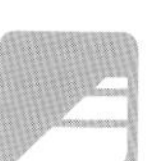 

## About...

This journey rises from Griffith Park's more populated areas, up past the famous Griffith Observatory and into wilderness, or "high country," along a rugged back road. Here, you can explore Griffith Park's south-facing slopes and upper reaches. An alternative route, via Vista del Valle (intermittently closed for maintenance), allows cyclists to experience Mount Hollywood's northern slopes—best ridden on hybrid or mountain bikes and definitely recommended for its tranquility and varied landscapes.

This adventurous ride begins at Ferndell Park, home to more than 50 species of ferns and tropical plants along a stream. A short way up Western Canyon, you'll emerge from a canopy of Sycamores onto sunny hillsides, thick with the eucalyptus, scrub oak and chaparral that typify Southern California's open terrain.

As the route meanders up the canyon, splendid views unfold, revealing the Griffith Observatory, perched on a ridge to your right. This Art Deco landmark, open to the public, houses a superb planetarium, telescopes, and an education center dedicated to astronomy. The observatory is itself a star—famously appearing in *Rebel Without a Cause*, alongside James Dean, in *The Terminator*, *The Rocketeer* and many other films (as well as multiple TV shows).

From the observatory, you pass through a short tunnel. Once around a couple of turns, you've begun the best part of the ride: into the park's rustic interior. Mount Hollywood Drive, completely car-free, is like a rugged country road, gradually ascending the pass between Mount Hollywood and Mount Lee. Pines and oaks shade the way. From the summit, you descend to the park's other side before looping back up the hill again. Keep your eyes peeled for wild things: deer, coyotes, snakes, red-tailed hawks soaring above and even ultra-reclusive bobcats.

### Vista del Valle Option

This alternative ascent (three miles longer, with 200 additional feet of climbing) explores Mount Hollywood's more remote northern flank. Vista del Valle winds upward, opening fleeting panoramas of the northern valleys and mountains. Charred tree stumps along the roadside—the aftermath of a massive brushfire—contrast strikingly with the green hillsides on the ridge's Fern Dell side. Heavy rains washed out a patch of Vista del Valle's paved surface, leaving a stretch of dirt road. So, a hybrid or mountain bike would be best here.

One of this ride's delights is The Trails Café, nestled in Fern Dell, just before the journey's end, offering the perfect spot for well-deserved refueling and relaxation. In addition to homemade pies, quiches and cookies, the savory and sweet menu offerings include fresh-squeezed lemonade, great coffee and avocado sandwiches. Amid aromas of baked goods, the shady patio—its rustic picnic tables nestled beneath trees strung with lanterns and whimsical ornaments—provides plenty of bohemian ambiance.

## Ride Log

0.0 Begin riding north on Fern Dell Dr.

0.4 The Trails Café.

2.0 Turn right on West Observatory Ave toward Griffith Observatory.

2.4 Griffith Observatory. Follow the circular drive past the observatory and down the short winding downhill on East Observatory Ave.

2.7 Turn left at the Y where East Observatory meets Vermont Canyon Rd.

2.8 Pass through the tunnel and turn right on Mt. Hollywood Dr.

2.9 Ride around the right end of the gate.

4.5 Continue straight over the summit. The descent has several sharp curves and there can be debris on the road, so be careful.

7.2 Griffith Park Dr. Dismount and walk around the right end of the gate and then turn right.

7.9 Mineral Wells picnic area.

## Ride Log continued...

P1 Griffith Observatory
P2 Griffith Park Merry-go-round
P3 Autry National Center
P4 Los Angeles Zoo
P5 Travel Town Museum
P6 Bronson Canyon Park & Caves
P7 Greek Theatre

B1 Safety Cycle Shop
1014 Western, Los Angeles
R1 Spokes 'n Stuff
4400 Crystal Springs Dr, Los Angeles

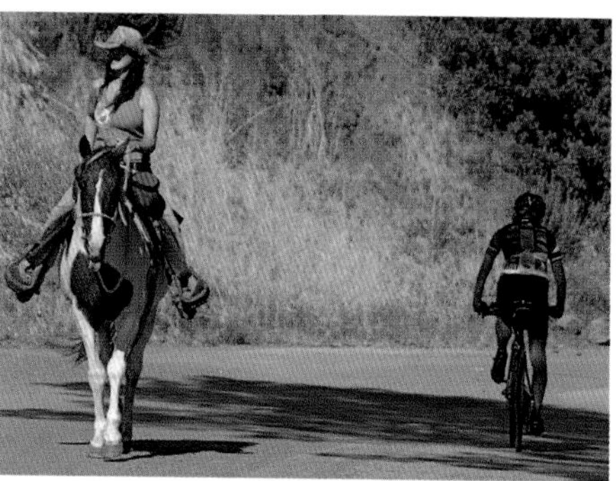

*Only cyclists, hikers and the occasional horse are allowed on Mount Hollywood Drive.*

**8.2** Wilson and Harding Golf Course clubhouse.

**9.1** Turn left on Crystal Springs Dr.

**10.2** Autry National Center and the Los Angeles Zoo.

**12.1** Travel Town. Continue up the hill.

**12.8** Turn right on Mt. Hollywood Dr. Walk around the left end of the gate.

**15.5** Continue straight over the summit.

**17.1** Turn right on West Observatory Ave and right on Western Canyon Rd.

**19.3** End of the ride.

### The Vista del Valle Option

**2.7** Turn right at the Y where East Observatory meets Vermont Canyon Rd.

**3.4** Turn left on Commonwealth Canyon Dr just past the Greek Theatre. Pass the tennis courts and Roosevelt Municipal Golf Course.

**4.0** Turn left on Vista del Valle. Dismount and walk around the left end of the gate.

**5.9** Dirt road begins.

**6.5** Paved road resumes.

**7.6** Turn right on Mt. Hollywood Dr. The descent has several sharp curves and there can be debris on the road, so be careful.

**10.2** Griffith Park Dr. Walk around the right end of the gate and turn right.

**10.9** Mineral Wells picnic area.

**11.2** Wilson and Harding Golf Course clubhouse.

**12.1** Turn left on Crystal Springs Dr.

**13.2** Autry National Center and the Los Angeles Zoo.

**15.1** Travel Town. Continue up the hill.

**15.8** Turn right on Mt. Hollywood Dr. Walk around the left end of the gate.

**18.5** Continue straight over the summit.

**20.1** Turn right on West Observatory Ave and right on Western Canyon Rd.

**22.3** End of ride.

### Mount Hollywood Drive - Vista del Valle

*Please note: the profile for Ride 35 is depicted in 300ft vertical increments due to unusually high elevation.*

Altitude ft: 1600, 1300, 1000, 700, 400
Distance miles: 0, 5, 10, 15, 20, 22.3

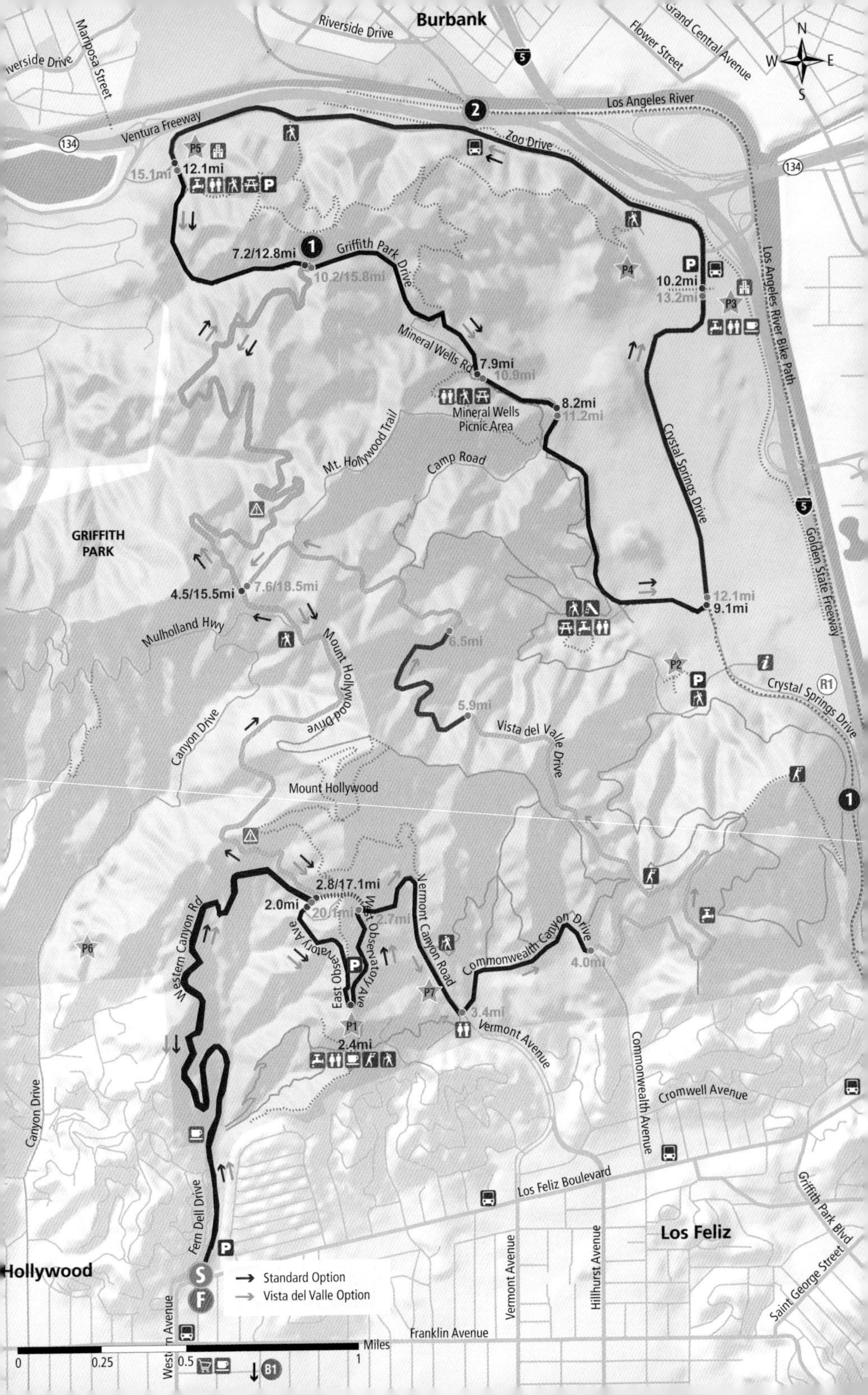
Burbank
Riverside Drive
Grand Central Avenue
Flower Street
Mariposa Street
Los Angeles River
Ventura Freeway
Zoo Drive
134
5
2
1
P5
P4
P3
P2
P1
P6
P7
R1
B1
15.1mi
12.1mi
7.2/12.8mi
10.2/15.8mi
Griffith Park Drive
Mineral Wells Rd
7.9mi
10.9mi
8.2mi
11.2mi
Mineral Wells Picnic Area
10.2mi
13.2mi
Los Angeles River Bike Path
Crystal Springs Drive
Mt. Hollywood Trail
Camp Road
GRIFFITH PARK
Golden State Freeway
4.5/15.5mi
7.6/18.5mi
12.1mi
9.1mi
Mulholland Hwy
Mount Hollywood Drive
6.5mi
5.9mi
Vista del Valle Drive
Canyon Drive
Mount Hollywood
2.8/17.1mi
2.0mi
20.1mi
2.7mi
West Observatory Ave
East Observatory Ave
Vermont Canyon Road
Commonwealth Canyon Drive
4.0mi
Western Canyon Rd
3.4mi
2.4mi
Vermont Avenue
Commonwealth Avenue
Cromwell Avenue
Los Feliz Boulevard
Canyon Drive
Fern Dell Drive
Los Feliz
Griffith Park Blvd
Hillhurst Avenue
Saint George Street
Hollywood
S
F
Standard Option
Vista del Valle Option
Western Avenue
Franklin Avenue
0
0.25
0.5
1
Miles
N
S
E
W

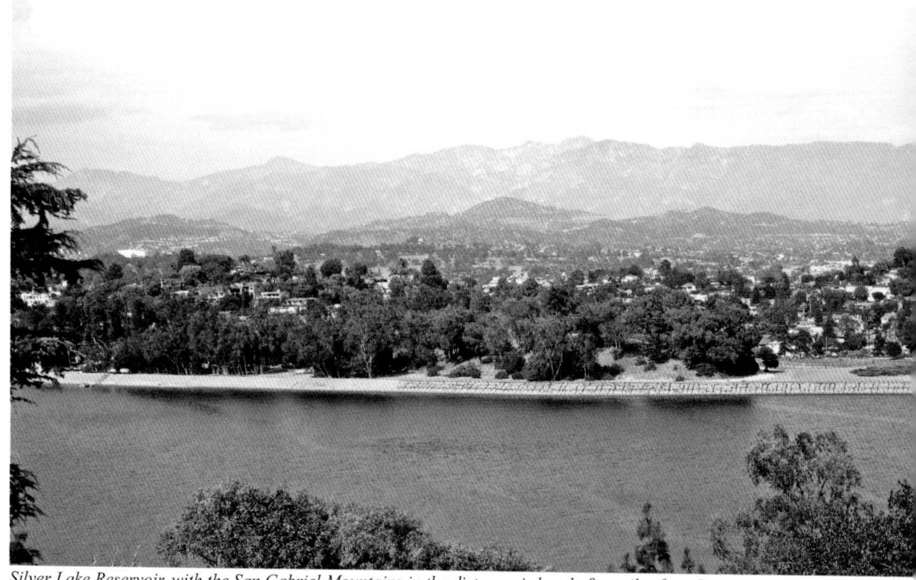

*Silver Lake Reservoir, with the San Gabriel Mountains in the distance, is barely five miles from Downtown L.A.*

## At a Glance

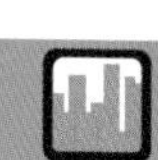

**Distance** 6.9 miles **Elevation Gain** 800 feet

### Terrain

This mostly flat ride has three short hills: along West Silver Lake Drive, Tesla Avenue, and Rowena Avenue. The pavement quality is good, except along Griffith Park Boulevard, where the concrete has cracked and bumpy spots.

### Traffic

Traffic is typically moderate. All the busy sections, except for Rowena Avenue, have bike lanes.

### How to Get There

Exit the 5 Freeway onto Los Feliz Boulevard, turn west and then, south onto Riverside Drive. Continue south about one mile, turn right onto Fletcher Drive, then left at the signal onto Glendale Boulevard and, finally, right onto Silver Lake Boulevard. Park along the lake front.

### Food and Drink

There's no shortage of cafés and other casual hangouts around Silver Lake, including Intelligentsia Coffee & Tea, at Sunset Junction, and Silverlake Coffee, on Glendale Boulevard. For supermarket goods (from prepared salads to energy bars), try Trader Joe's on Hyperion.

### Side Trip

To experience the interior of one of the neighborhood's many stellar Mid-Century Modern houses, consider touring the late architect Richard Neutra's own home, the VDL Research House, at 2300 Silver Lake Boulevard (open most Saturdays 11:00 a.m. to 3:00 p.m., **www.neutra.vdl.org**).

**Links to** 2

**Where to Bike Rating** 

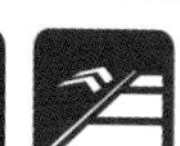  

# About...

As rides go, this one's fairly short: two quasi-concentric loops, totaling about seven miles around Silver Lake Reservoir and its surroundings. The little journey gives you a sense of this rapidly re-emerging neighborhood—now an epicenter of L.A. hip, with an eclectic creative crowd, lots of fun eateries, as well as one-of-a-kind shops selling Mid-Century Modern furnishings. This section of the city is also known for its houses of that same vintage, many by cutting-edge architects of the era.

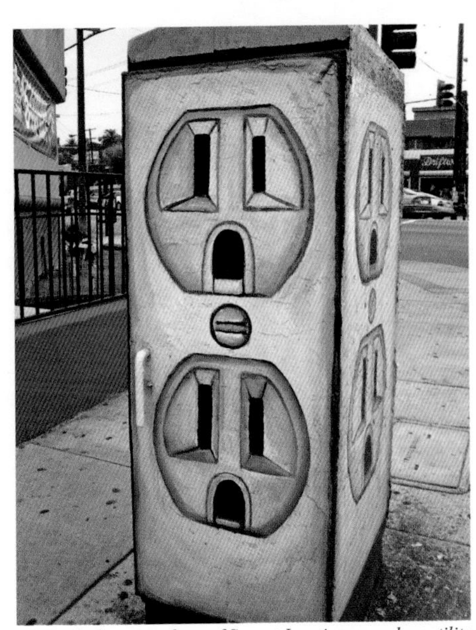

*In the funky atmosphere of Sunset Junction, an urban utility box masquerades as a giant electrical outlet.*

This ride, like the neighborhood, centers on the Silver Lake Reservoir—named not for its shimmering waters, but for Herman Silver, a member of the city's first Board of Water Commissioners. As you pedal along the lake, our opening loop, you'll get a taste of the distinctive character of this place—lush hillsides overlooking the water, yet only a few miles from Downtown. Some of the terrain is so steep that the pedestrian alleys are actually stairs. So, it's not surprising that *The Music Box*, a 1932 Academy Award winning cinematic short, featuring Laurel and Hardy moving a piano up hillside steps, was filmed here (you can visit the location: Place of Interest P1).

Along the route, you'll get a glimmer of the neighborhood's architectural riches. Though Spanish Mediterranean style is well represented here, the area is most famous for its trove of California Modernist homes, many by mid-20th century masters, including architects Richard Neutra, Rudolph Schindler and John Lautner. An entire street, albeit a short one, is called Neutra Place, and many Mid-Century Modernist gems stand in the vicinity—on or near Silver Lake Boulevard.

The reservoir's waters are definitely for looking not touching, keeping boating, swimming and fishing off limits, but venues for play and relaxation encircle this manmade lake (actually two adjoining basins). At its south end is a dog park, as well as the Silver Lake Recreation Center, with a basketball court and a playground with a sandbox. On the northeast side is Silver Lake Meadow, a passive park with grassy expanses, where you can unwind after a ride, toss a Frisbee, picnic or lie back and watch the clouds drift by. A 2.2-mile, packed-dirt jogging-and-walking path runs along this side of the water, connecting the meadow and recreation center.

From the lake's immediate vicinity, our route continues into a bigger loop around it. Though Silver Lake was out of fashion only a few years ago, it is now a destination with a high "hip quotient"—home to an artsy crowd. The stretches along Silver Lake Boulevard, Sunset Boulevard and the Rowena Corridor take you past plenty of fun eateries; one-of-a-kind shops selling such goods as vintage modern furniture; and venues hosting the neighborhood's hot indie and alternative rock scene.

# Ride Log

- P1 Sliver Lake Meadow
- P2 Neutra VDL Research House
- P3 Fargo Street—steepest in Los Angeles
- P4 Laurel and Hardy Park & Music Box Stairs
- P5 Bellevue Park
- P6 Sunset Junction
- P7 Shakespeare Bridge
- P8 Griffith Park

B

- B1 Coco's Variety Store
  2427 Riverside Dr, Los Angeles
- B2 Echo Park Cycles
  1932 Echo Park Blvd, Echo Park
- B3 Speedworkz Bike Shop
  3112 Sunset Blvd, Los Angeles
- B4 Golden Saddle Cyclery
  1618Lucile Ave, Los Angeles

*Cyclists of every ilk enjoy this area.*

**0.0** Begin in the vicinity of Silver Lake Meadow. Star riding south (the lake will be on your right) using th bike lane on Silver Lake Blvd.

**0.1** Pass the Neutra VDL Research House.

**0.7** Just past the Silver Lake dog park, turn right ont Van Pelt Pl and pass the Silver Lake Recreation Center

**0.8** Turn right onto West Silver Lake Dr.

**0.9** Continue to the right where West Silver Lake D crosses Redesdale Ave.

**1.7** Turn right onto Tesla Ave.

**1.9** Turn right onto Armstrong Ave.

**2.2** Turn right onto Silver Lake Blvd.

**2.9** Just past the Silver Lake dog park, continu straight (south) on Silver Lake Blvd.

**3.6** Angle to the right onto Parkman Ave.

**3.7** Turn right onto Sunset Blvd.

**4.2** Angle to the right (actually straight) onto Griffith Park Blvd. If you miss this turn and come to Edgecliff or Lucile avenues, turn right for one block to rejoi the route.

**5.5** Turn right onto Hyperion Ave. Bike lane ends.

**5.7** Turn right onto Rowena Ave.

**6.2** Rowena Ave merges with Glendale Blvd.

**6.5** Continue to the right on Glendale Blvd at the signal.

**6.7** Turn right onto Silver Lake Blvd.

**6.9** Arrive back at Silver Lake Meadow.

**Silver Lake**

Altitude ft: 550, 450, 350

Distance miles: 0, 1, 2, 3, 4, 5, 6, 6.9

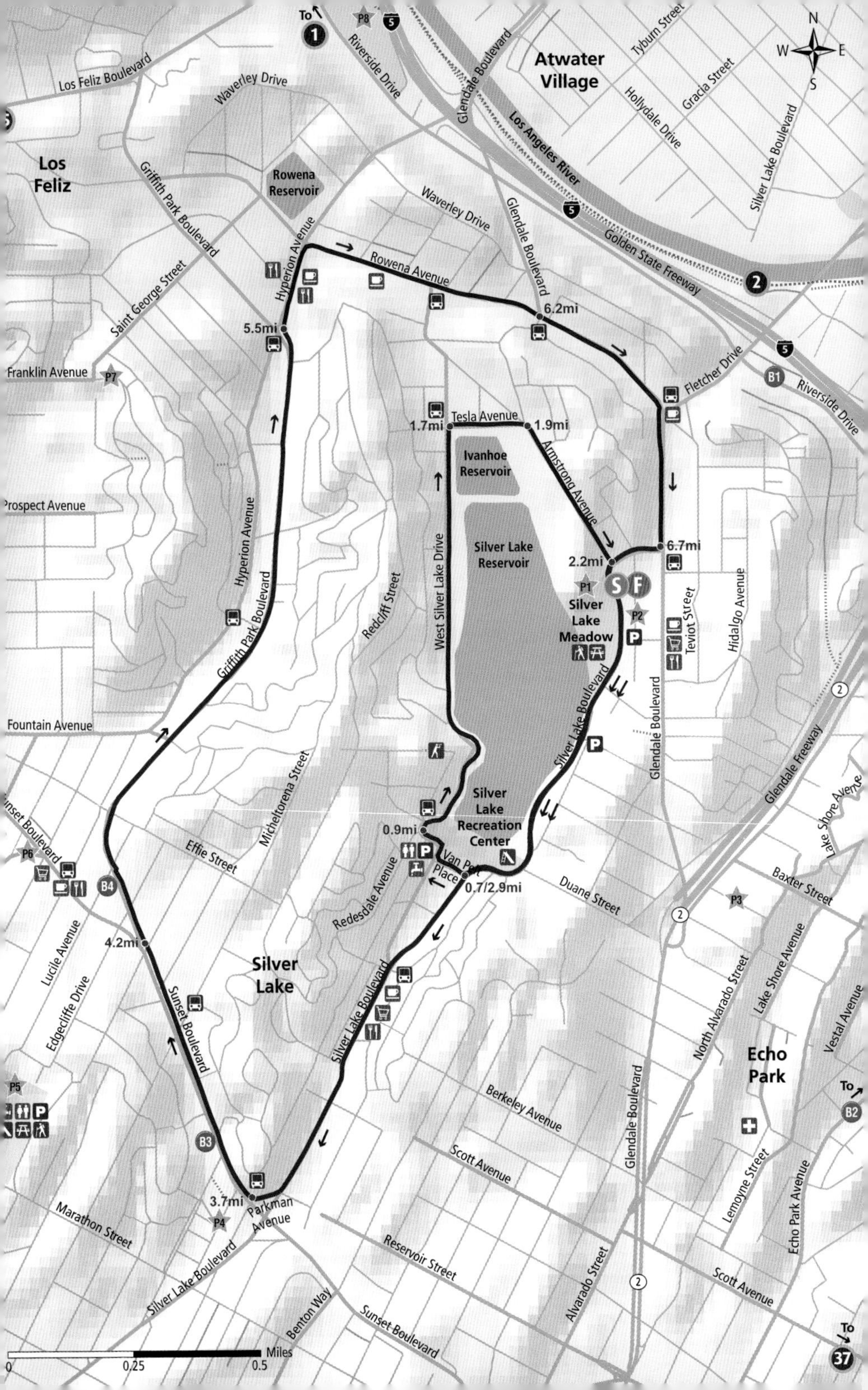

Atwater Village
Los Feliz
Silver Lake
Echo Park
Rowena Reservoir
Ivanhoe Reservoir
Silver Lake Reservoir
Silver Lake Meadow
Silver Lake Recreation Center
Los Angeles River
Golden State Freeway
Glendale Freeway
Los Feliz Boulevard
Waverley Drive
Riverside Drive
Glendale Boulevard
Tyburn Street
Gracia Street
Hollydale Drive
Silver Lake Boulevard
Griffith Park Boulevard
Saint George Street
Hyperion Avenue
Rowena Avenue
Fletcher Drive
Franklin Avenue
Tesla Avenue
Armstrong Avenue
Prospect Avenue
West Silver Lake Drive
Redcliff Street
Teviot Street
Hidalgo Avenue
Fountain Avenue
Micheltorena Street
Effie Street
Sunset Boulevard
Van Pelt Place
Redesdale Avenue
Duane Street
Baxter Street
Lake Shore Avenue
Lucile Avenue
Edgecliffe Drive
North Alvarado Street
Vestal Avenue
Berkeley Avenue
Scott Avenue
Lemoyne Street
Echo Park Avenue
Marathon Street
Parkman Avenue
Reservoir Street
Alvarado Street
Benton Way
To
0.7/2.9mi
0.9mi
1.7mi
1.9mi
2.2mi
3.7mi
4.2mi
5.5mi
6.2mi
6.7mi
Miles
0
0.25
0.5
N
S
E
W

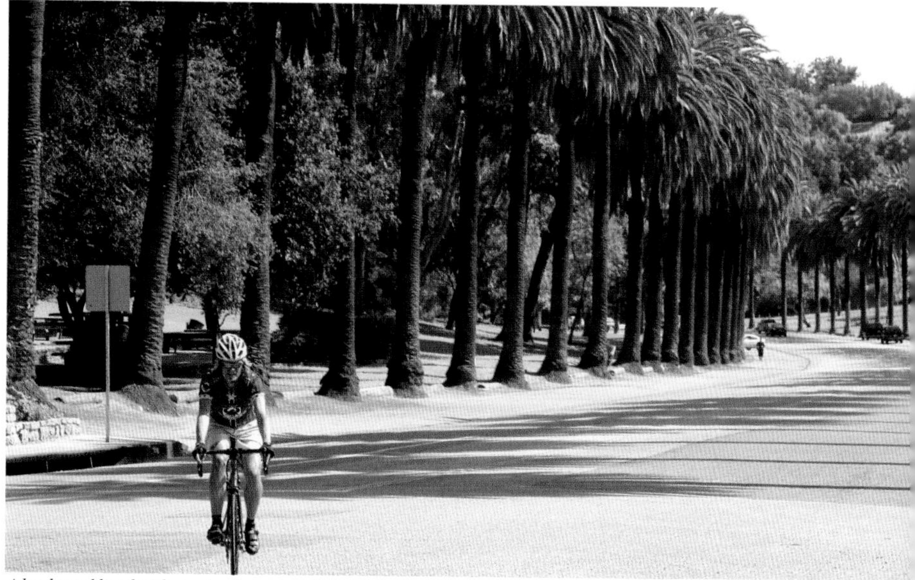

*A boulevard lined with regal palms curves through the park.*

## At a Glance

**Distance** 7.5 miles **Elevation Gain** 750 feet

### Terrain

Rolling terrain, punctuated by two moderate climbs, characterizes the ride. Inside the park, road conditions are fair, with some potholes and patches of loose surface (watch for them).

### Traffic

Traffic within the park is typically light, except when crowds descend on Dodgers Stadium. So, it's best to avoid cycling here immediately before or after a game (baseball season is April to October). Always be extra-vigilant at road crossings.

### How to Get There

From the 5 Freeway, exit at Stadium Way; or from the 110 Freeway, at Hill Street/Stadium Way. Follow signs to Grace E. Simons Lodge and park along Elysian Park Drive or nearby in one of the park's free lots. Metro Gold Line's Chinatown station is near Stadium Way, via College Street to Chavez Ravine.

### Food and Drink

The surrounding neighborhoods, such as Echo Park, reached via Elysian Park Avenue to Sunset, offer plenty of dining and snack options.

### Side Trip

It's an easy ride on North Broadway or Stadium Way to Chinatown, with its eclectic shops, cultural ambiance and authentic Asian cuisines, including Chinese, Cambodian, Thai and Vietnamese.

**Links to**   

**Where to Bike Rating** 

 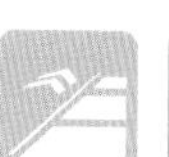  

# About...

In Greek mythology, the afterlife paradise of heroes and poets was known as the Elysian Fields (later inspiration for the Champs-Elysées in Paris). Los Angeles' Elysian Park, along the northern fringes of downtown, may not be an afterlife paradise, but it's surprisingly idyllic: a relatively undiscovered cycling realm with lush wooded hillsides, native chaparral, green meadows and unfolding vistas of the urban landscape below.

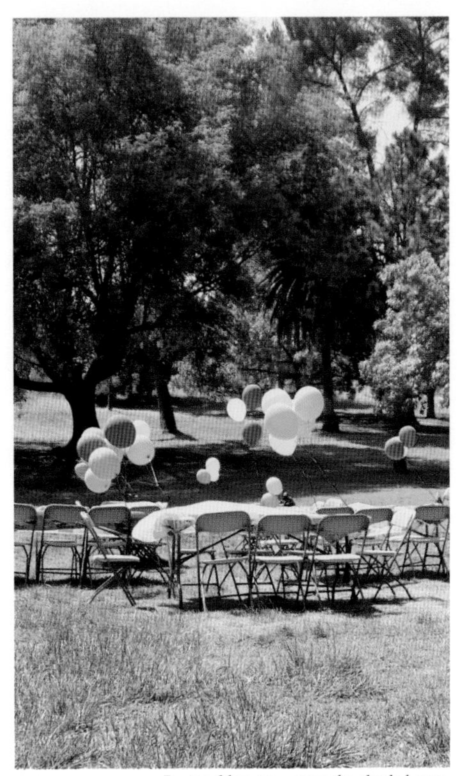

*Parties blossom across the shady lawns.*

The Pasadena Freeway heading north from Downtown Los Angeles passes through a series of 1930s era portals, four short tunnels bored through low, green, forested hills. As you enter these passageways—collectively know as the Figueroa Street Tunnels—you might wonder: What's up there? Though a mystery to many, it's a glimpse of Elysian Park, the city's oldest and second-largest park, encompassing some 600 acres of urban woodland.

Given the character of this undulant landscape, we could have easily named this ride "Trees and Overlooks." A remarkable little journey, it begins from the Chavez Ravine Arboretum (the oldest in Southern California), a canyon with more than 1,000 species of native and imported trees. You pedal through walnut woodlands before the winding route leads you among eucalyptus, pine, oaks and palms. Of particular note are the grove of deodar cedars, nestled in a glen between Point Grandview and Elysian Reservoir, and the grand allée of wild date palms along Stadium Way. The ride's concluding miles, on Elysian Park Drive, along the park's western edge, have the feel of a country road meandering amid stands of eucalyptus and native live oak, revealing views of the meadows below. Occasionally you will get glimpses of playgrounds and walking trails.

The park's many lookouts over the city are stunning. Early in the ride, after you cross Stadium Way and crest a modest hill, you'll be rewarded with the first of these urban vistas: Angel's Overlook. Further along the ridgeline road, past several turnouts with excellent views of the Elysian Valley and Glendale Narrows (juncture of the Los Angeles River and Arroyo Seco), you'll reach Point Grandview: one of the finest perches for gazing at the downtown skyline and, on a good air day, Long Beach and Catalina Island, in the distance to the south. From atop Park Row Drive Bridge, spanning the 110 Freeway, just past Elysian Reservoir, you'll see myriad taillights of cars heading toward downtown. Rejoice at not being down there. Finally, the Victory Memorial Grove overlook on Lilac Terrace, offers a spectacular view of the green hillsides of Chavez Ravine and Bishop Canyon, on the park's northern edge.

# Ride Log

0.0 From the intersection of Stadium Way and Elysian Park Dr, begin a short climb upward, following the signs pointing to "Northeast Little League."

0.4 Angels Point overlook.

0.9 Pass the Northeast L.A. Little League baseball diamonds at Elysian Fields.

1.4 Stay to the left on the upper road at the Y—the lower road leads to Solano Canyon Rd.

1.6 Turn left onto Grand View Dr toward Elysian Reservoir and Point Grandview overlook. This road has no sign, but it's the only one in this area turning left.

2.0 Point Grandview overlook.

2.8 Elysian Reservoir.

2.9 Turn left at Park Row St (follow signs pointing to the North Broadway entrance). If you're looking for a shorter ride without the second climb, turn right here, then left onto Solano Canyon Dr and rejoin the route at Academy Rd.

3.4 Turn right onto Elysian Park Dr.

3.6 Turn right onto North Broadway.

3.7 Turn right onto Solano Ave.

3.9 Turn left at Amador St and pass the entrance to Radio Hill Gardens (unless you're making the recommended excursion up to the gardens).

4.2 Turn right on Jarvis St at the stop sign and then, left onto Solano Ave. Merge onto Academy Rd.

4.9 Los Angeles Police Academy.

5.0 Turn right onto Academy Rd.

5.3 Continue on Academy (at the stop sign, you'll actually make a left to remain on Academy) then turn left onto Stadium Way.

5.9 Turn right onto Elysian Park Ave.

6.0 Turn right onto Lilac Terrace at the sign pointing to "Victory Memorial Grove at Elysian Park" and follow the road upward, making a sharp right turn through an open gate and passing Lilac Terrace Park.

6.4 Pass around the gate at the end of Lilac onto Elysian Park Dr.

6.7 Pass around a gate, cross Scott Ave, and pass around a second gate, continuing on Elysian Park Dr.

6.9 Pass around a gate, cross Academy Rd, and pass around a second gate, continuing on Elysian Park Dr.

7.3 Pass around a gate, pass Grace E. Simons Lodge.

7.5 Finish the ride at Stadium Way.

P1 Dodger Stadium
P2 Los Angeles Police Academy
P3 Chinatown
P4 Grace E Simmons Lodge
P5 Chavez Ravine Arboretum
P6 Memorial Victory Grove
P7 Avenue of the Palms
P8 Radio Hill Gardens
P9 Los Angeles Historic State Park
P10 Los Angeles River Center & Gardens

B1 Echo Park Cycles
1932 Echo Park Blvd, Echo Park
B2 Flying Pigeon L.A.
3714 N. Figueroa St, Los Angeles
B3 Bike Oven
3706 N. Figueroa St, Los Angeles

## Elysian Park

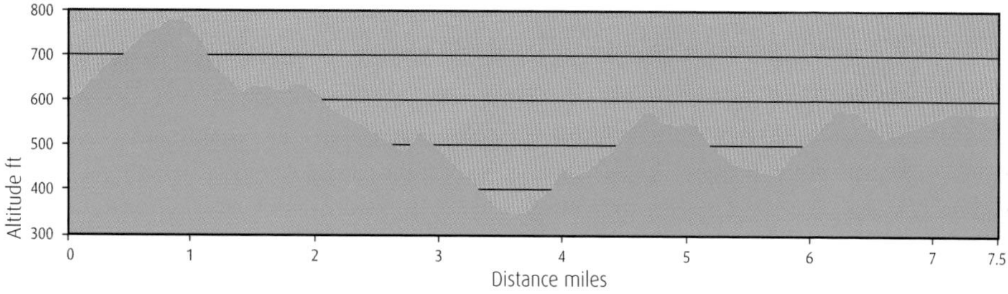

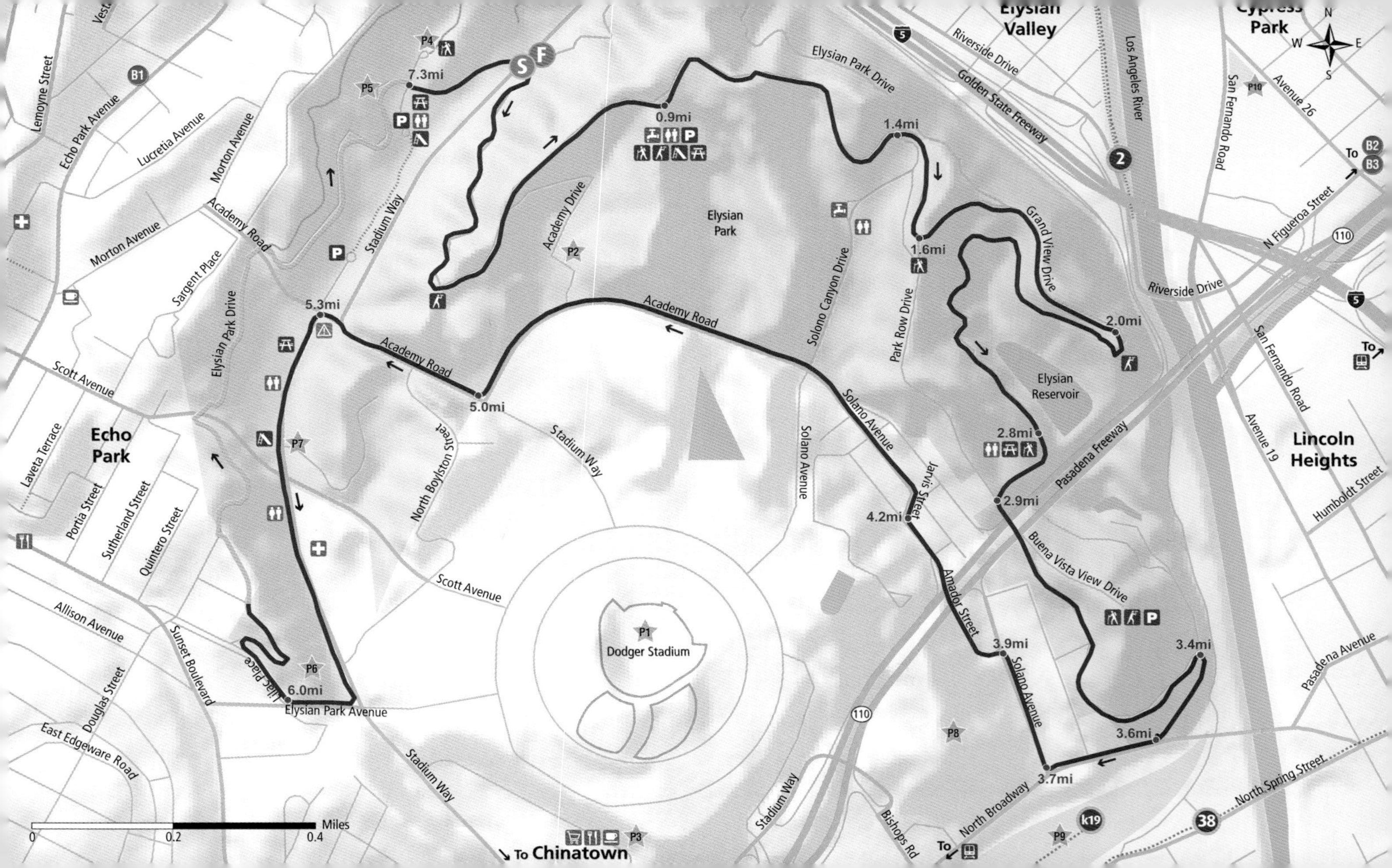
Elysian Valley
Cypress Park
Lincoln Heights
Echo Park
Elysian Park
Elysian Reservoir
Dodger Stadium
To Chinatown
Los Angeles River
Riverside Drive
Golden State Freeway
Elysian Park Drive
San Fernando Road
Avenue 26
N Figueroa Street
Grand View Drive
Park Row Drive
Solono Canyon Drive
Academy Drive
Academy Road
Stadium Way
Solano Avenue
Jarvis Street
Amador Street
Pasadena Freeway
Buena Vista View Drive
Avenue 19
Humboldt Street
Pasadena Avenue
North Spring Street
North Broadway
Bishops Rd
North Boylston Street
Scott Avenue
Elysian Park Avenue
Lilac Place
Sunset Boulevard
Allison Avenue
Douglas Street
East Edgeware Road
Quintero Street
Sutherland Street
Portia Street
Laveta Terrace
Sargent Place
Morton Avenue
Lucretia Avenue
Echo Park Avenue
Lemoyne Street
0.9mi
1.4mi
1.6mi
2.0mi
2.8mi
2.9mi
3.4mi
3.6mi
3.7mi
3.9mi
4.2mi
5.0mi
5.3mi
6.0mi
7.3mi
Miles
0
0.2
0.4

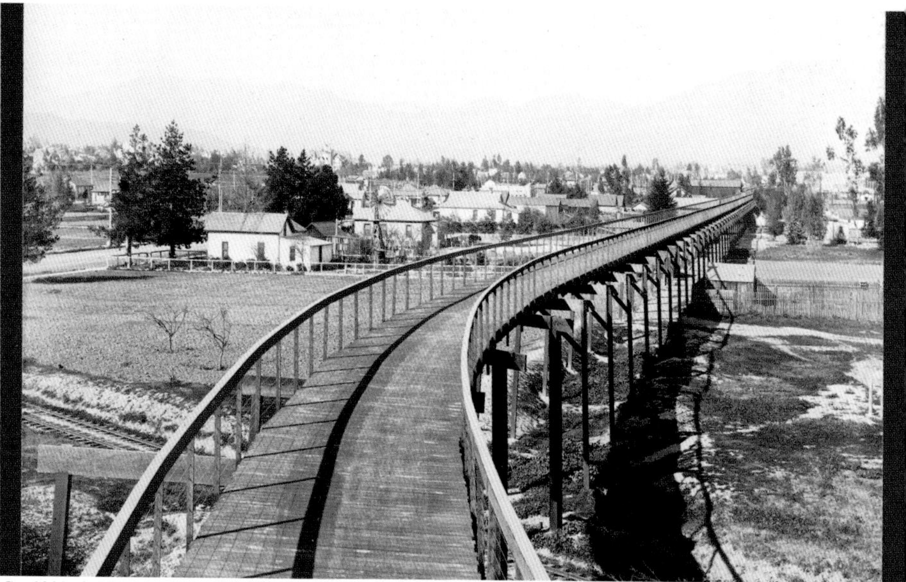

*Ca. 1900, the elevated tollway, made of pine painted green, was wide enough for four cyclists. (Photo coutesy of the Archives, Pasedena Museum of History.)*

## At a Glance

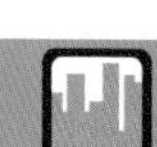

**Distance** 20.0 miles **Elevation Gain** 1,100 feet

### Terrain

Climbing gradually from Union Station to Pasadena, the route combines city streets with a streamside concrete bike path through Arroyo Seco. (After rainfall, leaves and twigs tend to clutter the path.)

### Traffic

The Arroyo Seco path is car-free. On the streets, traffic tends to be light, though more congested near Old Pasadena.

### How to Get There

Exit the 101 Freeway at Alameda Street or the 110 at Hill Street, then follow signs to Chinatown. Park in one of this neighborhood's many inexpensive lots (or in a lot near Union Station). Alternatively, travel to Union Station via Metro train (Red, Purple or Gold line) or bus.

### Food and Drink

Old Pasadena has plenty of refreshment options, from espresso bars to ice cream parlors. Near Union Station: Chinatown specializes in Asian cuisines and Olvera Street in Mexican fare. And Philippe's, the French-dipped Sandwich's alleged birthplace, is a block north of the station.

### Side Trip

The Heritage Square Museum, at Griffin Avenue and East Avenue 43, features a collection of eight Victorian homes, including the Octagon House. Old Pasadena offers museums, galleries, restaurants, unique shops and historic buildings.

**Links to** 2 15 37 41 K6 K19

**Where to Bike Rating** 

 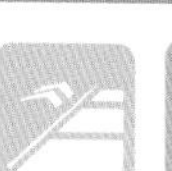  

# About...

Our California Cycleway ride emulates a long-defunct bicycle "highway," dreamed up by a cycling pioneer and promoter from Pasadena. Even more than 100 years later, this ride remains enjoyable and rewarding, connecting the many diversions in and between downtown Los Angeles and Pasadena. If you prefer a one-way ride, you can return to Union Station on Metro's Gold Line train.

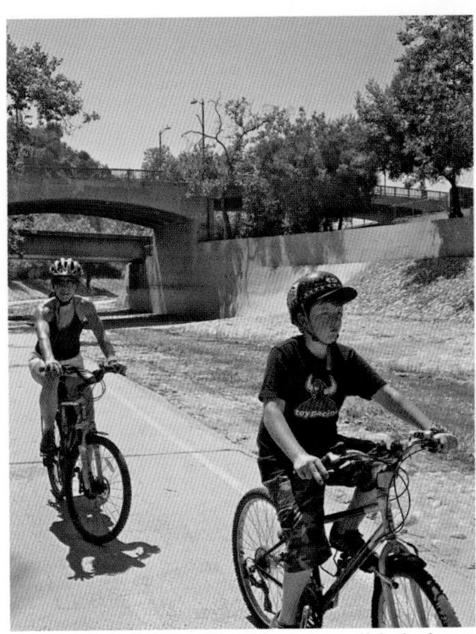

*Today's Arroyo Seco bike path parallels the former California Cycleway.*

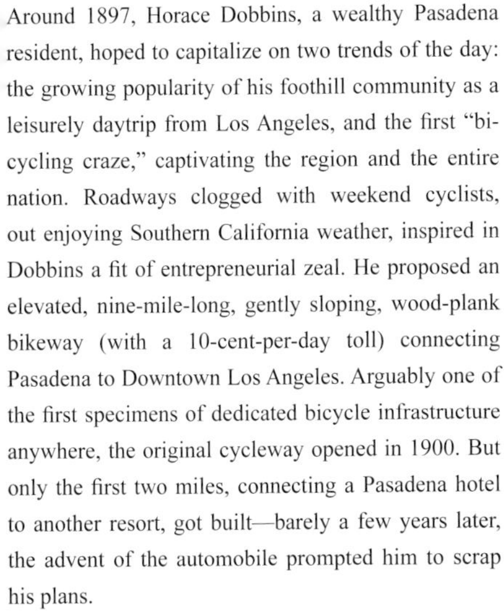

Around 1897, Horace Dobbins, a wealthy Pasadena resident, hoped to capitalize on two trends of the day: the growing popularity of his foothill community as a leisurely daytrip from Los Angeles, and the first "bicycling craze," captivating the region and the entire nation. Roadways clogged with weekend cyclists, out enjoying Southern California weather, inspired in Dobbins a fit of entrepreneurial zeal. He proposed an elevated, nine-mile-long, gently sloping, wood-plank bikeway (with a 10-cent-per-day toll) connecting Pasadena to Downtown Los Angeles. Arguably one of the first specimens of dedicated bicycle infrastructure anywhere, the original cycleway opened in 1900. But only the first two miles, connecting a Pasadena hotel to another resort, got built—barely a few years later, the advent of the automobile prompted him to scrap his plans.

In the spirit of Dobbins, our "Cycleway" begins at Union Station's transit hub, in Downtown Los Angeles, near his bikeway's intended southern terminus. From there, we follow streets amid old warehouses and rail lines before turning north along the eastern side of Arroyo Seco, in the Lincoln Heights neighborhood, full of vintage Craftsman-style bungalows. Our route soon joins a bike trail deeper in the Arroyo Seco, right along the water (see Kids' Ride 6). Dobbins's cycleway would have had a similar atmosphere: a shaded path paralleling a flowing creek.

Further north, crossing into Pasadena proper, our route continues along the arroyo's east side, through a neighborhood of gracious homes on quiet, tree-lined streets, making for tranquil, picturesque riding. (The houses on California Boulevard are especially grand.) After a short descent into Old Pasadena, our cycleway ride reaches its northern terminus, at Green Street and Fair Oaks Avenue—near the starting point of Dobbins's wooden bikeway, just behind the Moorish Colonial-style Castle Green apartments, formerly a hotel.

Whether you ride our cycleway from Downtown Los Angeles north or from Pasadena south, we encourage you to explore the neighborhoods around either end. If you run out of steam or time, you can always return via Metro's Gold Line from the Del Mar or Memorial Park stations in Pasadena, or, conversely, from Union Station in Los Angeles.

# Ride Log

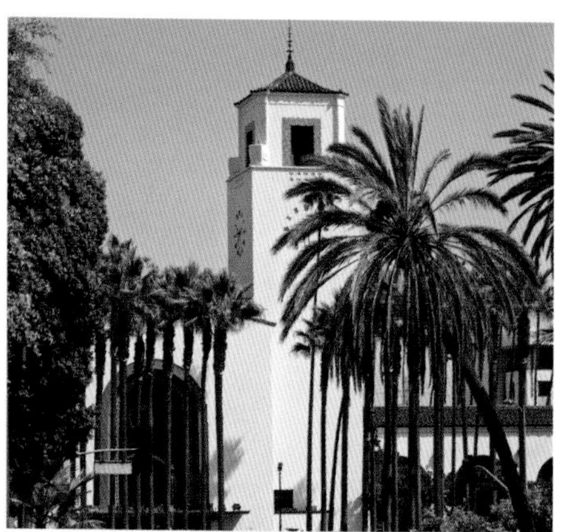

*Union Station, built in Downtown L.A. in 1939, punctuates the ride's start.*

**0.0** From Union Station, begin riding towards the mountains on North Alameda St, which becomes North Spring St at College St.

**1.5** Continue straight when North Spring merges with North Broadway.

**2.2** Turn left on Griffin Ave.

**4.1** Cross Griffin just past the soccer fields (to your left) and the Audubon Center (to your right). Watch the cross traffic in both directions. Follow the access ramp down through the gate to the concrete bike path near the bottom of Arroyo Seco. Continue north. If there is any possibility of rain or high water in the arroyo, do not use this bike path. Instead, continue on Griffin Ave/South Ave 52 for roughly 0.8 miles. Turn right on Figueroa St for 1.1 miles to York Blvd, then turn right and ride for 0.8 miles, rejoining the cycleway at Arroyo Dr.

**6.0** Leave Arroyo Seco via the access ramp where the bike path ends. Pass through the park and turn left on Marmion Way.

**6.2** Turn right on Pasadena Ave.

**6.5** Turn left on Arroyo Dr, which becomes South Arroyo Blvd at Columbia St.

**8.5** Turn right on California Blvd.

**8.7** Turn left on Grand Ave.

**9.3** Turn right on Green St.

**10.0** Arrive at the corner of Green and Raymond. The northern terminus of the first California Cycleway was behind the Castle Green Apartments—the Moorish Colonial style building occupying this corner. To return to Union Station, turn right on Raymond Ave.

**10.6** Turn right on California Blvd.

**11.6** Turn left on South Arroyo Blvd, which becomes Arroyo Dr at Columbia St.

**13.5** Merge right onto Pasadena Ave.

**13.8** Turn left on Arroyo Verde Rd at the signal, which becomes Marmion Way.

**13.9** Turn right into the park and then onto the Arroyo Seco Bike Path.

**15.8** Exit Arroyo Seco at the soccer fields.

**15.9** Turn right on Griffin Ave.

**17.9** Turn right on North Broadway. Continue on North Spring St at South 18th Ave.

**20.0** Union Station: end of the cycleway.

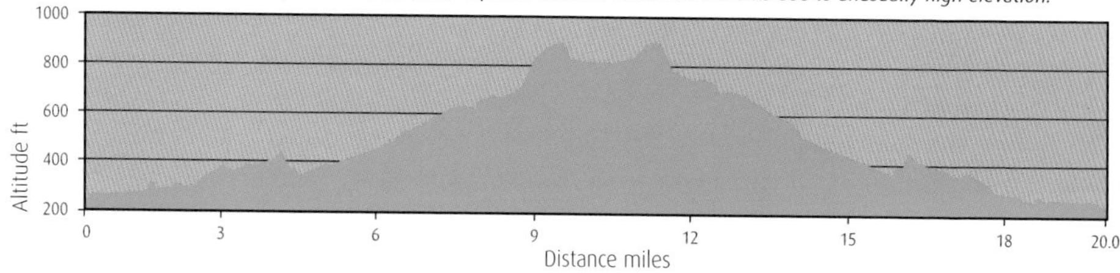

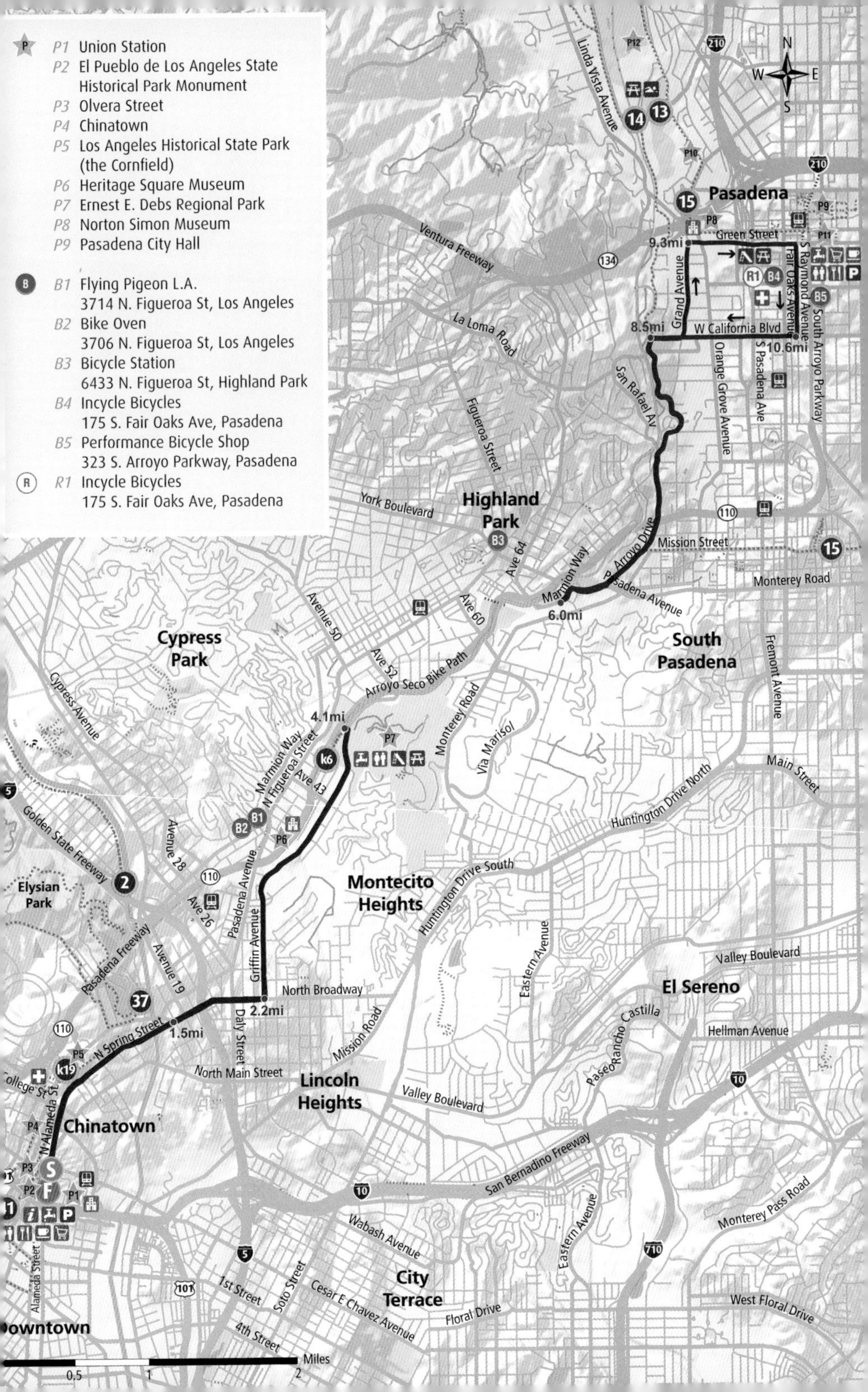
P1 Union Station
P2 El Pueblo de Los Angeles State Historical Park Monument
P3 Olvera Street
P4 Chinatown
P5 Los Angeles Historical State Park (the Cornfield)
P6 Heritage Square Museum
P7 Ernest E. Debs Regional Park
P8 Norton Simon Museum
P9 Pasadena City Hall
B1 Flying Pigeon L.A. 3714 N. Figueroa St, Los Angeles
B2 Bike Oven 3706 N. Figueroa St, Los Angeles
B3 Bicycle Station 6433 N. Figueroa St, Highland Park
B4 Incycle Bicycles 175 S. Fair Oaks Ave, Pasadena
B5 Performance Bicycle Shop 323 S. Arroyo Parkway, Pasadena
R1 Incycle Bicycles 175 S. Fair Oaks Ave, Pasadena
Pasadena
Highland Park
South Pasadena
Cypress Park
Montecito Heights
El Sereno
Lincoln Heights
Chinatown
City Terrace
Downtown
Elysian Park
Linda Vista Avenue
Ventura Freeway
La Loma Road
Figueroa Street
York Boulevard
Green Street
Grand Avenue
Fair Oaks Avenue
S Raymond Avenue
South Arroyo Parkway
W California Blvd
Orange Grove Avenue
S Pasadena Ave
San Rafael Av
Arroyo Drive
Marmion Way
Pasadena Avenue
Mission Street
Monterey Road
Fremont Avenue
Ave 64
Ave 60
Avenue 50
Ave 52
Arroyo Seco Bike Path
Ave 43
N Figueroa Street
Cypress Avenue
Golden State Freeway
Avenue 28
Pasadena Avenue
Ave 26
Griffin Avenue
Pasadena Freeway
Avenue 19
Via Marisol
Huntington Drive North
Huntington Drive South
Main Street
Eastern Avenue
Valley Boulevard
Rancho Castilla
Paseo
Hellman Avenue
North Broadway
N Spring Street
Daly Street
Mission Road
North Main Street
College St
N Alameda St
Alameda Street
San Bernadino Freeway
Monterey Pass Road
Wabash Avenue
Soto Street
1st Street
4th Street
Cesar E Chavez Avenue
Floral Drive
West Floral Drive
9.3mi
8.5mi
10.6mi
6.0mi
4.1mi
2.2mi
1.5mi
Miles
0.5
1
2

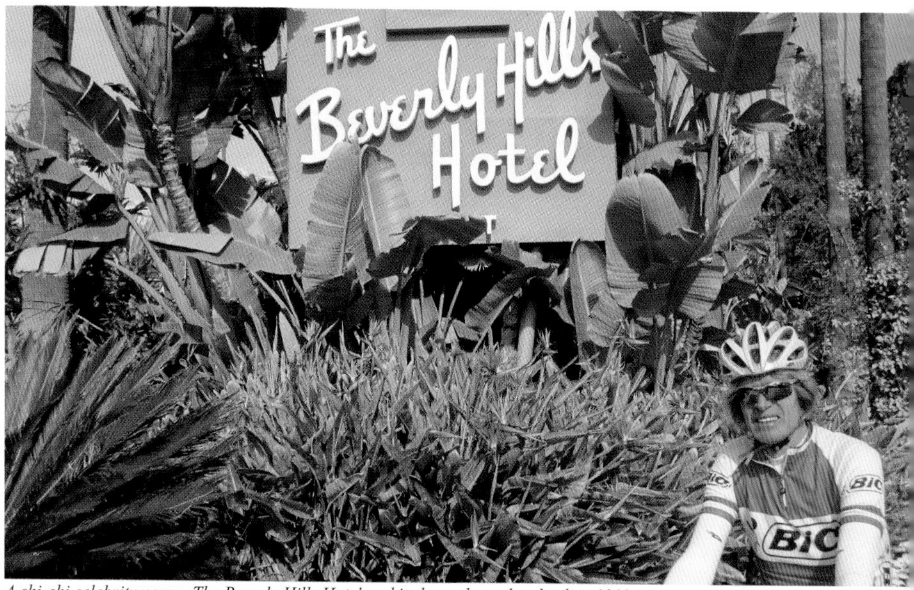


*A chi-chi celebrity venue, The Beverly Hills Hotel and its bungalows date back to 1912.*

## At a Glance

**Distance** 12.1 miles **Elevation Gain** 1,000 feet

### Terrain

Though much of the ride is on flats, its northern section has hills (hey, it's Beverly Hills).

### Traffic

The route follows quiet residential streets with few cars—except for the commercial blocks on Rodeo Drive and a short distance near City Hall, which sometimes have dense, but hardly high-speed, traffic.

### How to Get There

Exit the 405 Freeway at Santa Monica Boulevard, drive east approximately 2.5 miles and make a left onto Wilshire Boulevard. Turn right at Roxbury Drive and continue three blocks to Roxbury Memorial Park. From the Culver City Metro station, follow the first three miles of Ride 39.

### Food and Drink

From upscale dining to national chains, Santa Monica Boulevard has lots of eateries. Its coffee spots include Euro Caffe, between Rodeo and Camden drives.

### Side Trip

Greystone, a grand 1927 mansion with formal gardens, was built for oil tycoon Edward Doheny's son, who died there in a murder-suicide soon after the estate's completion. Now owned by the City of Beverly Hills, the property is open to the public as a city park, except during special events (daily, 10 a.m. to 5 p.m., PST, or until 6 p.m., PDT). From Loma Vista Drive turn left to Greystone's gates.

**Links to** 33 40

**Where to Bike Rating** 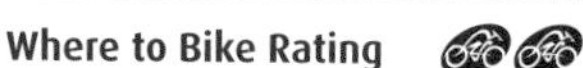

 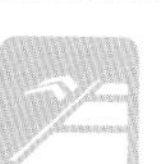  

# About...

This spin through Beverly Hills, world capitol of glamour, offers not merely a vicarious brush with lifestyles of the rich and famous—but also, simply, a chance to enjoy shady, gracious residential streets with remarkably few cars. With some notable architecture and green spaces en route, the journey sweeps by legendary hotels and mansions of stars of the silver screen (and airwaves), down Rodeo Drive with its swanky boutiques and past Beverly Hills' aptly opulent City Hall.

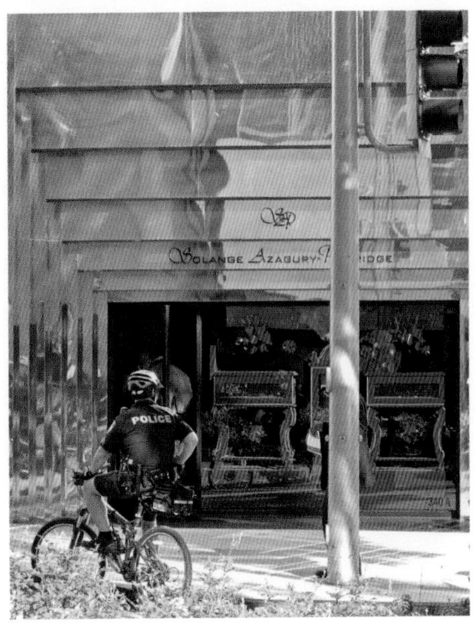

*A Beverly Hills bicycle cop contemplates a gemlike boutique on Rodeo Drive.*

In 1906, on exceptionally fertile ground for lima bean cultivation, the 5.7-square-mile city of Beverly Hills was founded—now a palm-studded enclave of affluence. Though we can't promise sightings of Hollywood glitterati (many live elsewhere, or cherish their privacy behind high hedges and tinted car windows), we can offer a pleasurable taste of this posh area. The major arteries here notoriously lack bike lanes, but many of Beverly Hills' lush residential streets are sparsely trafficked and refreshingly bikeable.

Early in our journey, we proceed up the gilded commercial stretch of Rodeo Drive, where Versace and Chanel await siliconed-cheek-by-liposuctioned-jowl with Harry Winston and Tiffany's. Gemlike boutiques with architectural pedigrees include number 333, Anderton Court (1952) by Frank Lloyd Wright, and number 343, Prada (2004) by OMA Rem Koolhaas. The Italianate 1928 Beverly Wilshire Hotel was home to Elvis, John Lennon and Richard Gere's character in *Pretty Woman*.

Onward through a leafy residential neighborhood, past the fanciful Spadena (or Witch's) House at Walden Drive and Carmelita Avenue. With its lopsided, pointy roof, artfully distressed paint and quirky windows, the 1921 building, now a private home, originally stood on a Culver City movie lot.

Loads of stars have lived in Beverly Hills. Take Carolwood Drive, right en route: Michael Jackson rented (and unfortunately died at) number 100; purportedly Mick Jagger holed up at 135; Burt Reynolds, Marilyn Monroe, Tony Curtis and Sony and Cher at 141; Elvis at 144; Barbra Streisand at 301; Clark Gable and Carole Lombard at 325; Walt Disney at 355; Gregory Peck at 375—the list rolls on across the neighborhood. If you're eager to ride a "star tour"—though most celebrity hideaways are, by design, hard to see—pick up a "star map" from a sidewalk vendor on Sunset or Hollywood Boulevard, but no vouching for accuracy.

The fairy godmother of Beverly Hills mansions—which transformed an agricultural backwater into a glamorous "playground"—was Pickfair, the fabled 1920s estate of silent film idols Mary Pickford and Douglas Fairbanks: 1143 Summit Drive. Alas, its 65 acres were subdivided and the house replaced by a McMansion. To experience similar vintage grounds, swing by Greystone (see: Side Trip), or Virginia Robinson Gardens (Places of Interest **7**). Finally, you'll pass Beverly Hills City Hall, a towering 1932 pseudo-Spanish extravaganza, flaunting Hollywood fantasy even in the civic realm.

# Ride Log

0.0 Depart from Roxbury Memorial Park and ride north along Roxbury Dr.
0.5 Turn right onto Charleville Blvd.
0.7 Turn left onto Rodeo Dr.
0.9 Cross Wilshire Blvd and then, continue on Rodeo.
1.5 Turn left onto Carmelita Ave.
1.9 Turn right onto Walden Dr.
2.3 Cross Lomitas Ave then, angle to the right onto Whittier Dr.
2.7 Cross Sunset Blvd.
2.9 Cross Lexington Rd.
3.0 Turn left onto Monovale Rd, which becomes Carolwood Dr.
3.7 Turn right onto Brooklawn Dr, at the bottom of a hill, then right onto Angelo Dr.
4.1 Turn left onto Benedict Canyon Rd. Cross traffic does not stop, so exercise caution when turning here.
4.2 Turn right onto Tower Rd, then right onto San Ysidro Dr.
4.7 Turn right onto Pickfair Way, which then becomes Summit Dr.
4.9 Stay to the right at the Y intersection with Carolyn Way.
5.1 Turn left onto Cove Way.
5.5 Turn left onto Hartford Way and then, left onto Lexington Rd.
6.0 Turn right onto Rexford Dr.
6.6 Turn left onto Elevado Ave.
6.7 Turn left onto Alpine Dr.
6.9 Turn right onto Lomitas Ave.
7.0 Turn left onto Foothill Rd.
7.4 Turn right onto Doheny Rd.
7.8 Turn left onto Loma Vista Dr. Be prepared for a short, steep climb.
7.9 Turn right onto Robert Ln.
8.1 Turn right onto Hillcrest Rd.
8.9 Turn right onto Carmelita Ave.
9.3 Turn right onto Alpine Dr.
9.6 Turn left onto Elevado Ave.
9.7 Turn left onto Rexford Dr.
10.2 Cross Santa Monica Blvd and pass City Hall.
10.6 Turn right onto Clifton Way.
10.7 Turn right onto Crescent Dr.
10.9 Turn left onto Brighton Way (a one-way street).
11.3 Turn left onto Bedford Dr (a one-way street).
11.4 Cross Wilshire Blvd (a dog-leg to the right).
11.5 Turn right onto Charleville Blvd.
11.6 Turn left onto Roxbury Dr.
12.1 Cross Olympic Blvd and arrive at Roxbury Memorial Park. End of ride.

P1 Century City Center
P2 Beverly Wilshire Hotel
P3 Rodeo Drive
P4 Beverly Gardens Park
P5 Spadena House
P6 Playboy Mansion
P7 Virginia Robinson Gardens
P8 Beverly Hills Hotel
P9 Will Rogers Memorial Park
P10 Coldwater Canyon Park
P11 Greystone Park & Mansion
P12 Beverly Hills City Hall
P13 Academy of Motion Picture Arts & Sciences
P14 Paley Center for Media
P15 The Museum of Tolerance

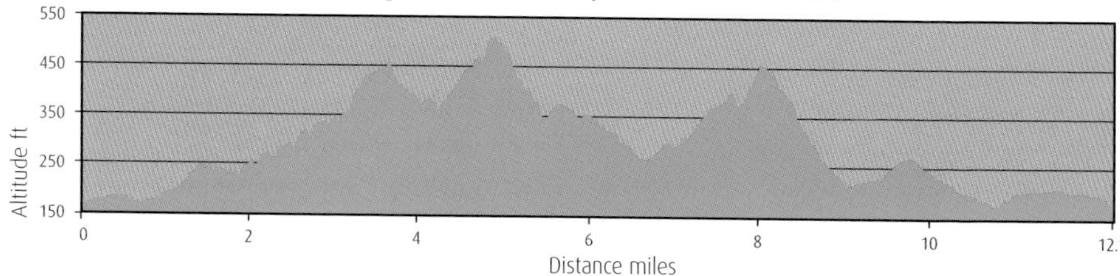

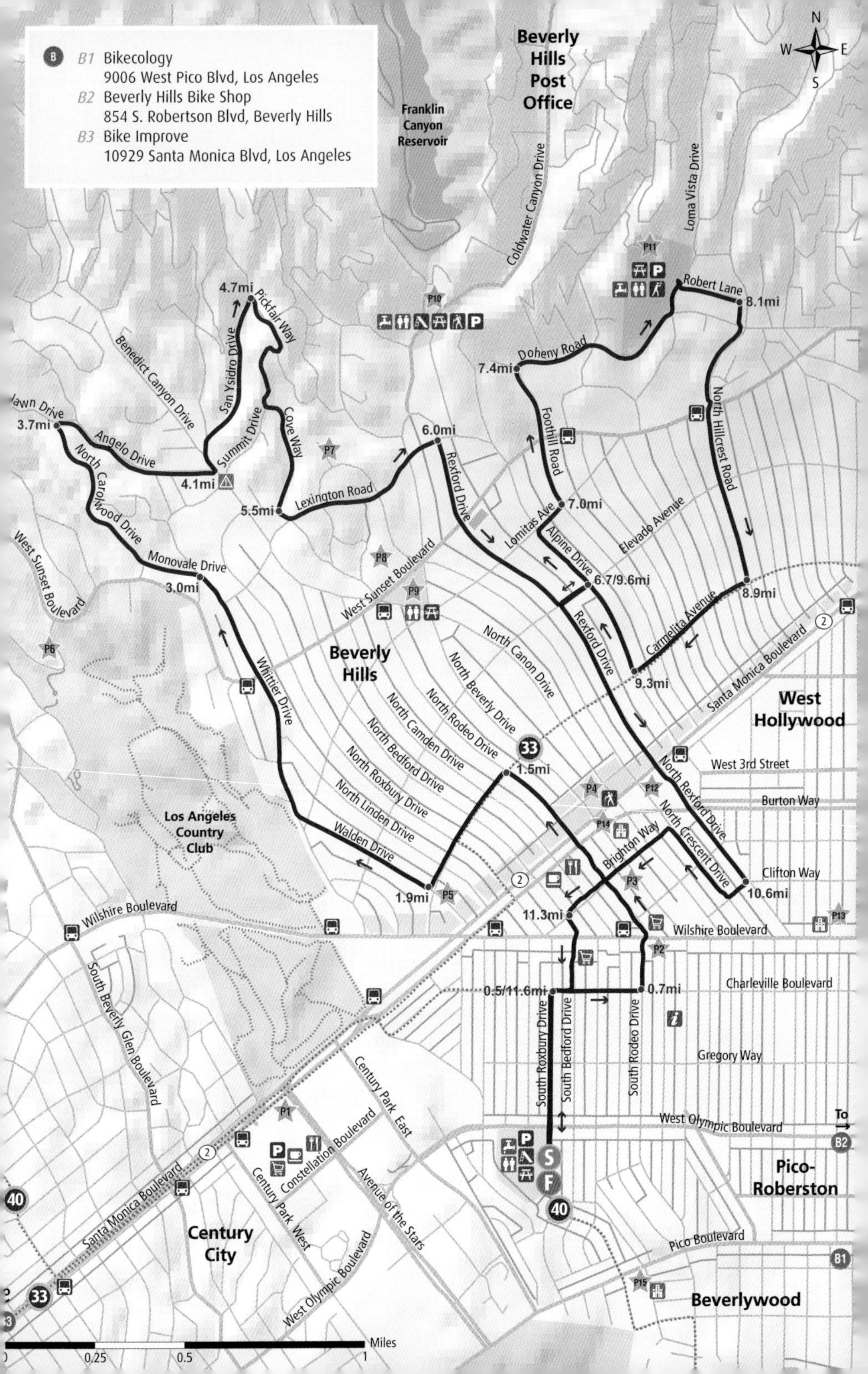

B1 Bikecology
9006 West Pico Blvd, Los Angeles
B2 Beverly Hills Bike Shop
854 S. Robertson Blvd, Beverly Hills
B3 Bike Improve
10929 Santa Monica Blvd, Los Angeles
Beverly Hills Post Office
Franklin Canyon Reservoir
Coldwater Canyon Drive
Loma Vista Drive
Robert Lane
8.1mi
Doheny Road
7.4mi
Pickfair Way
4.7mi
San Ysidro Drive
Benedict Canyon Drive
Cove Way
Summit Drive
Angelo Drive
3.7mi
4.1mi
North Carolwood Drive
Lexington Road
5.5mi
6.0mi
Rexford Drive
Foothill Road
7.0mi
North Hillcrest Road
Lomitas Ave
Alpine Drive
Elevado Avenue
6.7/9.6mi
8.9mi
Carmelita Avenue
9.3mi
Monovale Drive
3.0mi
West Sunset Boulevard
Whittier Drive
Beverly Hills
North Canon Drive
North Beverly Drive
North Rodeo Drive
North Camden Drive
North Bedford Drive
North Roxbury Drive
North Linden Drive
Walden Drive
1.5mi
1.9mi
Los Angeles Country Club
Santa Monica Boulevard
West Hollywood
West 3rd Street
Burton Way
North Rexford Drive
North Crescent Drive
Brighton Way
Clifton Way
10.6mi
11.3mi
Wilshire Boulevard
0.5/11.6mi
0.7mi
Charleville Boulevard
South Roxbury Drive
South Bedford Drive
South Rodeo Drive
Gregory Way
West Olympic Boulevard
To B2
South Beverly Glen Boulevard
Century Park East
Constellation Boulevard
Century Park West
Avenue of the Stars
Pico-Roberston
Century City
West Olympic Boulevard
Pico Boulevard
Beverlywood
Miles
0.25
0.5
1

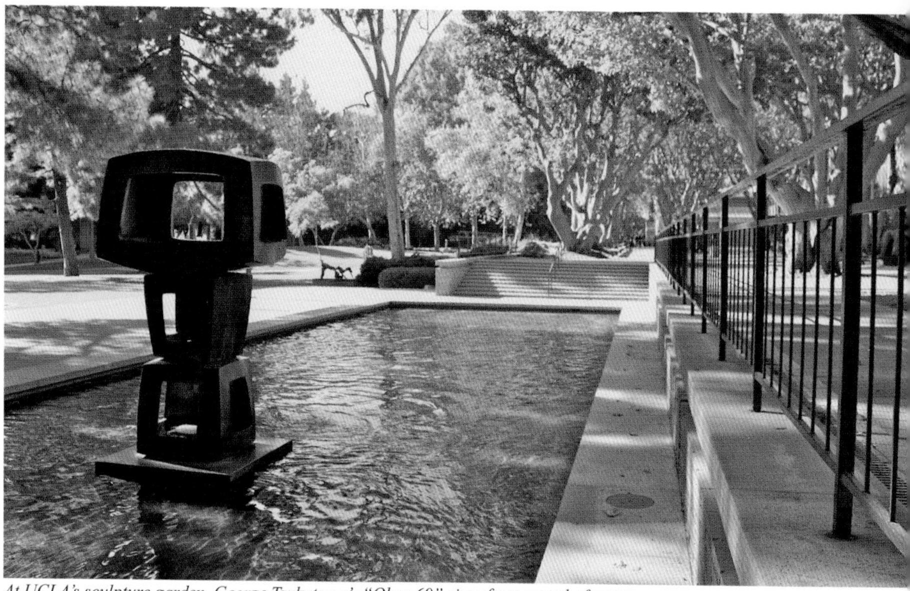

*At UCLA's sculpture garden, George Tsukatawa's "Obos 69" rises from a pool of water.*

## At a Glance

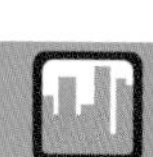

**Distance** 16.1 miles **Elevation Gain** 800 feet

### Terrain

Between Culver City and UCLA, the ride is mostly flat, apart from a few long, mild grades and a medium-intensity climb from Santa Monica Boulevard to the campus. The return trip is gradually downhill.

### Traffic

The route goes through quiet, low-traffic residential neighborhoods, except for two short high-traffic areas: Venice Boulevard at the Culver City Metro station and Santa Monica Boulevard through Century City.

### How to Get There

Board any Metro train to Downtown and transfer at Union Station or Seventh Street/Metro Center to the Expo Line. Disembark at Culver City (Expo Line's interim terminus until 2015). By car, exit the 10 Freeway at Robertson Boulevard and follow signs to Venice Boulevard and Expo Line parking (free).

### Food and Drink

Mid-ride, head into Westwood Village, a quintessential college town with lots of food and drink spots, from Jerry's Deli to Westwood Brewery.

### Side Trip

Visit the UCLA Hammer Museum, founded by late Occidental Petroleum CEO Armand Hammer. The permanent collection includes works by Rembrandt, Titian, Chardin and Daumier, Impressionist and Post-Impressionist paintings, contemporary art on paper and the UCLA Film & Television Archive. The museum is at Westwood and Wilshire boulevards. (Visit: **www.hammer.ucla.edu**.)

**Links to** 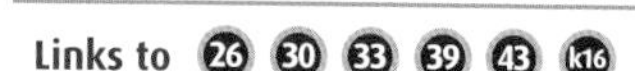


**Where to Bike Rating** 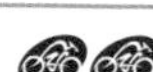

## About...

Whether you're a local or a tourist—visiting Westwood and the museums and gardens of UCLA—or a commuter to campus, this route allows you to connect to the university's offerings from Los Angeles's evolving and far-reaching light rail system. The ride begins at the Culver City Expo station (until 2015, the terminus of the new Expo Line) and meanders through mostly residential neighborhoods to the campus, with its forests, lawns, historic architecture, artwork, libraries and wealth of other publicly accessible resources.

In the 1950s, at the dawn of the tailfin, big outrageous cars and Southern California's booming freeway network, the vestiges of passenger light rail service on L.A.'s West Side sputtered to a final halt, choked by dwindling ridership. Soon, trolleys throughout L.A. were history. But now light rail is enjoying a comeback here, prompted by soaring fuel prices, clogged freeways and environmental foreboding. From L.A.'s newest light rail route, the Expo Line, this ride proposes an easy 5.7-mile connector to the UCLA campus, a place notoriously expensive for parking but great to explore by bike. Our ride makes a campus loop before returning to Culver City. It's a journey suitable for commuters to UCLA, as well as visitors perusing such campus highlights as the Fowler Museum, Franklin D. Murphy Sculpture Garden and Mildred E. Mathias Botanical Gardens.

This route winds from Culver City's Expo station through low-key residential streets in Castle Heights and Beverlywood, crosses a quiet corner of Beverly Hills and proceeds on Santa Monica Boulevard for 1.2 miles. Once on Westholme Avenue, you'll ascend through a pleasant residential neighborhood to UCLA.

This is one of the University of California's flagship campuses—spanning 419 rolling, wooded acres.

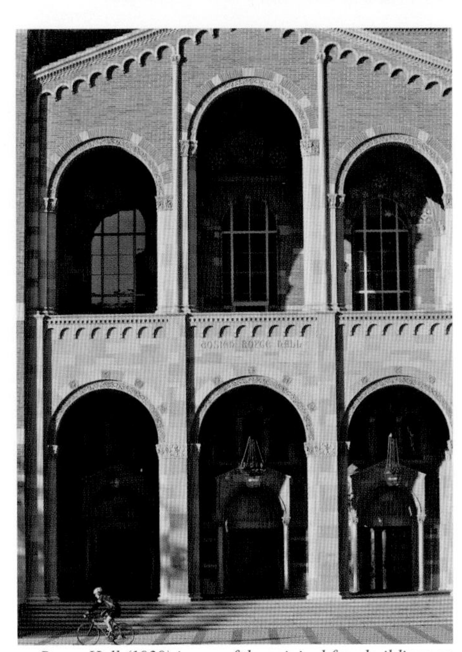

*Royce Hall (1929) is one of the original four buildings on UCLA's current campus.*

Founded in 1919, UCLA is a public research university with 163 buildings, seven professional schools, major teaching hospitals and nearly 40,000 students. Our loop nears a quad with the campus's four original buildings, including Royce Hall and Powell Library, rendered in Romanesque-revival style. Up the road, at the sculpture garden, you can wander (or lounge on the grass) among some 70 works by the likes of Rodin, Miró, Noguchi, David Smith and Richard Serra. But to really smell the flowers, stop by the seven lush acres of UCLA's botanical gardens: its bird and butterfly garden, its areas devoted to California, Australian and Hawaiian native plants, respectively, and much more. Or swing by the Fowler Museum for art and culture of Africa, Asia and the Americas. On-campus museums and gardens are admission free (for hours, see: **www.happenings.ucla.edu/arts**).

Once back in Culver City, you can hop the light rail to points near and far—Downtown L.A., Pasadena or Long Beach. You can take the Expo Line to UCLA's rival: USC. Or if you're feeling really energetic, you can even get there by bike (see Ride 43).

# Ride Log

- *P1* The Museum of Tolerance
- *P2* Roxbury Memorial Park
- *P3* Rodeo Drive
- *P4* Century City Center
- *P5* Hannah Carter Japanese Garden
- *P6* Murphy Sculpture Garden
- *P7* Fowler Museum of Cultural History
- *P8* Mildred E. Mathais Botanical Garden
- *P9* Inverted Fountain
- *P10* Regency Village Theatre (Fox Theater, 1931)
- *P11* Hammer Museum
- *P12* Museum of Jurassic Technology

**0.0** Starting from the Expo Line station, cross Venice Blvd at the crosswalk and commence riding west.
**0.4** Turn right onto Main St/Bagely Ave.
**0.7** Turn left onto Harlow Ave after crossing under the 10 Freeway.
**0.9** Turn right onto Castle Heights Ave as Harlow ends.
**2.1** Turn right onto Beverwil Dr.
**2.6** Turn left onto Cashio St at the signal.
**2.7** Turn right onto Roxbury Dr as Cashio ends.
**3.3** Pass Roxbury Memorial Park and then, cross Olympic Blvd.
**3.7** Turn left onto Charleville Blvd.
**4.1** Angle to the left onto Durant Dr.
**4.2** Turn right onto Moreno Dr, cross South Santa Monica at the signal and angle left onto Santa Monica Blvd westbound. Join the bike lane. Note: This artery has no bike lane for a short distance, so feel free to ride this section of the boulevard on its broad sidewalk.
**5.4** Turn right onto Westholme Ave.
**6.0** Cross Wilshire Blvd.
**6.7** Cross Hilgard Ave and enter the UCLA campus.
**6.8** Turn right onto Charles E. Young Dr South.
**6.9** Turn right onto Circle Dr East.
**7.4** Turn left onto Charles E. Young Dr North.
**7.6** Turn right onto Royce Dr.
**7.7** Turn left onto Charles E. Young Dr North.
**8.2** Turn left onto Charles E. Young Dr West at the stop sign.
**8.7** Turn left onto Charles E. Young Dr South at Ronald Reagan Medical Center.
**9.3** Turn right onto Westholme Ave.
**10.0** Cross Wilshire Blvd.
**10.7** Turn left onto Santa Monica Blvd.
**11.7** Continue straight using the far right lane marked "Santa Monica Blvd Local Access Only" at Century Park East.
**11.8** Turn right onto Moreno Dr, then left onto Druant Dr.
**12.1** Angle to the right onto Charleville Blvd.
**12.3** Turn right onto Roxbury Dr.
**12.7** Cross Olympic Blvd, pass Roxbury Memorial Park.
**13.3** Turn left onto Cashio as Roxbury Dr ends.
**13.5** Turn right onto Beverwil Dr at the signal.
**13.9** Turn left onto Castle Heights Ave at the stop sign.
**15.1** Turn left onto Harlow as Castle Heights Ave ends.
**15.4** Turn right onto Bagely Ave and cross under the 405 Freeway.
**15.8** Turn left onto Venice Blvd at the signal, joining the bike lane.
**16.1** Arrive back at the Expo Line station. End of ride.

### The UCLA Connection

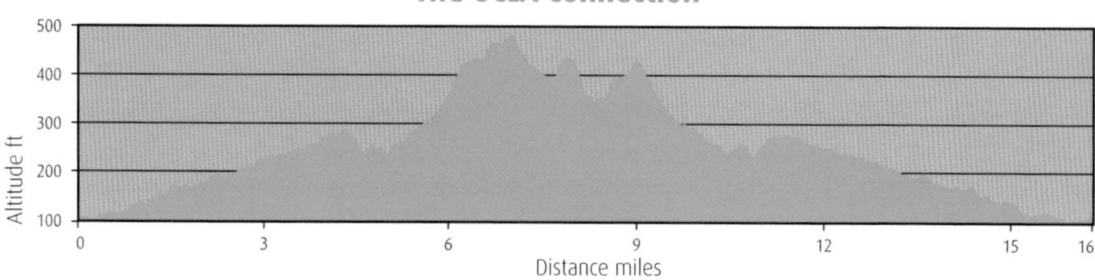

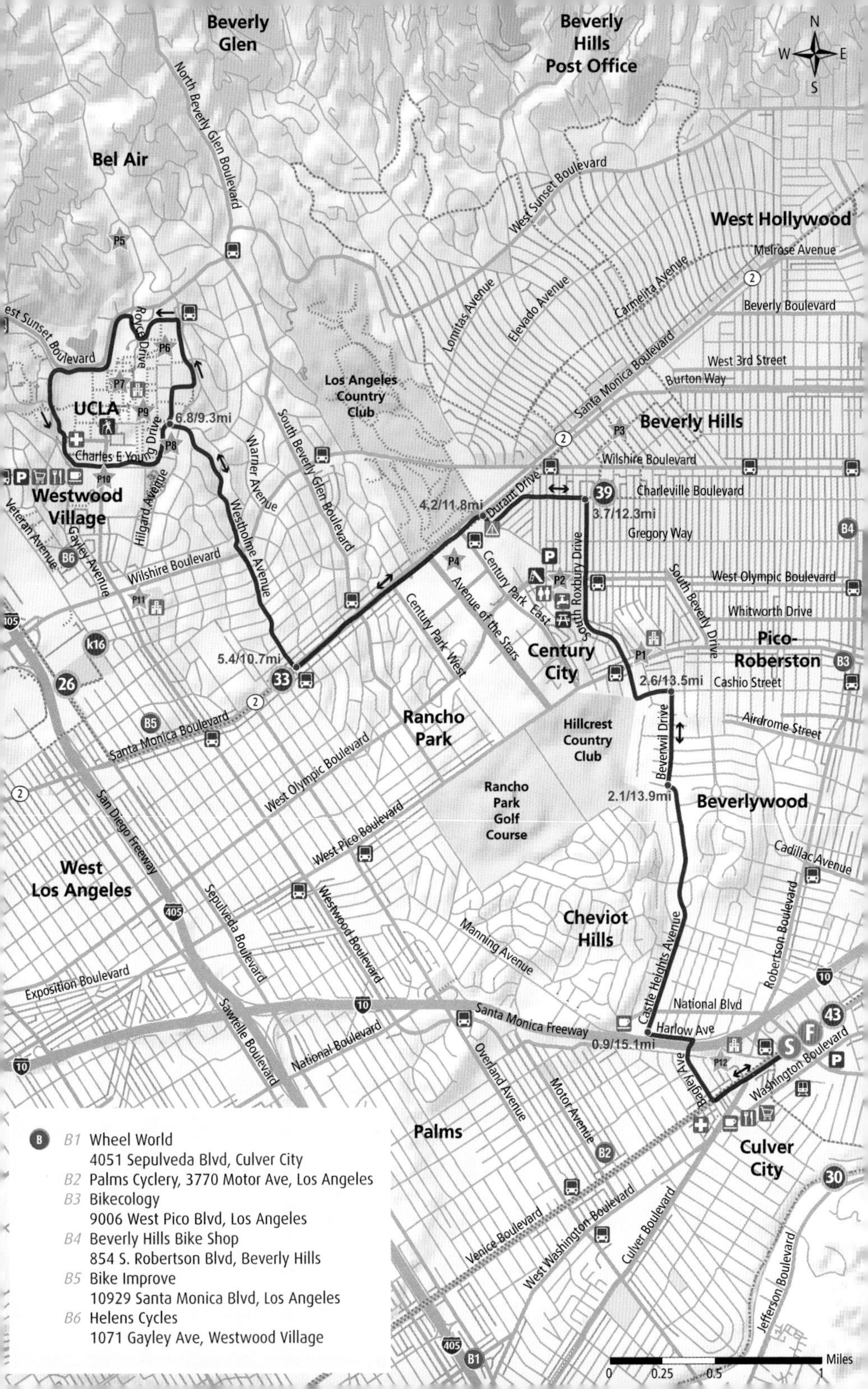

Beverly Glen
Beverly Hills Post Office
N
W
E
S
North Beverly Glen Boulevard
Bel Air
West Sunset Boulevard
West Hollywood
Melrose Avenue
P5
Beverly Boulevard
Carmelita Avenue
Elevado Avenue
Lomitas Avenue
Royce Drive
P6
West 3rd Street
Burton Way
Santa Monica Boulevard
Los Angeles Country Club
P7
UCLA
P9
6.8/9.3mi
P3
Beverly Hills
Hilgard Avenue
Young Drive
Charles E Young
P8
Warner Avenue
South Beverly Glen Boulevard
Wilshire Boulevard
P10
Westwood Village
Westholme Avenue
Durant Drive
39
Charleville Boulevard
4.2/11.8mi
3.7/12.3mi
Gregory Way
Veteran Avenue
Gayley Avenue
B4
B6
Wilshire Boulevard
P4
Century Park East
P2
South Roxbury Drive
South Beverly Drive
West Olympic Boulevard
P11
Avenue of the Stars
Century Park West
Whitworth Drive
405
k16
Century City
P1
Pico-Roberston
B3
5.4/10.7mi
33
26
2.6/13.5mi
Cashio Street
Rancho Park
Airdrome Street
B5
Santa Monica Boulevard
Hillcrest Country Club
Beverwil Drive
West Olympic Boulevard
Rancho Park Golf Course
2.1/13.9mi
Beverlywood
San Diego Freeway
West Pico Boulevard
Cadillac Avenue
West Los Angeles
Westwood Boulevard
Sepulveda Boulevard
Cheviot Hills
Robertson Boulevard
Manning Avenue
Castle Heights Avenue
Exposition Boulevard
10
National Blvd
43
Santa Monica Freeway
Harlow Ave
Sawtelle Boulevard
National Boulevard
Overland Avenue
0.9/15.1mi
S
F
P12
Bagley Ave
Washington Boulevard
Motor Avenue
Palms
Culver City
B2
30
Venice Boulevard
West Washington Boulevard
Culver Boulevard
Jefferson Boulevard
B1
B1 Wheel World
4051 Sepulveda Blvd, Culver City
B2 Palms Cyclery, 3770 Motor Ave, Los Angeles
B3 Bikecology
9006 West Pico Blvd, Los Angeles
B4 Beverly Hills Bike Shop
854 S. Robertson Blvd, Beverly Hills
B5 Bike Improve
10929 Santa Monica Blvd, Los Angeles
B6 Helens Cycles
1071 Gayley Ave, Westwood Village
Miles
0
0.25
0.5
1

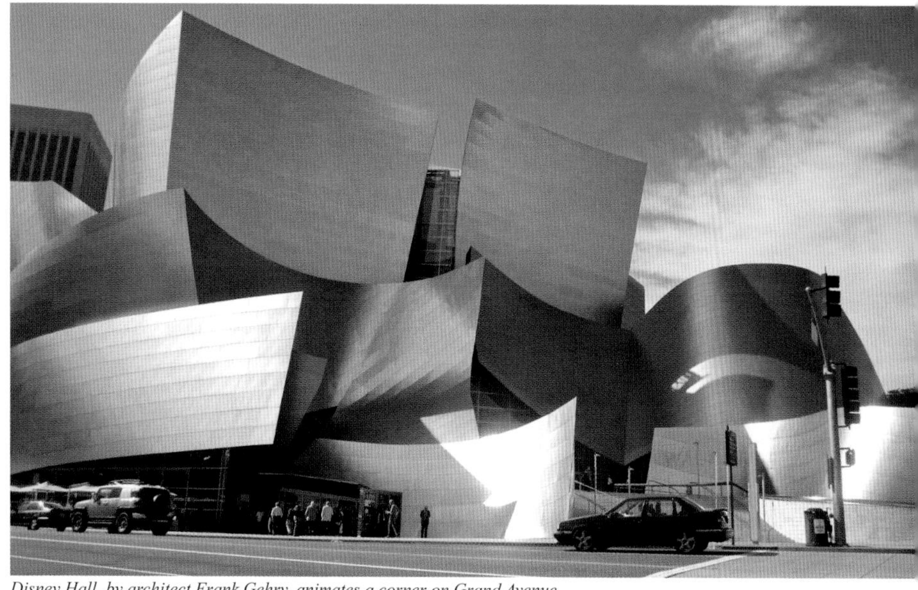

*Disney Hall, by architect Frank Gehry, animates a corner on Grand Avenue.*

## At a Glance

**Distance** 12.3 miles **Elevation Gain** 1,200 feet

### Terrain

Near the start, you'll need to tackle Bunker Hill, so, yes, that's climbing, but the remainder of the tour is flat.

### Traffic

Because this is an urban ride on city streets, traffic is part of the mix (heaviest on weekdays).

### How to Get There

Exit the 101 Freeway at Alameda Street, or the 110 Freeway at Hill Street, and follow signs to Chinatown. Park in one of the neighborhood's many inexpensive lots (typically $3 to $5 per day). Or travel to Union Station via Metro train (Red, Purple or Gold line) or bus.

### Food and Drink

"Fueling" options en route are almost endless: Cole's Pacific Electric Buffet (1908), the Original Pantry Café (open 24 hours since 1924), Nickel Diner, Grand Central Market, Philippe's Home of the Original French Dipped Sandwich, Chinatown eateries and many others.

### Side Trip

Historic Theatre Row, Broadway between Third and Ninth streets, had the world's largest collection of movie theaters around 1931. The ornate marquees remain, but these majestic theaters are mostly closed. Some are stores for cheap goods, while a few survivors show Spanish-language films and occasional mainstream releases to promote preservation efforts. These six blocks recall the heyday of the Silver Screen.

**Links to** 38 42 43 k19

**Where to Bike Rating** 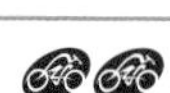

  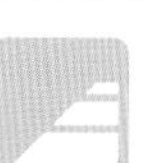 

# About...

Downtown L.A. grew from a small Spanish settlement, founded in 1781, near Olvera Street. In the area's Golden Age, the 1920s and '30s, department stores, theaters and posh hotels rose here, creating a commercial, cultural and transit hub for Southern California. Decades after a post-war exodus to the suburbs, Downtown is experiencing some resurgence, with outmoded office buildings becoming residential lofts and hip dining and entertainment venues gradually taking root. The historic legacy and recent changes make this an interesting place to tour, especially with the city's nascent and growing "cyclophilia."

Downtown L.A. is so packed with landmarks and interesting venues, we're providing a running list of our top picks. Organized by area, it's a menu, or smorgasbord, of hot and noteworthy places, listed in the order you'll encounter them en route, just over your handlebars:

## Bunker Hill

The Chinatown Gateway: Dragons over Broadway mark this threshold to a neighborhood full of restaurants and shops. The Cathedral of Our Lady of the Angeles (2002), designed by Rafael Moneo: L.A.'s Roman Catholic Archdiocese. The Music Center complex: Ahmanson Theatre, Mark Taper Forum, Dorothy Chandler Pavilion (home to L.A.'s opera) and Walt Disney Concert Hall (2003), the famous undulant steel-clad building by Frank Gehry. The Museum of Contemporary Art, or MOCA (1986): designed by Arata Isozaki. Millennium Biltmore (1923): a grand old hotel. Bunker Hill Steps (1991): by landscape architect Lawrence Halprin. Los Angeles Central Library (1926): designed in Egyptian Revival-style by Bertram Grosvenor Goodhue with carvings, murals, and much more. Maguire Gardens (1993): by Lawrence Halprin.

## Financial District

Jewelry, flower, fabric, and fashion districts: Each has its own enclave. Los Angeles Convention Center. Staples Center: home court to the Lakers and Clippers; home ice to the Kings. L.A. Live and the Nokia Theatre.

## Historic Core

Vibiana (1876): events and performance space, formerly the Cathedral of St. Vibiana and Archdiocese of Los Angeles. The Geffen Contemporary at MOCA: recent art in a former warehouse. Little Tokyo Historic District: includes the Japanese American National Museum and Higashi Honganji Buddhist Temple. Million Dollar Theatre (1918): one of the country's first movie palaces. Bradbury Building (1893): with its ornate wrought-iron court and cage elevators, the interior appeared in *Blade Runner*. Angels Flight: funicular railroad (25 cents each way). Grand Central Market (1917): an open-air emporium with fresh produce, meats, exotic spices and ethnic eats. City Hall (1928): a beacon in L.A., with a 27th-floor observation deck.

## El Pueblo

Chinese American Museum. Plaza Firehouse Museum: in an 1884 firehouse. Italian American Museum. Olvera Street: birthplace of Los Angeles, with 27 historic structures and a Mexican open-air marketplace. U.S. Post Office Terminal Annex (1940): a Spanish Colonial-style confection by Gilbert Stanley Underwood. Union Station (1939): by John and Donald Parkinson, with others, in Mission Revival style. And Chinatown.

Whew! Given downtown L.A.'s weekday pedestrian and vehicular traffic, this ride is best on weekends, ideally before noon.

# Ride Log

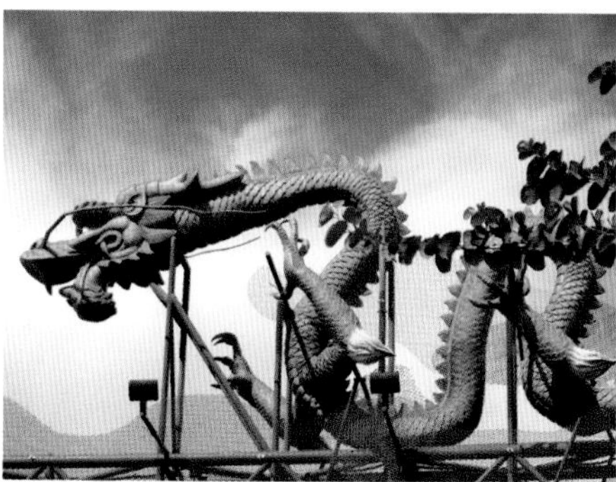
Golden dragons—fierce but smiling—form a gateway into Chinatown.

P1 Echo Park Lake
P2 Vista Hermosa Park
P3 MacArthur Park
P4 Pershing Square
P5 Los Angeles Historic Theatre District
P6 Hope Grand Park
P7 Los Angeles State Historic Park
P8 Elysian Park

B1 Downtown L.A. Bicycles
425 Broadway, Los Angeles
B2 El Maestro Bicycle Shop
806 Main St, Los Angeles

0.0 From Alpine St in Chinatown begin riding south on Broadway.

0.6 Turn right onto Temple St.

1.4 Turn left onto Boylston St after passing under the 110 Freeway.

1.6 Turn right onto Colton St.

1.8 Turn left onto Toluca St.

2.0 Just before Second St, turn right, ride up the ramp and merge onto First St.

2.7 Turn right onto Grand Ave.

3.2 Turn right onto Fifth St.

3.4 Turn right onto Figueroa St.

3.5 Turn right onto Fourth St.

3.6 Turn right onto Flower St (runs one-way).

3.9 Turn left onto Seventh St.

4.7 Turn right onto Wall St.

5.4 Turn right onto Pico Blvd.

6.5 Turn right onto L.A. Live Way.

6.7 Turn right on Chick Hearn Ct.

7.0 Turn left onto Figueroa St.

7.5 Turn right onto Seventh St.

8.1 Turn left onto Main St.

8.9 Turn right onto First St.

9.2 Turn right onto Central Ave.

9.4 Turn right onto Third St.

10.1 Turn left onto Hill St.

10.2 Turn left onto Fourth St (runs one-way).

10.4 Turn left onto Main St (runs one-way).

11.3 Turn right onto Cesar E Chavez Ave.

11.4 Turn right onto Union Station.

11.6 Cross Alameda St onto Los Angeles St.

11.7 Turn right onto Arcadia St.

11.8 Turn right onto Main St.

12.1 Turn left onto Cesar E Chavez Ave then, righ onto Spring St.

12.3 Turn left onto Alpine St. Arrive at Broadway. Enc of tour.

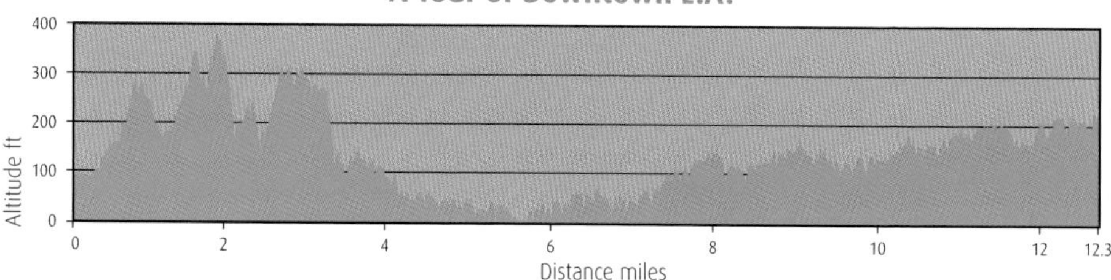

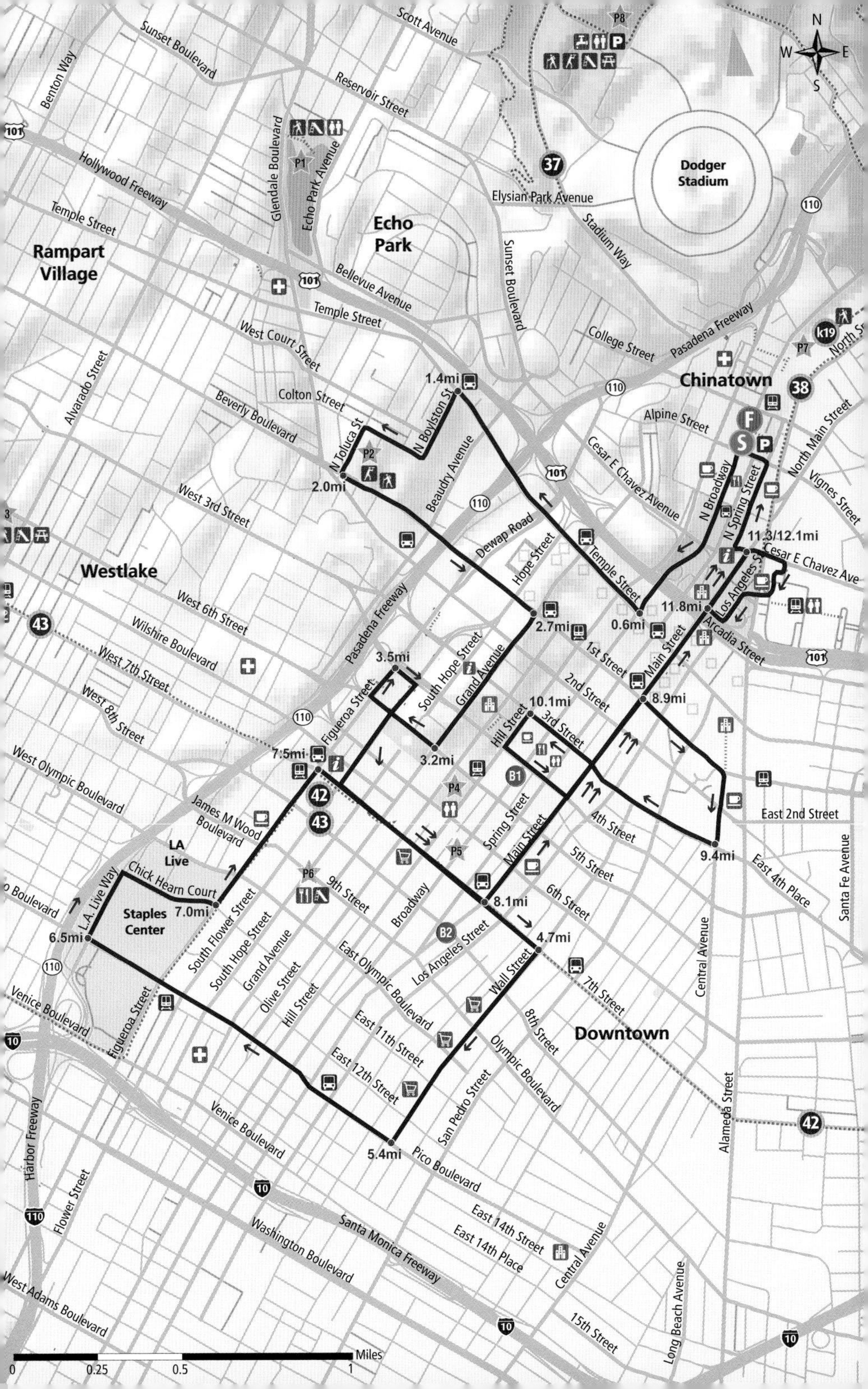

Dodger Stadium
Echo Park
Rampart Village
Westlake
Chinatown
Downtown
LA Live
Staples Center
Scott Avenue
Sunset Boulevard
Reservoir Street
Benton Way
Hollywood Freeway
Temple Street
Glendale Boulevard
Echo Park Avenue
Elysian Park Avenue
Stadium Way
Bellevue Avenue
West Court Street
College Street
Pasadena Freeway
Alvarado Street
Colton Street
Beverly Boulevard
N Toluca St
N Boylston St
Beaudry Avenue
Alpine Street
Cesar E Chavez Avenue
N Broadway
N Spring Street
North Main Street
Vignes Street
West 3rd Street
Dewap Road
Hope Street
Temple Street
Cesar E Chavez Ave
Los Angeles St
West 6th Street
Wilshire Boulevard
West 7th Street
West 8th Street
1st Street
Main Street
Arcadia Street
2nd Street
South Hope Street
Grand Avenue
Figueroa Street
Hill Street
3rd Street
West Olympic Boulevard
James M Wood Boulevard
Spring Street
Main Street
4th Street
East 2nd Street
Chick Hearn Court
L.A. Live Way
South Flower Street
9th Street
Broadway
5th Street
6th Street
East 4th Place
Santa Fe Avenue
South Hope Street
Grand Avenue
Olive Street
Hill Street
East Olympic Boulevard
Los Angeles Street
Wall Street
7th Street
Central Avenue
Venice Boulevard
Figueroa Street
East 11th Street
East 12th Street
8th Street
Olympic Boulevard
San Pedro Street
Alameda Street
Venice Boulevard
Pico Boulevard
Harbor Freeway
Flower Street
East 14th Street
East 14th Place
Central Avenue
Washington Boulevard
Santa Monica Freeway
West Adams Boulevard
15th Street
Long Beach Avenue
1.4mi
2.0mi
2.7mi
0.6mi
11.3/12.1mi
11.8mi
3.5mi
3.2mi
8.9mi
10.1mi
7.5mi
9.4mi
7.0mi
6.5mi
8.1mi
4.7mi
5.4mi
P1
P2
P4
P5
P6
P7
P8
B1
B2
37
38
42
43
k19
F
S
P
101
110
10
N
E
S
W
Miles
0
0.25
0.5
1

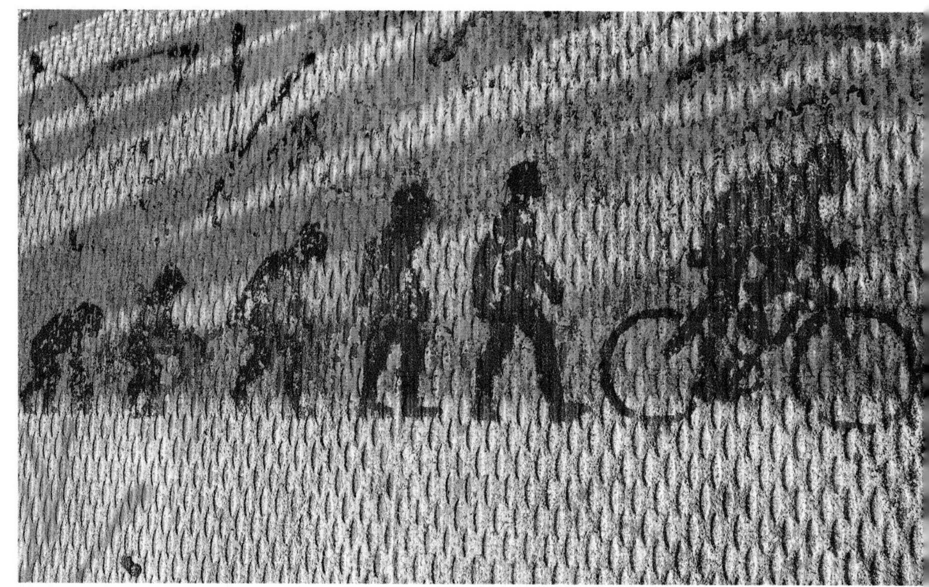

*Evolution: from ape to... cyclist.*

## At a Glance

**Distance** 25.1 miles **Elevation Gain** 1,000 feet

### Terrain

This ride has two small hills: first, over the Seventh Street Bridge and then, leading up to Boyle Heights. After that, it's flat all the way to Long Beach. Late day, on-shore headwinds can blow northward off the ocean.

### Traffic

Expect urban street traffic conditions as far south as Vernon. Then, the ride continues on car-free river bike trails.

### How to Get There

Exit the 110 Freeway at Sixth Street in Downtown L.A. and make a right onto Flower Street. Park in one of the inexpensive ($5 to $8 per day) lots on Eighth, Ninth or 10th Street, west of Flower. Or, by train: Take the Metro Red, Blue, Purple or Expo line to the Seventh Street/Metro Center station.

### Food and Drink

You'll find plenty of food shops and eateries on Long Beach's Pine Avenue, as well as its Shoreline Village.

### Side Trip

Explore downtown Long Beach via protected bike lanes on Broadway (one-way eastbound) and Third Street (one-way westbound), which will take you all the way to Alamitos Avenue, a happening street in the East Village Arts District.

**Where to Bike Rating** 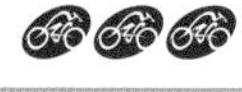

  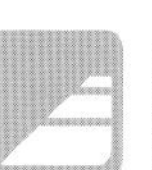 

# About...

Suppose you're near Downtown L.A., hankering for a day in Long Beach to soak up its arts, cycling and foodie scene. You happily ride down, cutting through industrial zones before joining river bike trails for a long, carefree spin to Long Beach. But, after a day exploring the waterfront or East Village Arts District, you may not have the legs, or daylight, to pedal back. What to do? Here's the perfect solution: Go ahead, linger after dark and then, you (and your bike) can hop Metro's Blue Line train home.

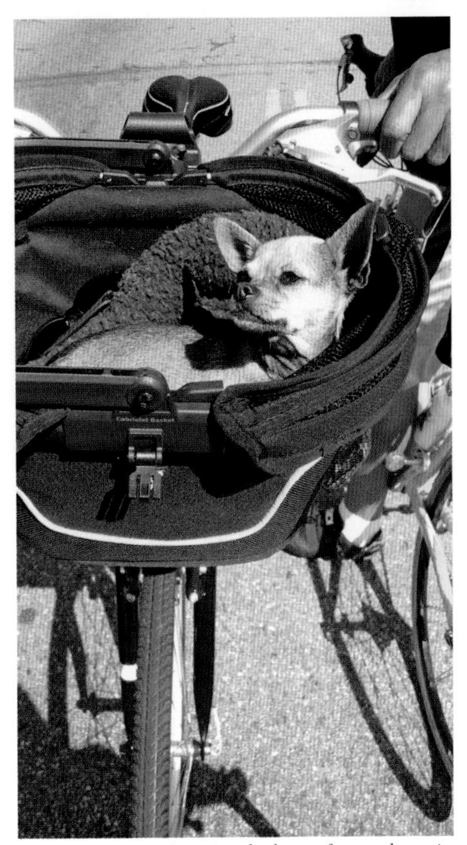

*A pup-in-a-basket out for an urban spin.*

Making its escape from Downtown L.A., this route passes through a series of urban layers—across the Jewelry, Floral, Fashion and Produce districts, by aging warehouses and graffiti-peppered industrial structures. Then, you turn through a modest gate onto the main attraction: a 17-mile-long, straight shot into downtown Long Beach on a car-free bicycle expressway, the L.A. River and LARIO bike trails. Turn your pedals, and let 'er rip (or enjoy a leisurely pace, if you prefer). The paths run along the banks of concrete-channelized, often dry, rivers. Not exactly the bounty of nature, alas, but as you approach the ocean, you'll see where clusters of reeds, other greenery and abundant birdlife are beginning to reclaim this waterway.

This route to Long Beach may someday be part of a folk legend—thanks to a recent rivalry between man and machine, specifically bicyclist and airplane. In July 2011, when part of the 405 Freeway was briefly closed for construction, Jet Blue airline mounted a clever publicity stunt to bypass that closure (and the anticipated "Carmaggedon"). The carrier offered $4.00 fares for the barely 35-mile flight between Burbank and Long Beach. Naturally, a throw-down soon took form: six bicyclists from L.A.'s street-smart Wolfpack Hustle vs. a Jet Blue flight. The cyclists and one airline passenger all left a designated house in Burbank at the same time. While the jetsetter traveled by taxi to the airport, arriving the requisite one hour before departure, and, at the other end, caught a taxi from Long Beach's airport to its aquarium, the Wolfpack riders took off on their velos. Their route began on city streets, followed essentially by our Ride 2 through Griffith Park, then back on streets to Vernon and, finally, onto these very river paths all the way south the aquarium. The Wolfpack "flew" (so to speak)—and won by more than an hour.

When you're ready to return, you can fly back north on your bike by simply reversing the southbound route. Or else, board a Metro Blue Line train for a 45-minute ride to the Seventh Street/Metro Center station. The fare's only a buck and a half.

## Ride Log

**0.0** Begin riding southeast on Seventh St from the Seventh St/Metro Center station.
**1.5** Cross Alameda St.
**2.2** Cross the Los Angeles River on the Seventh St Bridge.
**2.6** Turn right onto Boyle St.
**3.3** Turn left onto Olympic Blvd.
**3.9** Turn right onto Grande Vista Ave, which becomes Downey Rd south of Washington Blvd.
**5.4** Turn left onto District Blvd. Be careful of the railroad tracks.
**6.1** District bends to the right.
**6.8** Cross Atlantic Blvd.
**6.9** Enter the South County L.A. River Bike Trail through the gate on the left side of District Blvd (be prepared for a short, steep entry ramp).
**7.7** Pass Maywood Riverfront Park.
**9.6** Pass Cudahy City Park.
**11.7** Pass under Imperial Hwy, make a U-turn, then a right and cross to the river's east bank via the sidewalk on the south side of Imperial (where it bridges over the river).
**11.7** Join the LARIO Bikeway.
**12.6** Pass Hollydale Community Park.
**14.4** Pass Ralph C. Dills Park.
**16.4** Pass Deforest Park.
**19.9** Pass Wrigley Greenbelt. (The Wardlow station for Metro's Blue Line is four blocks east of the river here—a "bail out" option, in case you need it).
**23.6** Turn left past Golden Shores RV Park and exit the LARIO Bikeway. Continue past Golden Shore Marine Biological Reserve, Palm Beach Park and the Catalina Express terminal.
**24.1** The path turns left, running parallel to the shipping channel.
**24.2** Turn left and cross Golden Shore at Shoreline Aquatic Park.
**24.6** Cross Shoreline Dr, turn right and then, continue on Long Beach Bikeway 17.
**24.8** Ride across Pine Ave using the bicycle crosswalk, then turn left at Rainbow Lagoon and ride up the small hill.
**25.0** Cross Ocean Blvd.
**25.1** Arrive at the Metro Blue line transit mall at First St and Pine Ave.

(R) *R1* Downtown LA Bicycles
1626 Hill St, Downtown L. A.
*R2* Wheel Fun Rentals
419 Shoreline Village Dr, Long Beach
*R3* Alfredo's Beach Club, 700 Shoreline Dr (Alamitos Beach), Long Beach

**For riders returning via the Blue Line:** Board the train at Long Beach's First Street or Transit Mall stations. Take the train to Seventh Street/Metro Center station, in Downtown L.A. (but if you parked near the Convention Center, exit one stop earlier, at Pico station). If you are returning by bike, reverse the southbound route back to Downtown. *Don't forget to cross to the west bank of the Los Angeles River at Imperial Hwy via the sidewalk (where it bridges over the river).*

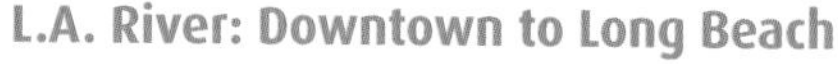


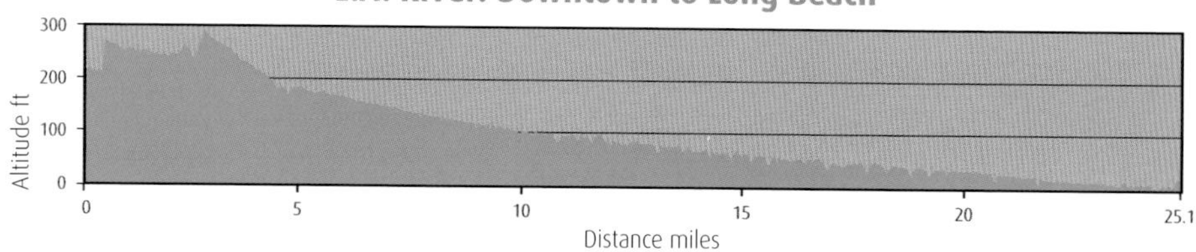

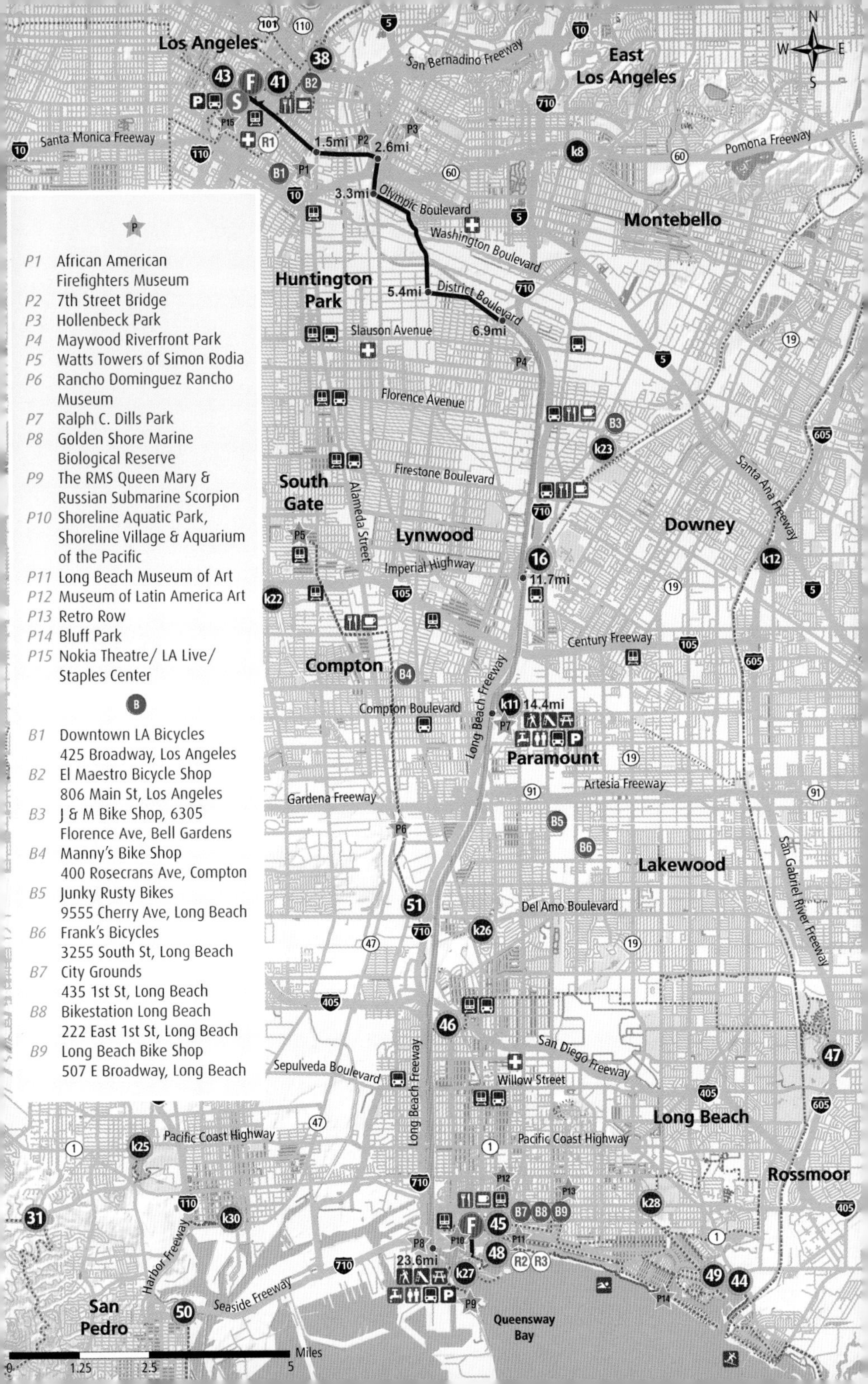

P1 African American Firefighters Museum
P2 7th Street Bridge
P3 Hollenbeck Park
P4 Maywood Riverfront Park
P5 Watts Towers of Simon Rodia
P6 Rancho Dominguez Rancho Museum
P7 Ralph C. Dills Park
P8 Golden Shore Marine Biological Reserve
P9 The RMS Queen Mary & Russian Submarine Scorpion
P10 Shoreline Aquatic Park, Shoreline Village & Aquarium of the Pacific
P11 Long Beach Museum of Art
P12 Museum of Latin America Art
P13 Retro Row
P14 Bluff Park
P15 Nokia Theatre/ LA Live/ Staples Center
B1 Downtown LA Bicycles 425 Broadway, Los Angeles
B2 El Maestro Bicycle Shop 806 Main St, Los Angeles
B3 J & M Bike Shop, 6305 Florence Ave, Bell Gardens
B4 Manny's Bike Shop 400 Rosecrans Ave, Compton
B5 Junky Rusty Bikes 9555 Cherry Ave, Long Beach
B6 Frank's Bicycles 3255 South St, Long Beach
B7 City Grounds 435 1st St, Long Beach
B8 Bikestation Long Beach 222 East 1st St, Long Beach
B9 Long Beach Bike Shop 507 E Broadway, Long Beach
Los Angeles
East Los Angeles
Montebello
Huntington Park
South Gate
Lynwood
Downey
Compton
Paramount
Lakewood
Long Beach
Rossmoor
San Pedro
Queensway Bay
San Bernadino Freeway
Santa Monica Freeway
Pomona Freeway
Olympic Boulevard
Washington Boulevard
District Boulevard
Slauson Avenue
Florence Avenue
Firestone Boulevard
Alameda Street
Imperial Highway
Century Freeway
Santa Ana Freeway
Long Beach Freeway
Compton Boulevard
Artesia Freeway
Gardena Freeway
San Gabriel River Freeway
Del Amo Boulevard
San Diego Freeway
Sepulveda Boulevard
Willow Street
Pacific Coast Highway
Harbor Freeway
Seaside Freeway
1.5mi
2.6mi
3.3mi
5.4mi
6.9mi
11.7mi
14.4mi
23.6mi
Miles
0
1.25
2.5
5
N
S
E
W

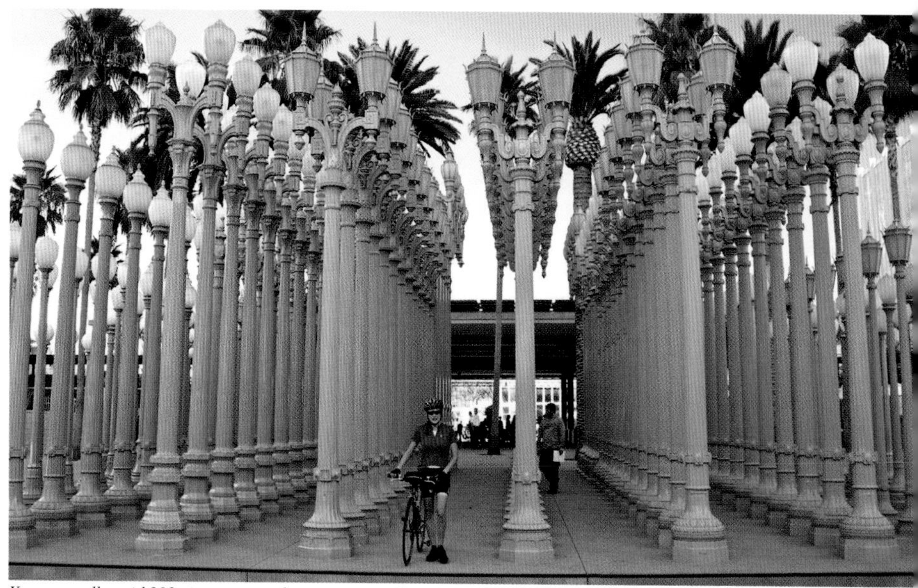

*You can walk amid 202 vintage street lamps in artist Chris Burden's 2008 work "Urban Lights," in front of LACMA.*

## At a Glance

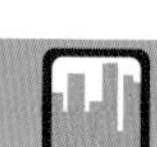

**Distance** 31.7 miles **Elevation Gain** 1,300 feet

### Terrain

This fairly flat route has a few little hills. Pavement is rough in spots, mostly along Fourth Street and Venice Boulevard.

### Traffic

Even with its long bike lanes and a cyclist-friendly "bike boulevard," the shuffle is an intense urban riding experience, with traffic nearby.

### How to Get There

Exit the 110 Freeway at Sixth Street and turn right onto Flower Street. West of Flower, off Eighth, Ninth and 10th streets, are inexpensive parking lots ($5 to $8 per day). Or, by train, take the Red, Blue, Purple or Expo Metro line to the Seventh Street/Metro Center station.

### Food and Drink

Several neighborhoods en route, including Koreatown and Little Ethiopia, may entice you with ethnic cuisines. Around MacArthur Park, you'll find everything from Langer's Delicatessen to Hot Mama's Tamales Café, as well as plenty of food trucks.

### Side Trip

Make a short detour to Museum Row, which includes the Los Angeles County Museum of Art (LACMA), Craft and Folk Art Museum, A+D Architecture and Design Museum and La Brea Tar Pits. (From Cochran Avenue, turn right onto Eighth Street and then, right onto Spaulding Avenue. Cross Wilshire Boulevard to the epicenter: LACMA.) The museums have bike racks.

**Links to** 25 27 28 30 40 41 42

**Where to Bike Rating** 

# About...

From skyscrapers to surf, the "shuffle" cuts a broad swath across L.A., tracing a route from Downtown to Venice Beach. Instead of putting riders onto full-throttle city streets, this journey capitalizes on three recent additions to L.A.'s bikeway system: the Fourth Street Bike Boulevard, plus new cycling lanes on Seventh Street and along the Expo Line. These improvements make it easier and safer to explore diverse neighborhoods en route, including MacArthur Park and Miracle Mile. Never far from public transportation, you can always hop a bus or train for a stretch.

Just west of the Seventh Street/Metro Center station, you'll roll onto one of L.A.'s newest bike lanes. In 2010, the city council updated its biking plan, and by the summer of 2011, this street was "striped" for cyclists. Then, almost overnight, the city center became safer and more accessible to riders.

In a mile, you'll reach MacArthur Park, inspiration for the 1968 song by the same name. The park's ups and downs have been extreme. In the 19th century, it was surrounded by luxury hotels and dubbed the "Champs Elysées of L.A." During much of the '80s and '90s, however, it became an epicenter of gang crime. But since 2002, it's seen dramatic clean-up and revitalization. Paddleboats have returned to its lake, the fountain flows again, families flock here for music events and eclectic food vendors add spice to the scene, particularly along the park's periphery.

After passing the legendary Park Plaza Hotel and Lafayette Park, you'll join the new Fourth Street Bike Boulevard—more than 3.5 miles of safe, quiet residential streets with road-surface "sharrows" (chevron-and-bicycle icons) and intersections controlled by four-way stop signs. The "Boulevard" ends near Museum Row and the Farmers' Market, with its hub of eateries, shops and fresh produce vendors. After pedaling within easy reach of the oozing La Brea Tar Pits, which swallowed up many Ice Age mammals, you'll continue on residential streets to Venice Boulevard: an eight-mile straight shot to the ocean.

For a shorter ride, instead of continuing all the way to the beach, you can turn around in Culver City—ideally, after a latte in one of its downtown cafés. But if you choose to go all the way to Venice Beach, you can peruse the boardwalk there or take a spin along the beach to Santa Monica (Ride 27).

The trip back retraces Venice Boulevard to Culver City and then, cuts through a residential neighborhood to join the new bike lane along Metro's Expo Line. Just before hitting this Expo segment, be sure to check out the Hayden Tract's architectural experiments by Eric Owen Moss, including his black Stealth Building, Umbrella and Samitaur Tower.

The bike lane ends near Exposition Park, the Museum of Natural History and Coliseum stadium. From here, cross Exposition Boulevard and traverse the University of Southern California (USC) campus (slowly, please) before returning to the Seventh Street/Metro Center station.

# Ride Log

0.0 Starting from the intersection of Figueroa St and Seventh St, ride west, past the Wilshire Grand Hotel.

1.2 Pass MacArthur Park.

1.3 Turn right onto Park View St.

1.6 Turn left onto Sixth St.

2.0 Turn right onto Occidental Blvd/Hoover St. Stay to the left on Hoover St.

2.2 Turn left onto the Fourth St Bicycle Boulevard.

3.6 Cross Western Ave.

5.6 Cross La Brea Ave.

5.8 Turn left onto Cochran Ave just before Fourth St ends at Park La Brea.

6.1 Cross Wilshire Blvd.

6.5 Cross Olympic Blvd.

6.7 Turn left onto Edgewood Pl.

6.9 Turn right onto Redondo Blvd.

## Ride Log continued...

7.4 Cross Pico Blvd.
7.6 Turn right onto Venice Blvd, joining the bike lane.
9.2 Cross under the 10 Freeway.
10.2 Cross Robertson Blvd.
12.1 Cross Sepulveda Blvd.
14.5 Cross Lincoln Blvd/Pacific Coast Hwy.
15.8 Arrive at Venice Beach. Begin the return to Downtown by riding east along Venice Blvd. If you want to return on public transportation, ride to Venice Way and Pacific Ave and board the 733 Express Bus to Downtown.
17.1 Cross Lincoln Blvd/Pacific Coast Hwy.
19.5 Cross Sepulveda Blvd.
21.4 Turn right onto Robertson Blvd. In Culver City, it becomes Higuera St.
22.1 Turn left onto Hayden Place.
22.5 Turn right onto National Blvd. Approach the traffic light at Jefferson from the rightmost left-turn lane.
22.7 As you make the turn toward Jefferson, enter the bike lane running parallel to Metro's elevated tracks.
23.0 Cross La Cienega Blvd using the crosswalk, then join the bike lane.
24.5 Turn right onto Harcourt Ave, following the "Bike Route" signs.
24.6 Turn left onto Exposition Blvd, rejoining the bike lane.
26.5 Use the crosswalk where Exposition Blvd merges with Rodeo Rd.
27.8 Cross Vermont Ave.
28.1 Use the crosswalk at the west end of the USC/ Exposition Park station. Continue straight through the USC on Trousdale Pkwy/University Ave.
28.5 Angle to the left, cross Jefferson Blvd using the crosswalk and begin riding north on the bike lane along Hoover St.
29.9 Turn right onto Venice Blvd.
30.8 Turn left onto Figueroa St, just past the Los Angeles Convention Center.
31.3 Pass Nokia Theatre/L.A. Live.
31.7 Arrive back at the Seventh Street Metro Center station. End of ride.

B
B1 Downtown LA Bicycles
1626 Hill St, Downtown L. A.
B2 El Maestro Bicycle Shop
806 Main St, Downtown L. A.
B3 Rolling Cowboys Bicycle Shop
3505 Pico Blvd, Mid City
B4 Bicycle Kitchen
706 N. Heliotrope Dr, Los Angeles
B5 Palms Cycle, 3770 Motor Ave, Palms
B6 Wheel World Cycles
4051 Sepulveda Blvd, Culver City
B7 Bikerowave
12255 Venice Blvd, Los Angeles
B8 Helen's Cycles
2472 Lincoln Blvd, Marina del Rey
B9 MDR Bike Company
4051 Lincoln Blvd, Marina del Rey
B10 LA Bicycles, 3219 Hoover St, USC

R
R1 Downtown LA Bicycles
1626 Hill St, Downtown L. A.
R2 Perry's Café & Rentals, several locations on the Marvin Braude Bike Trail
R2 Venice Bike & Skates
21 Washington Blvd, Marina del Rey
R4 Spokes N' Stuff, 4200 Admiralty Way
Marina del Rey (rental only)

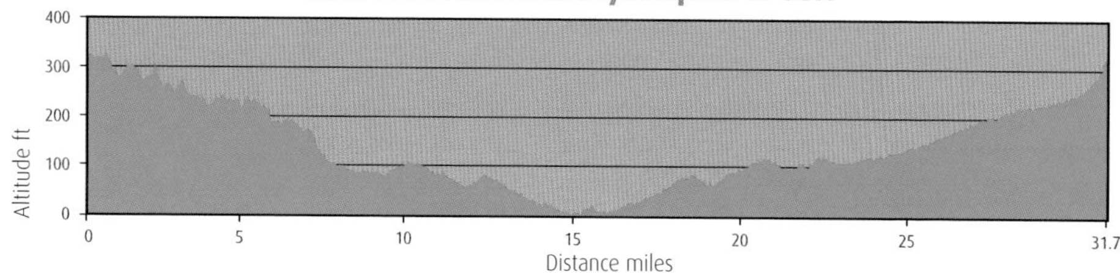

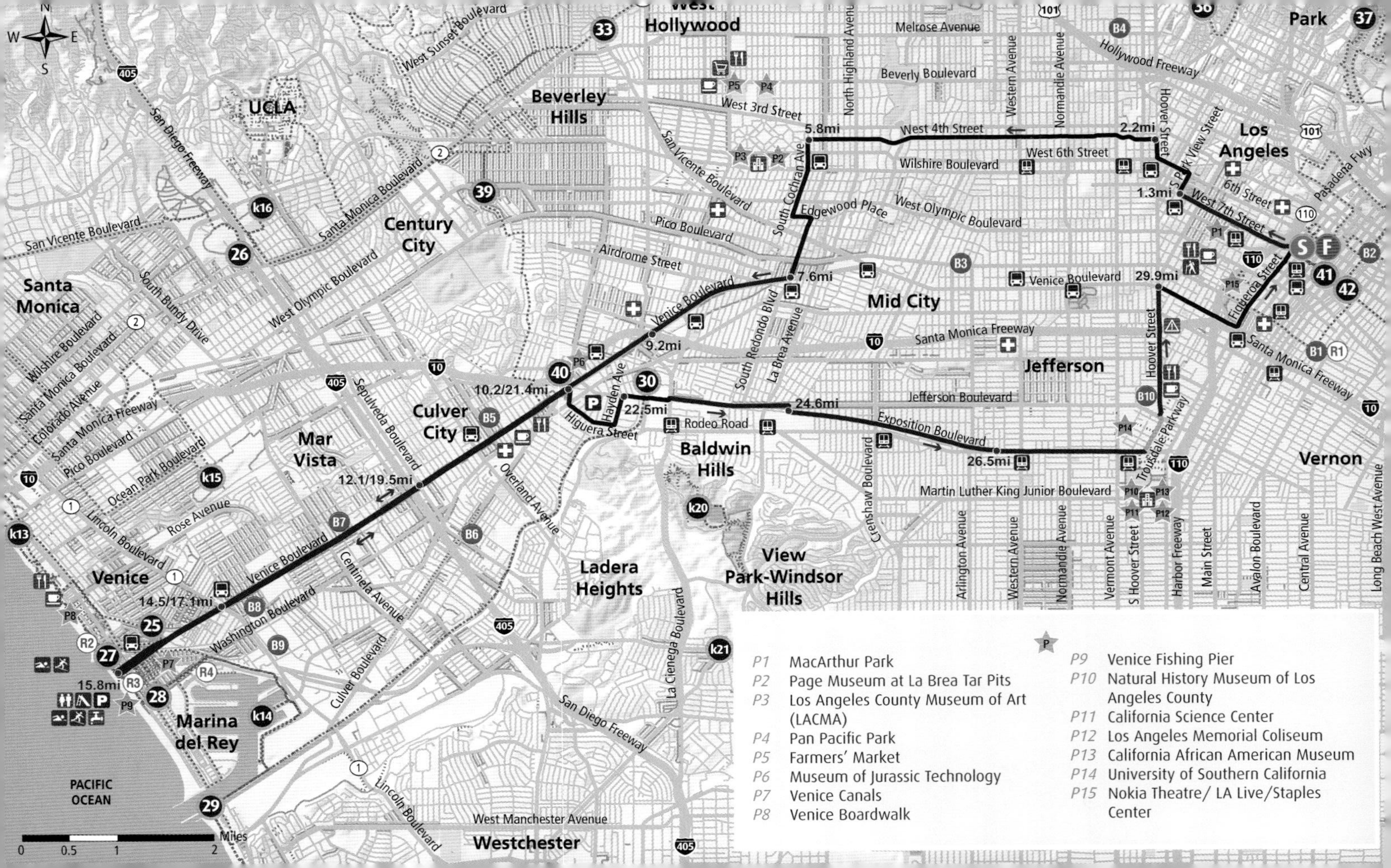
West Hollywood
Beverley Hills
UCLA
Century City
Santa Monica
Venice
Marina del Rey
PACIFIC OCEAN
Mar Vista
Culver City
Baldwin Hills
Ladera Heights
View Park-Windsor Hills
Westchester
Mid City
Jefferson
Los Angeles
Vernon
Park
West Sunset Boulevard
San Diego Freeway
Santa Monica Boulevard
San Vicente Boulevard
West Olympic Boulevard
South Bundy Drive
Wilshire Boulevard
Colorado Avenue
Santa Monica Freeway
Pico Boulevard
Ocean Park Boulevard
Lincoln Boulevard
Rose Avenue
Venice Boulevard
Washington Boulevard
Centinela Avenue
Sepulveda Boulevard
Culver Boulevard
Overland Avenue
Higuera Street
Hayden Ave
Rodeo Road
La Cienega Boulevard
West Manchester Avenue
Airdrome Street
Edgewood Place
South Cochran Ave
South Redondo Blvd
La Brea Avenue
Crenshaw Boulevard
Jefferson Boulevard
Exposition Boulevard
Martin Luther King Junior Boulevard
Arlington Avenue
Western Avenue
Normandie Avenue
Vermont Avenue
S Hoover Street
Harbor Freeway
Main Street
Avalon Boulevard
Central Avenue
Long Beach West Avenue
Trousdale Parkway
Hoover Street
Figueroa Street
Melrose Avenue
Beverly Boulevard
West 3rd Street
North Highland Avenue
West 4th Street
West 6th Street
Hollywood Freeway
S Park View Street
West 7th Street
6th Street
Pasadena Fwy
15.8mi
14.5/17.1mi
12.1/19.5mi
10.2/21.4mi
9.2mi
7.6mi
5.8mi
2.2mi
1.3mi
29.9mi
26.5mi
24.6mi
22.5mi
Miles
0
0.5
1
2
P1 MacArthur Park
P2 Page Museum at La Brea Tar Pits
P3 Los Angeles County Museum of Art (LACMA)
P4 Pan Pacific Park
P5 Farmers' Market
P6 Museum of Jurassic Technology
P7 Venice Canals
P8 Venice Boardwalk
P9 Venice Fishing Pier
P10 Natural History Museum of Los Angeles County
P11 California Science Center
P12 Los Angeles Memorial Coliseum
P13 California African American Museum
P14 University of Southern California
P15 Nokia Theatre/ LA Live/Staples Center

# Long Beach

The Long Beach area has many great ingredients: beaches, history, parks, museums, rivers, marinas, loads of eateries, a hip arts district, cool architecture, a fascinating commercial port, a small amusement park, a faux-Italian canals neighborhood—and a commitment to progressive cycling infrastructure. Maybe the only thing missing is mountains—no dramatic elevation change here.

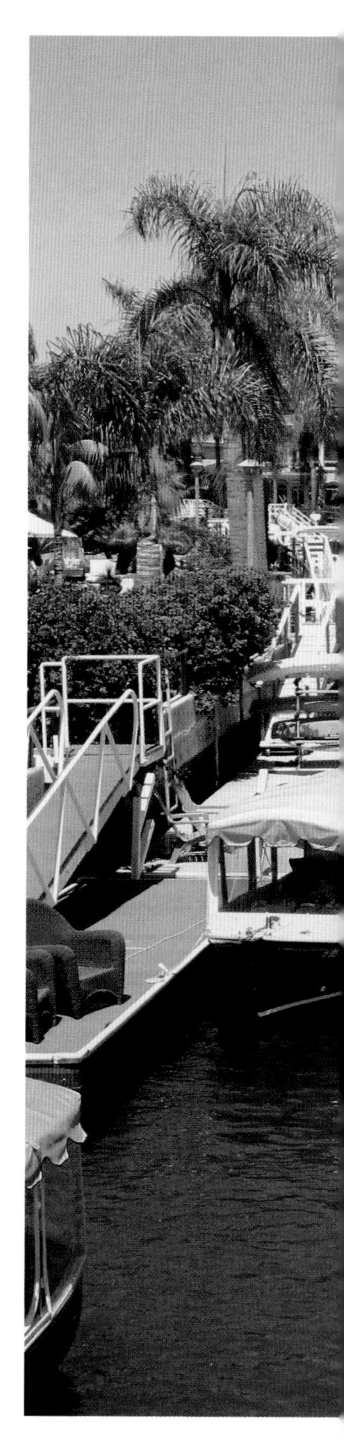

More than any other Southern California city, Long Beach has funneled resources, energy and ideas into developing innovative cycling infrastructure (spanning over 270 miles so far). It has L.A. County's first "bike boulevard," a street with traffic-calming features; the first physically separated bike lanes, or "cycletracks," west of New York; and Southern California's first traffic-intersection green boxes to protect cyclists from turning cars. A recipient of the League of American Bicyclists' Bronze bike-friendly-community rating, Long Beach remains a work in progress—its "velophilic" enthusiasm evident in the dozens of whimsical bike-rack styles all over town.

As California's fifth largest city, Long Beach spans 52 square miles, and this chapter extends even further. To the west, our San Pedro Waterfront ride explores the adjacent port city of San Pedro, its beaches, Victorian lighthouse, Korean hilltop bell and temple-like structure, and (coupled with Long Beach harbor) one of the world's largest shipping ports, with tall, praying-mantis cranes hoisting containers from freighters. At the coast's opposite end, we recommend a foray into Orange County via our Surf City USA spin.

The name Long Beach says a lot, and our Coastal ride sweeps along that great shoreline, with highlights including the Queen Mary, a 1930s ocean liner now permanently moored as a hotel-entertainment venue. But, rest assured, there's also plenty to explore inland. On the Long Beach Arts & Craftsmen route, check out the East Village arts scene and Retro Row vintage shopping, with lots of Art Deco architecture and Craftsman-style bungalows en route. The Marine Stadium ride goes from a 1932 Olympics rowing venue to the Naples neighborhood's quaint canals and bridges and onto a Cal State campus with a Japanese garden and huge, blue pyramid. Our El Dorado double-loop winds through a verdant park, and the Long Beach Periferico makes a grand ring around the city, with access to all the other rides.

A final spin beginning in Long Beach heads north to an iconic grassroots masterwork: the extraordinary Watts Towers of Simon Rodia (amazing to behold—every time).

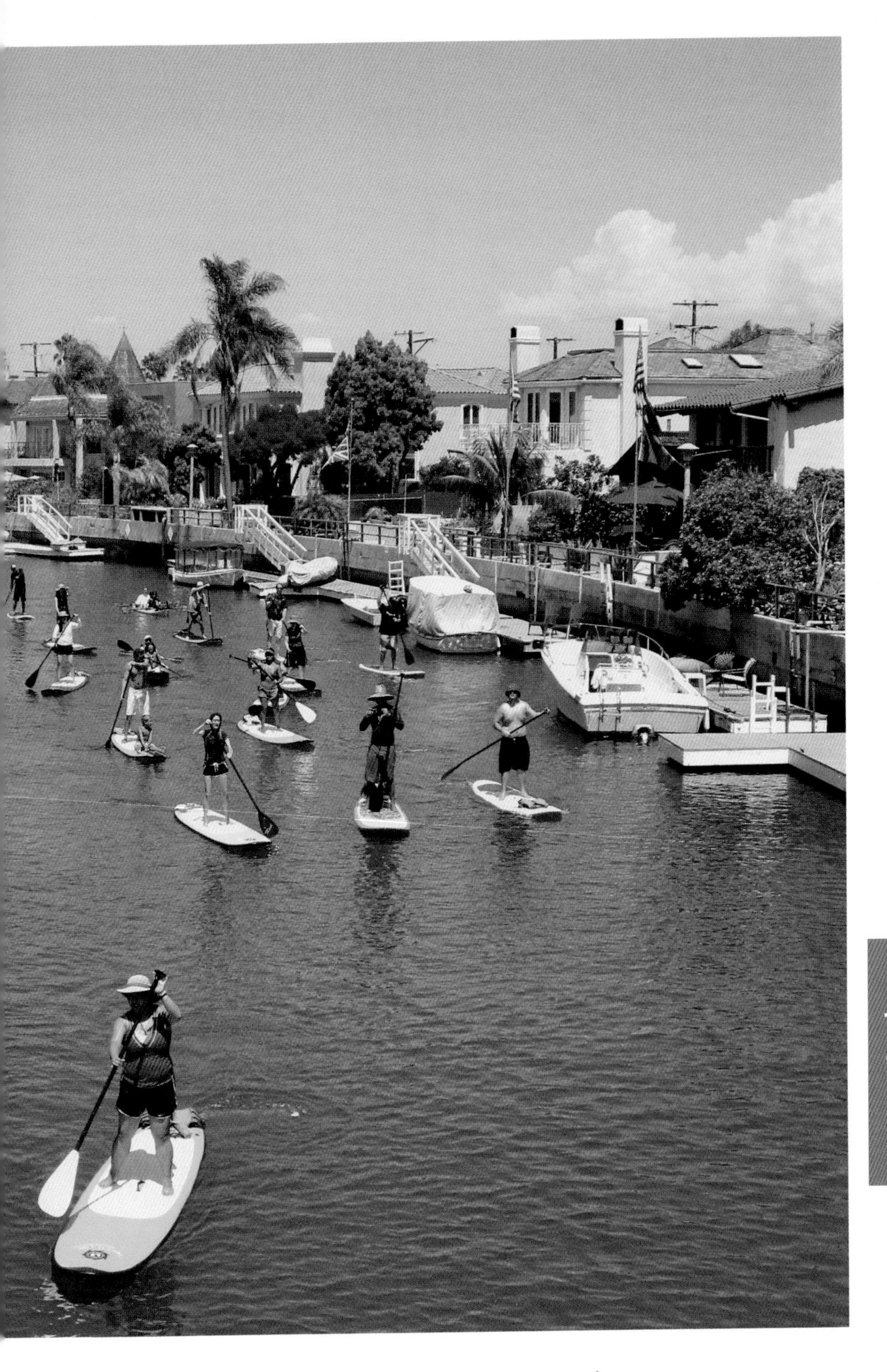

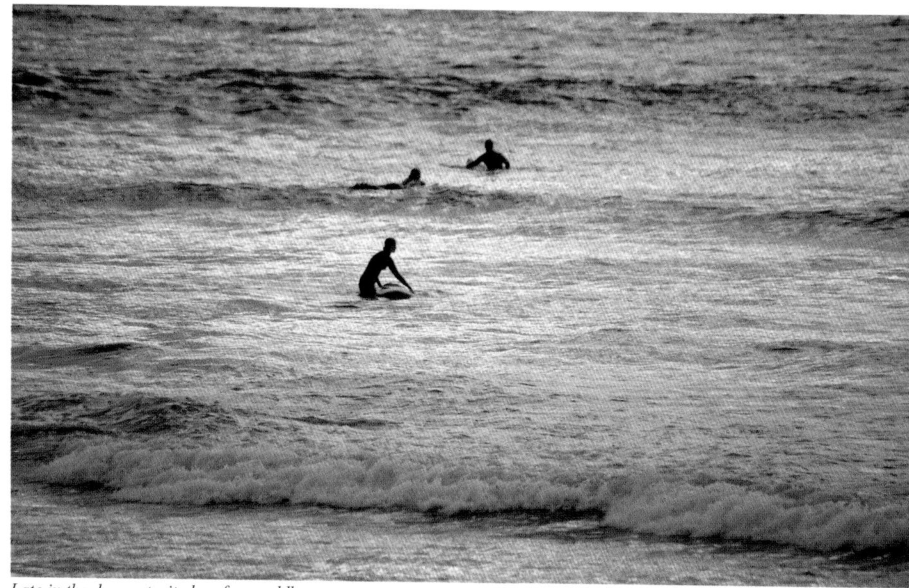

*Late in the day, wetsuited surfers paddle out.*

## At a Glance

**Distance** 21.1 miles **Elevation Gain** 300 feet

### Terrain

Except for small grade changes on the bridge over the Anaheim Bay Inlet and near Dog Beach, this ride's pretty flat. Watch for sand on the path south of Warner Avenue.

### Traffic

The ride begins on quiet streets and bike lanes, partly along the Pacific Coast Highway, and then, from Sunset Beach south, continues on the Huntington Beach Bike Path (be prepared to share it with pedestrians).

### How to Get There

From the 405 or 605 Freeway south, exit at Seal Beach Boulevard. Continue south and turn right onto Westminster Avenue/Second Street and then, left onto Marina Drive to free marina parking near Joe's Crab Shack.

### Food and Drink

You'll find plenty of eateries around the Huntington Beach Pier. Near the ride's end, Bogart's Coffee House, in Seal Beach, offers a laid-back hang-out amid aromas of java.

### Side Trip

With all the cool surfing beaches on this ride, a stop at the International Surf Museum is definitely in order. Many of the exhibits focus on surfing's history, artifacts and memorabilia, as well as wave-rider-themed art. (The museum is two blocks inland from the Huntington Beach Pier; open daily: **www.surfingmuseum.org**.)

**Links to**  

**Where to Bike Rating** 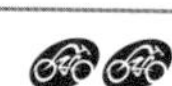

## About...

Take your passport along on this ride because you'll be crossing the border into Orange County. After exiting L.A. County and venturing into Seal Beach, you'll follow the shoreline south along a long stretch of So Cal beaches, where surfers rip the waves year round. You'll then turn around at the pier in Huntington Beach, the city that trademarked the name "Surf City USA," so it could capitalize on that lifestyle.

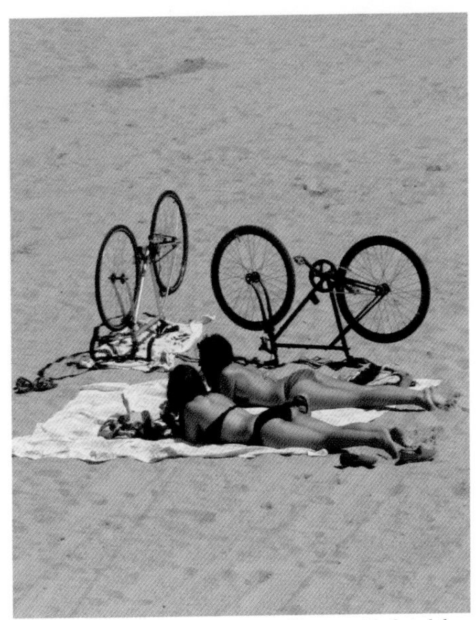

*Catching the rays: sunworshippers with their bikes.*

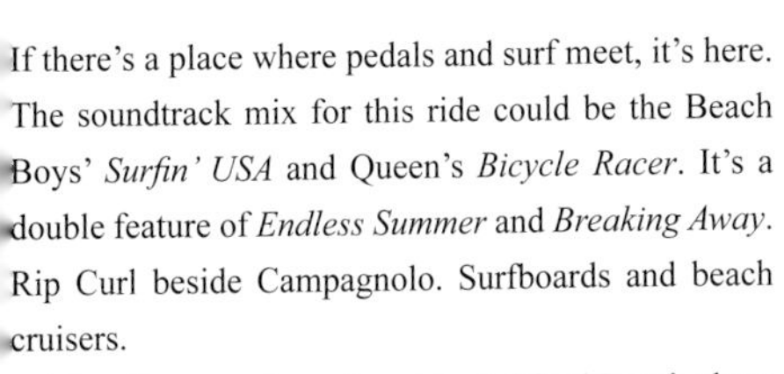

If there's a place where pedals and surf meet, it's here. The soundtrack mix for this ride could be the Beach Boys' *Surfin' USA* and Queen's *Bicycle Racer*. It's a double feature of *Endless Summer* and *Breaking Away*. Rip Curl beside Campagnolo. Surfboards and beach cruisers.

The ride starts through residential Seal Beach along Electric Avenue—once a Pacific Electric Trolley corridor, now a median park with a Red Car trolley fully restored and turned into a museum. After a short bit in the bike lane of Pacific Coast Highway (PCH), past the Seal Beach National Wildlife Refuge, Anaheim Bay and funky Sunset Beach Water Tower House (you'll know it when you see it), you turn toward the ocean.

As you ride along Pacific Avenue, you won't immediately experience the full-frontal beach because of a row of houses. You may be tempted to duck down an end-of-street access point to get your feet sandy. From here on, the route parallels a succession of beaches, beginning with Sunset County Beach, one of Southern California's widest. At the end of Sunset, you'll jump on the Huntington Beach Bike Path for a long, carefree ride past famous surf spots at Bolsa Chica State Beach, Huntington Beach and Huntington State Beach. Near the middle of this stretch, you'll pass Dog Beach, one of the few public shorelines around where Labradoodles, Schnauzers, mutts and other pups can legally frolic in the surf and sand. Some even ride the waves.

Bicycling here is like catching a wave that seems to roll on forever—just cruise along and enjoy. When you reach our turnaround point at Huntington Beach Pier, also known as Surf City Pier, you may be inspired to linger, catch some rays, watch the surfers, have a snack, buy a tacky T-shirt or some cotton candy or just kick back and take in the beach life.

Your return trip can either retrace the outbound route or deviate from it slightly, as our ride log suggests, by picking up PCH's bike lanes earlier for a spin through the Sunset Beach commercial district, with its surf shops and eclectic drive-up burger and taco joints. Then, as you descend the ramp from the bridge over Anaheim Bay Inlet, you'll breeze past the marina's quays and panoramic wetlands, where brightly clad kayakers often ply the briny waters.

*While Ride 44 has not been deemed kid-friendly in its entirety, it does include substantial sections which are entirely safe for family use.*

# Ride Log

**0.0** From the parking lot's exit in front of Joe's Crab Shack, turn right onto Marina Dr.

**0.1** Marina Dr bends to the right.

**0.6** Turn left as Marina Dr ends and cross the San Gabriel River.

**1.1** Turn right on Sixth St, then left onto Electric Ave.

**1.8** Turn left onto Seal Beach Blvd.

**2.1** Turn right onto Pacific Coast Hwy, joining the bike lane.

**3.7** Turn right onto Anderson St (at the quirky Sunset Beach Water Tower house).

**3.8** Turn left onto Pacific Ave.

**5.0** Pacific ends at Warner Ave. Cross the sidewalk, ride half way around the roundabout and begin riding south on the Huntington Beach Bike Trail.

**7.5** The bike path turns left, then right at a restroom facility and then crosses the inlet to Bolsa Chica lagoon.

**8.3** Pass Huntington Beach Dog Beach.

**10.4** Arrive at Huntington Beach Pier. To get to Main St, the Pier and Pacific Coast Hwy, ride up through the parking lot on northwest side of the pier. Return along the bike trail.

**15.6** Arrive at the end of the Huntington Beach Bike Trail. Turn right, following the roundabout to Warner Ave.

**15.7** Turn left onto Pacific Coast Hwy.

**18.6** Turn left onto Seal Beach Blvd.

**18.9** Continue straight on Ocean Ave.

**19.4** Pass Seal Beach's pier and Main St.

**19.8** Turn left into First St and enter the parking lot for Rivers End Café.

**20.0** Join the San Gabriel River near the front of the café and ride north.

**20.3** Turn left onto Marina Dr. Watch for cross traffic.

**20.4** Turn right after crossing the San Gabriel River.

**21.1** Turn left into the Joe's Crab Shack parking area. End of ride.

*P1* Electric Avenue Median Park
*P2* Seal Beach National Wildlife Refuge
*P3* Bolsa Chica Ecological Reserve
*P4* International Surfing Museum
411 Olive Ave, Huntington Beach
*P5* Huntington Beach Pier
*P6* Seal Beach Pier and Eisenhower Park

*B1* Sports Authority
6346 Pacific Coast Hwy, Long Beach
*B2* Main Street Cyclery
317 Main St, Seal Beach
*B3* Kings Bicycle Store
1190 Pacific Coast Hwy, Seal Beach
*B4* Outspoken
16400 Pacific Coast Hwy, Huntington Beach
*B5* JAX Bicycle Center
401 Main St, Huntington Beach
*B6* Surf City Cyclery
7470 Edinger Ave, Huntington Beach
*B7* Huntington Beach Bicycles
15862 Springdale St, Huntington Beach

R
*R1* Outspoken
16400 Pacific Coast Hwy, Huntington Beach
*R2* Zack's Surf City
Huntington Beach Pier
*R3* Wheel Fun Rentals at Hilton
Waterfront Beach Resort, 21100 Pacific Coast Hwy, Huntington Beach

**Surf City USA**

Altitude ft
100
0
0 3 6 9 12 15 18 21.1
Distance miles

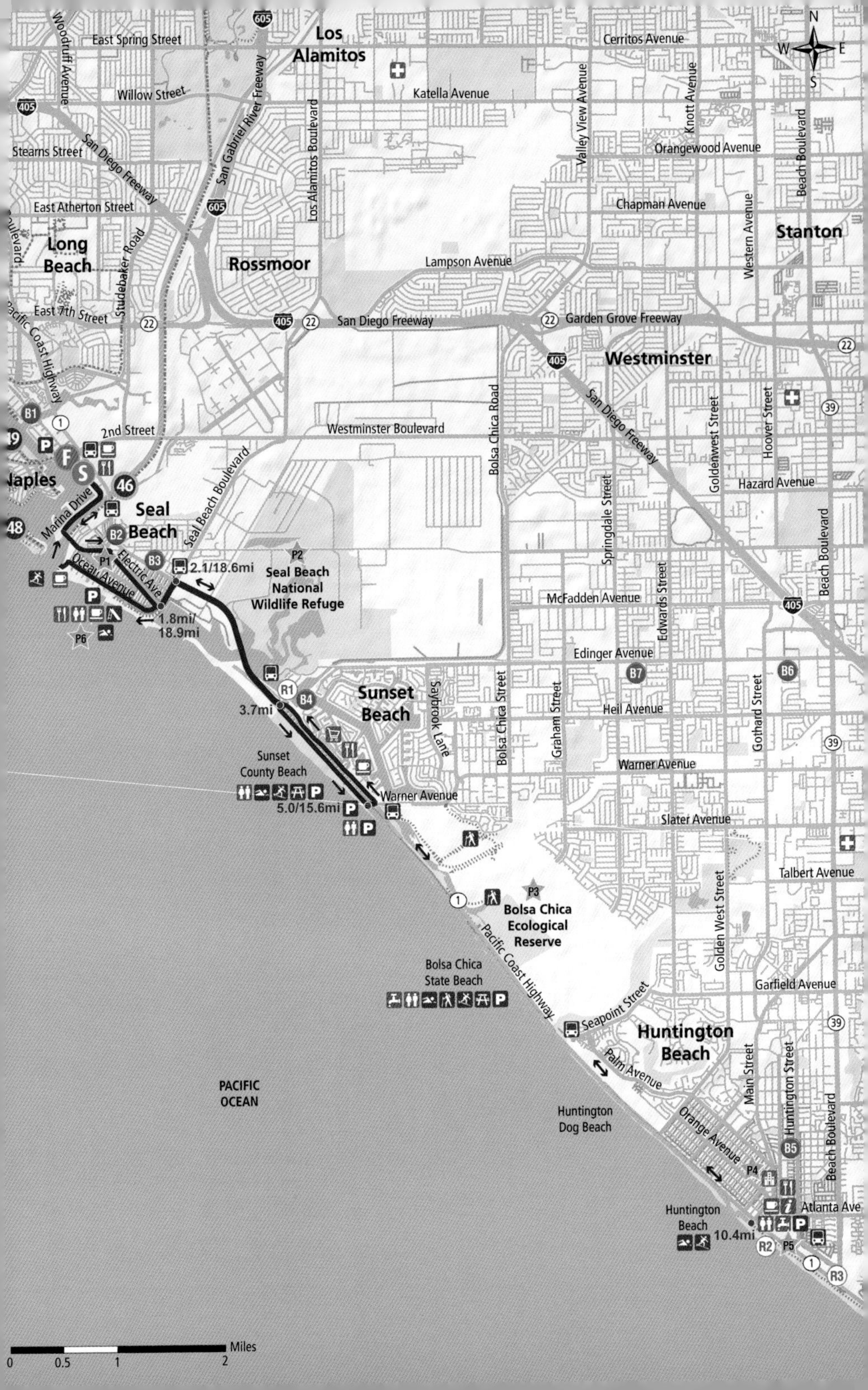

Los Alamitos
Rossmoor
Long Beach
Naples
Seal Beach
Sunset Beach
Westminster
Stanton
Huntington Beach
East Spring Street
Willow Street
Stearns Street
East Atherton Street
East 7th Street
2nd Street
Woodruff Avenue
Studebaker Road
San Diego Freeway
San Gabriel River Freeway
Los Alamitos Boulevard
Cerritos Avenue
Katella Avenue
Orangewood Avenue
Chapman Avenue
Lampson Avenue
Garden Grove Freeway
Valley View Avenue
Knott Avenue
Western Avenue
Beach Boulevard
Westminster Boulevard
Bolsa Chica Road
Goldenwest Street
Hoover Street
Hazard Avenue
Springdale Street
Edwards Street
McFadden Avenue
Edinger Avenue
Heil Avenue
Warner Avenue
Slater Avenue
Talbert Avenue
Garfield Avenue
Gothard Street
Graham Street
Bolsa Chica Street
Saybrook Lane
Golden West Street
Main Street
Huntington Street
Atlanta Ave
Seapoint Street
Palm Avenue
Orange Avenue
Pacific Coast Highway
Marina Drive
Electric Ave
Ocean Avenue
Seal Beach Boulevard
Seal Beach National Wildlife Refuge
Bolsa Chica Ecological Reserve
Sunset County Beach
Bolsa Chica State Beach
Huntington Dog Beach
Huntington Beach
PACIFIC OCEAN
2.1/18.6mi
1.8mi/ 18.9mi
3.7mi
5.0/15.6mi
10.4mi
B1
B2
B3
B4
B5
B6
B7
P1
P2
P3
P4
P5
P6
R1
R2
R3
46
48
Miles
0
0.5
1
2
N
S
E
W

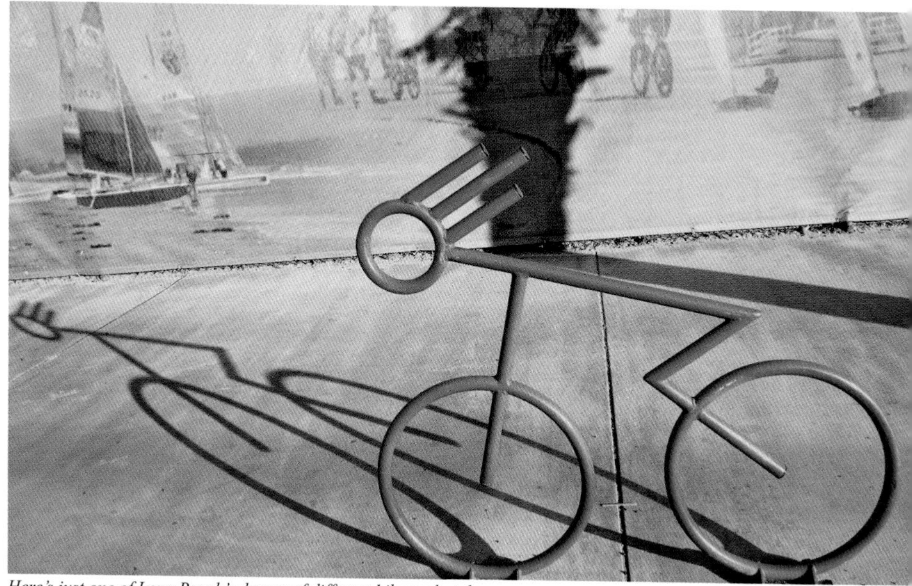

*Here's just one of Long Beach's dozens of different bike rack styles.*

## At a Glance

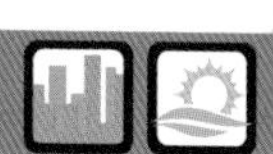

**Distance** 10.9 miles **Elevation Gain** 400 feet

### Terrain

The ride is flat except for a wee climb up Nieto Avenue onto Vista Street in Belmont Heights.

### Traffic

Other than a few blocks around Belmont Shores and Retro Row, this ride is a combo of bike lanes; a "bike boulevard" (on Vista Street); and a "separated bikeway" (on Third Street and Broadway), buffered from traffic by a row of parked cars.

### How to Get There

From the 710 Freeway, take Broadway through downtown Long Beach and two miles beyond it to Bixby Park. Park here or on adjacent streets. Alternatively, take Metro Blue Line south to the Long Beach Transit Mall and bicycle east on Broadway and then, First Street to the park.

### Food and Drink

Among the many East Village refueling spots are atmospheric coffee houses (such as the Village Grind and vegetarian joints including Steamed and the Zephyr Vegetarian Café.

### Side Trip

The Museum of Latin American Art's (MoLAA) sculpture garden and galleries has art from 20 Latin American countries (**www.molaa.com**). Another top option is the Long Beach Museum of Art—with ceramics, early 20th century European art, California modern and contemporary art, and more. (**www.lbma.org**).

**Links to** 42 46 48 49 k27

**Where to Bike Rating** 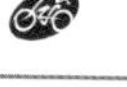

  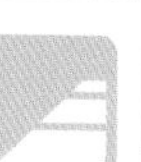 

## About...

On this easy spin, you'll get a good sense of Long Beach's inland offerings: from the city's progressive bicycling infrastructure to its art scene and Retro Row vintage shopping avenue. Along the way, the city's bounty of residential architecture comes into view, with Art Deco or streamlined Moderne confections and a medley of Craftsman-style bungalows and larger homes—especially in and around Belmont Heights, along Vista, First and Second streets—rivaling the more famous clusters in Pasadena.

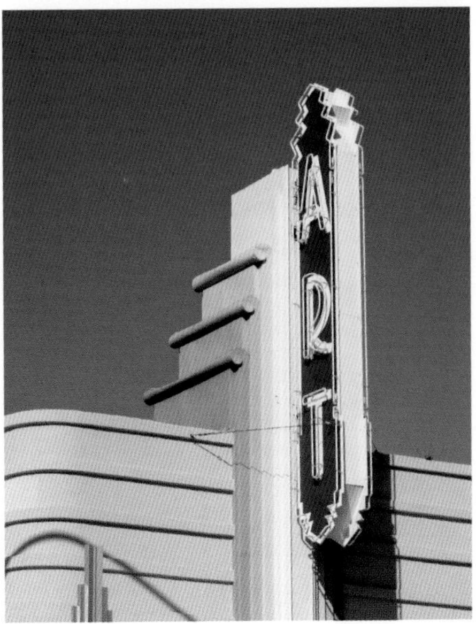


*On Retro Row: The restored 1920s Art Theater is now an artsy film, concert and event venue.*

More than any other Southern California city, Long Beach has committed resources, ideas and energy to urban bicycling solutions. This leisurely loop through eclectic inland neighborhoods gives you a taste of its recent innovations and experiments—including a "bicycle boulevard"; physically separated bike lanes, or "cycletracks"; and traffic-intersection green boxes to protect cyclists from turning cars. As you pedal along, watch for abundant bike racks, in at least 27 whimsical styles, evoking flying cyclists, high-wheelers, palms, waves, ice cream cones, carrots, sunflowers or guitars. The list goes on.

Our ride begins from Bixby Park, heading east through Belmont Shores' shopping district to Belmont Heights, a quiet, well-to-do neighborhood with vintage Craftsman cottages. The loop's eastern end connects with additional fun excursions: Naples's quaint canals, just across the Second Street Bridge from Belmont Shores (Ride 49); or Long Beach's shoreline bike path, reached by continuing straight on Termino Avenue around the Belmont Plaza Olympic Pool (Ride 48).

But back to our loop: In Belmont Heights, 1.5 miles of residential Vista Street are now L. A. County's first "bicycle boulevard." More common in the Netherlands or Berkeley, California, it's a street with traffic-calming measures for shared bike-and-car lanes. To slow and diminish traffic, Vista incorporates eight new roundabouts. The result: relaxed riding—safe enough for children pedaling to nearby elementary schools.

Next stop: Fourth Street's Retro Row with its hip, kitsch shops—featuring vintage attire, mid-century furnishings and skate boards—alongside small restaurants, coffee houses and wine bars. At the heart of the strip is the1920s Art Theater, serving up art films, first-run releases, live concerts and more.

The route jogs over to Third Street and later onto Broadway: two streets with a "separated bike lane," buffered from traffic by a curb-edged row of parked cars. This recent Long Beach addition even has bicycle traffic lights.

Onward through the emerging East Village Arts District, with galleries, Art Deco apartment buildings, street art, and bohemian restaurants and shops. Swing by the nearby Latin American Art Museum or explore Elm Street's outdoor artwork and galleries. Finally, coast along First Street's bike lanes back to the start.

Long Beach has earned a Bronze bike-friendly rating from the League of American Bicyclists. Yes, we know, Davis, California, is already Platinum and San Francisco Gold — but Long Beach's future cycling oasis is still a grand work in progress.

# Ride Log

B1 Jones Bicycles
5332 East 2nd St, Belmont Shores
B2 City Grounds, 435 1st St, Long Beach
B3 Bikestation Long Beach
222 East 1st St, Long Beach
B4 The Hub Community Bike Center
1730 Long Beach Blvd, Long Beach
R1 Wheel Fun Rentals
419 Shoreline Village Dr, Long Beach
R2 Wheel Fun Rentals
RMS Queen Mary, Long Beach
R3 Alfredo's Beach Club, 700 Shoreline Dr
(Alamitos Beach), Long Beach

P1 Long Beach Museum of Art
P2 Bluff Park
P3 Belmont Plaza Olympic Pool
P4 Naples
P5 Marine Stadium and Mothers Beach
P6 Retro Row
P7 Museum of Latin America Art
P8 East Village Arts Park
P9 Long Beach Performing Arts Center
P10 Long Beach Convention and Entertainment Center
P11 The Pike at Rainbow Harbor
P12 Shoreline Village
P13 Aquarium of the Pacific
P14 Shoreline Aquatic Park
P15 The RMS Queen Mary & Russian Submarine Scorpion
P16 Golden Shore Marine Biological Reserve

**0.0** From Bixby Park, begin riding east on First St.

**0.8** Cross Redondo Ave.

**1.2** Turn right onto Termino Ave.

**1.4** Cross Ocean Blvd, then turn left onto Olympic Plaza in front of the Belmont Plaza Olympic Pool.

**1.5** Turn left onto Bennett Ave and exit the parking area by turning right onto Ocean Blvd.

**2.3** Turn left onto 54th Pl, which then becomes Bay Shore Ave.

**2.7** Turn left onto Second St, joining the green bike lane.

**3.3** Turn right onto Livingston Dr.

**3.7** Turn left onto Nieto Ave as Livingston meets Broadway.

**3.8** Turn left onto the Vista Street Bike Blvd.

**4.9** Cross Redondo Ave.

**5.1** Turn left onto Obispo Ave then right onto Vista St.

**5.3** Turn left onto Temple Ave where Vista ends, cross Broadway, then turn right onto Second St.

**5.8** Turn right onto Junipero Ave.

**6.2** Turn left onto Fourth St.

**6.4** Turn left onto Cherry Ave.

**6.6** Turn right onto Third St, joining the bike lane.

**7.4** Cross Alamitos Ave then continue west using the protected bike lane running along the left side of Third. Carefully cross the street as traffic permits or use the crosswalk at Alamitos Ave. Obey the bicycle traffic signals.

**8.5** Turn left onto Maine Ave then left onto Broadway. The protected bike lane runs along Broadway's left side.

**9.7** Turn right onto Alamitos Ave.

**9.8** Turn left onto First St. Use the crosswalk if traffic conditions warrant. Join the bike lane

**10.9** Arrive back at Bixby Park. End of ride.

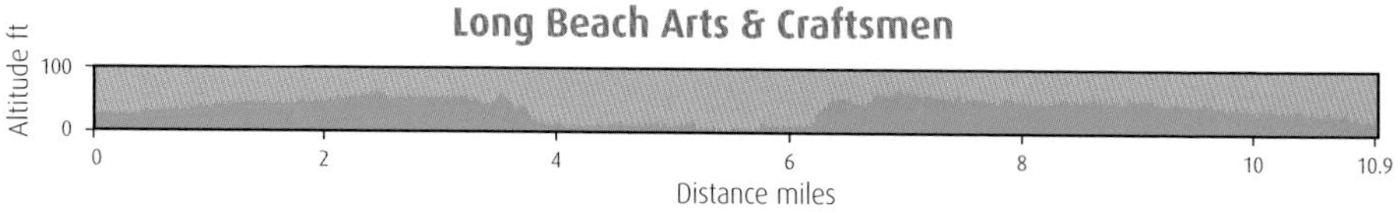

## Long Beach Arts & Craftsmen

Altitude ft: 0, 100
Distance miles: 0, 2, 4, 6, 8, 10, 10.9

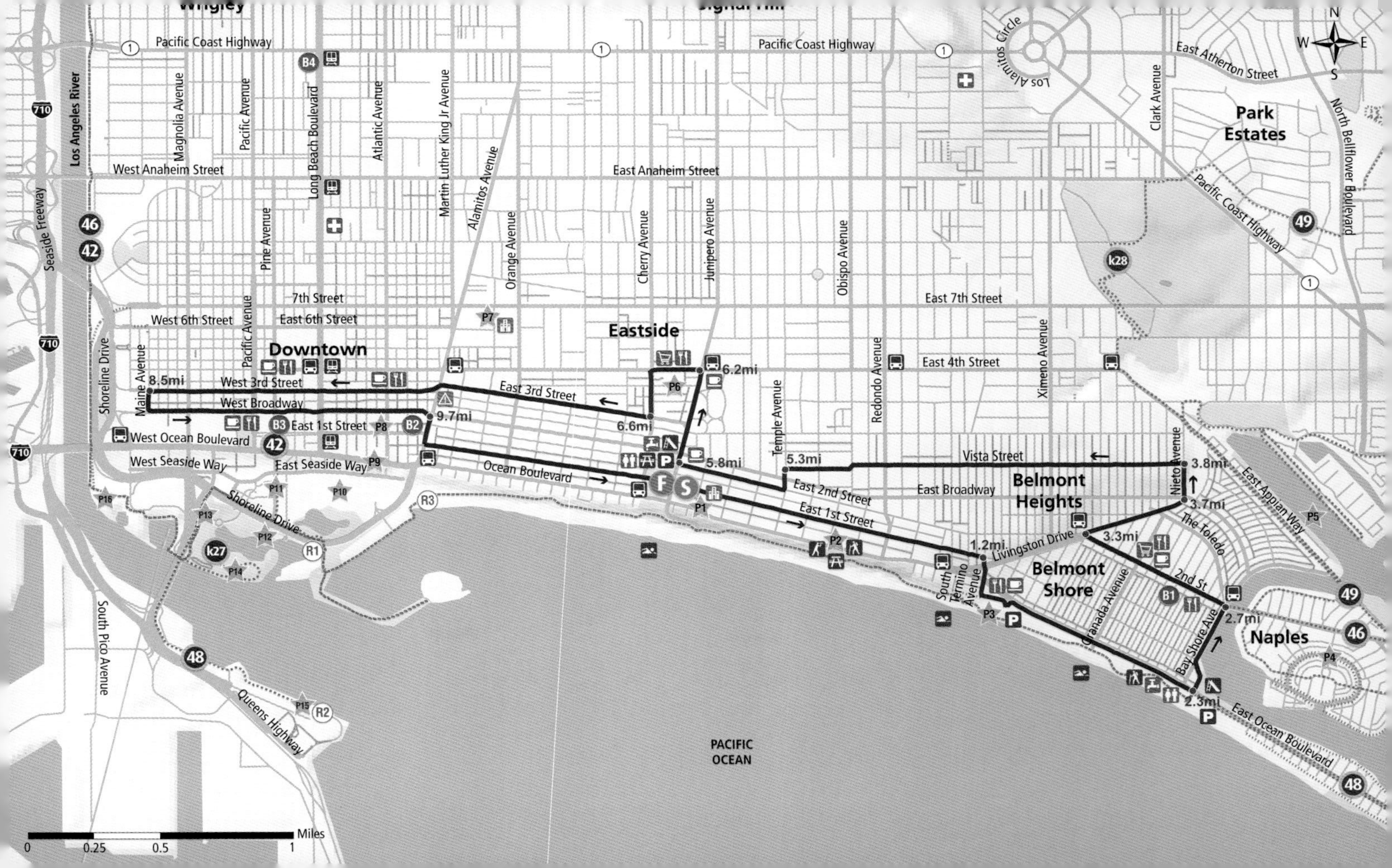

Pacific Coast Highway
Los Angeles River
Seaside Freeway
Magnolia Avenue
Pacific Avenue
Long Beach Boulevard
Atlantic Avenue
Martin Luther King Jr Avenue
Alamitos Avenue
Orange Avenue
Cherry Avenue
Junipero Avenue
Obispo Avenue
Temple Avenue
Redondo Avenue
Ximeno Avenue
Los Alamitos Circle
Clark Avenue
East Atherton Street
North Bellflower Boulevard
Park Estates
West Anaheim Street
East Anaheim Street
Pine Avenue
7th Street
East 7th Street
West 6th Street
East 6th Street
Eastside
Downtown
East 4th Street
Shoreline Drive
Maine Avenue
8.5mi
West 3rd Street
West Broadway
East 3rd Street
6.2mi
6.6mi
9.7mi
East 1st Street
West Ocean Boulevard
West Seaside Way
East Seaside Way
Ocean Boulevard
5.8mi
5.3mi
Vista Street
3.8mi
Nieto Avenue
East Broadway
East 2nd Street
Belmont Heights
3.7mi
East Appian Way
The Toledo
3.3mi
Livingston Drive
1.2mi
East 1st Street
South Termino Avenue
Belmont Shore
Granada Avenue
2nd St
2.7mi
Naples
Bay Shore Ave
2.3mi
East Ocean Boulevard
South Pico Avenue
Queens Highway
PACIFIC OCEAN
Miles
0
0.25
0.5
1

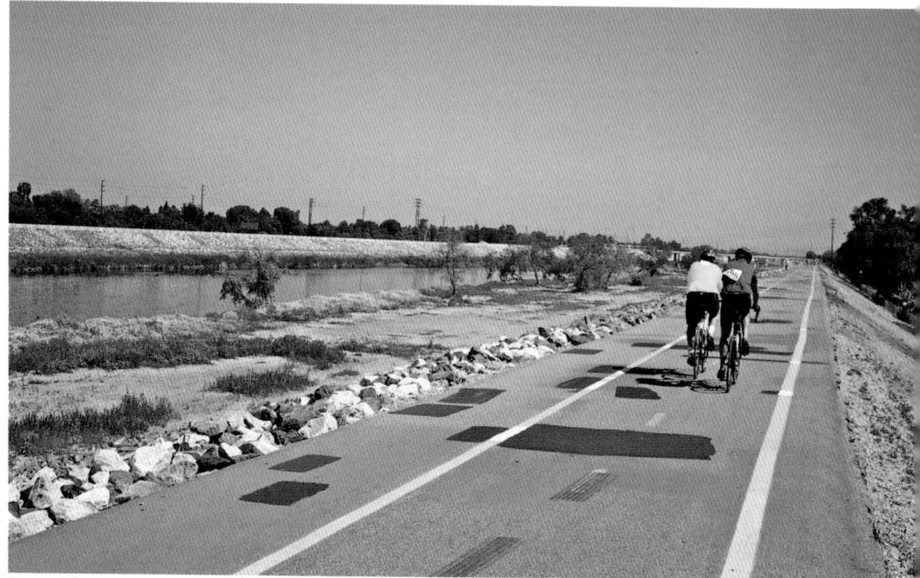

*River riding.*

## At a Glance

**Distance** 25.6 miles **Elevation Gain** 1,000 feet

### Terrain

This ring around Long Beach is flat except for brief grade changes where the river bikeways occasionally pass under a major street. Alternating between concrete and asphalt, the riding surfaces are typically in excellent condition.

### Traffic

Our "Periferico" features many miles on car-free bike paths, supplemented by bike lanes and a few blocks of uncategorized riding along quiet residential streets.

### How to Get There

From the 405 or 710 freeways, exit onto Pacific Place, Wardlow Road or Long Beach Boulevard. Continue to Metro's parking lot at Pacific Place and Wardlow Road. You'll also find plenty of on-street parking nearby. Alternatively, reach the Wardlow station via the Metro Blue Line.

### Food and Drink

Downtown Long Beach (along Pine Avenue), the Pike, Belmont Shores and Shoreline Village have plenty of eateries and coffeehouses.

### Side Trip

Retro Row, on Fourth Street between Junipero and Cherry avenues, is a vintage shopping district, offering hip used clothing and furniture—fun kitsch galore. The district also has many refreshment options, including Portfolio Coffee, at the Row's east end, serving up delish desserts and coffee. (From the Periferico route, turn right at Junipero and ride north about three quarters of a mile to Fourth.)

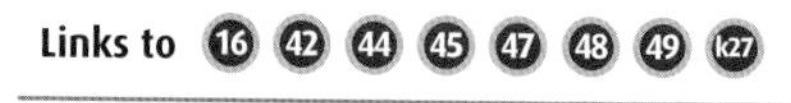


**Where to Bike Rating** 

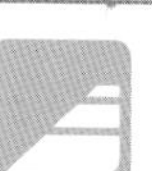

# About...

Many great metropolises, Paris, London, Mexico City and Washington, D.C., have ring roads with exciting names—Boulevard Périphérique, London Orbital, Anillo Periferico or Capitol Beltway—designed, at least in theory, to speed drivers around town while, ideally, reducing city-center congestion. Our Long Beach Bicycle Periferico borrows that idea, but with a spin. This ring is not necessarily about zipping across town, though you could, but about a car-free journey amid the features encircling the city—from river bikeways and residential districts to green spaces and oceanfront.

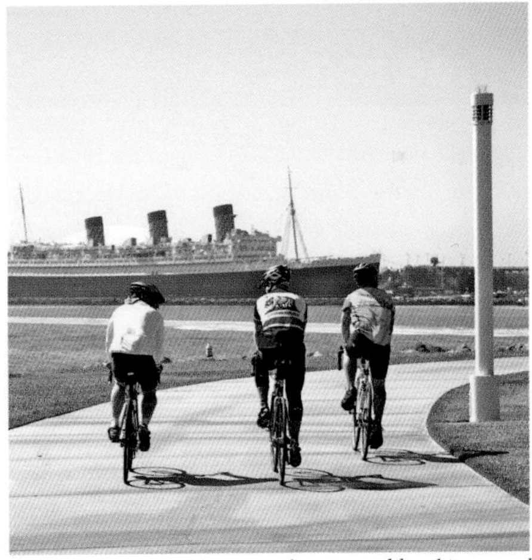

*The Queen Mary oceanliner-turned-hotel is moored permanently in Long Beach.*

Of course, a ring has no beginning or end—you can join it in many places. We suggest picking up this perimeter loop at Long Beach's northwest corner for its proximity to the Metro system, freeways and parking. From there, you'll roll along bike lanes in quiet, residential Bixby Knolls, named for early landowner-developers.

Once across Cherry Avenue, the ride continues near the airport and the center of local industrial history. For more than 70 years, Douglas Aircraft Company (later McDonald Douglas and eventually part of Boeing) manufactured planes here, including prop fighters and bombers and classic commercial aircraft, from the DC-3 through to DC-100. At the still active airport, the terminal—petite by modern standards—is a 1941 landmark that has appeared in Hollywood films. (In 1911, the very first transcontinental flight had actually landed in Long Beach, but on its sandy shores—the beach was the local runway until this airport was built.)

The ride turns at Rosie the Riveter Park, honoring the women who assembled World War II warbirds. You then spin by Veteran's Memorial Stadium, site of an antiques flea market (the third Sunday of each month) and home football field to Long Beach City College and several high schools. Soon, you'll pedal through Heartwell Park, with its amateur soccer and little league games and picnicking families. The park's safe paths, past a little lake, are well suited to leisurely cyclists of all ages.

Next: the San Gabriel River Bike Trail, a long, car-free straightaway roughly paralleling Long Beach's eastern boundary. From the trail, you can access El Dorado Park (Ride 47), Marine Stadium/CSULB (Ride 49), Alamitos Bay and Orange County (Ride 44).

The oceanfront bike path is the ride's southern edge: miles of protected beach, bordering attractions from Belmont Shores and Marine Park and to downtown Long Beach Shoreline Village and the RMS Queen Mary.

Finally, on the northbound leg, along the Los Angeles River Bikeway, near Long Beach's western boundary, you'll pass a curious residential neighborhood at mile 24: Wrigley Park, named for the chewing gum magnate and early Long Beach developer. Visible from the bike path, it's a quirky stretch of mid-century modern, ranch-style "chalets" (the Alps meet So Cal). Have a look over your right shoulder as you sail back to the start.

*While Ride 46 has not been deemed kid-friendly in its entirety, it does include substantial sections which are entirely safe for family use.*

# Ride Log

**0.0** Make your way to the south end of the Blue Line platform, on the sidewalk between the tracks and Cedar Ave. Begin riding east along Little Wardlow Rd (paralleling Wardlow, but separated by a wide curb).
**0.1** Turn left onto Pacific Ave.
**0.6** Turn right onto Bixby Rd, joining the bike lane.
**2.3** Turn left onto Industry Ave.
**2.4** Turn right onto Cover St, joining the bike lane.
**3.5** Ride around the Douglas Park traffic circle onto Worsham Ave.
**3.7** Turn left onto Conant St.
**4.4** Turn left on Clark Ave.
**4.9** Turn right into Heartwell Park just before Carson St. Follow the bike path through the park. Exercise caution when crossing Bellflower Blvd, Woodruff Ave and Palo Verde Ave.
**6.5** Cross Palo Verde, continuing on the bike path running parallel to the sidewalk along Carson St.
**7.3** Turn right, descend an access ramp, cross a small steel truss bridge, then turn right onto the San Gabriel River Bikeway.
**8.2** Pass El Dorado Park (Ride 47).
**9.9** Cross from the west to east bank of the San Gabriel River using the bridge. Continue south toward the ocean.
**13.7** Arrive at the Marina Dr bridge just before the ocean, exit the bike path, turn right and continue on Marina Dr.
**14.8** Turn left onto Second St. Exercise caution where automobiles exit from Second onto Appian Way.
**15.8** Turn left onto Bay Shore Ave, which then becomes 54th Pl.
**16.2** Cross Ocean Blvd, then join the Shoreline Pedestrian/Bicycle Path.
**19.8** Turn right onto the bikeway paralleling Shoreline Village Dr.
**20.0** Cross Shoreline Dr and continue along the bike way past Rainbow Lagoon Park.
**20.2** Cross Pine Ave.
**20.4** Turn left at Queens Way, crossing Shoreline Dr.
**20.6** Cross Aquarium Way, then angle left on the bike path along Golden Shore. Follow the arrow pointing to "Los Angeles River Trail."
**20.7** Cross Golden Shore using the crosswalk
**21.0** Pass the Catalina Express ferry terminal.
**21.2** Turn left just before Golden Shore RV Park, then right onto the Los Angeles River Bike Trail.
**25.1** Exit the Angeles River Bike Trail at Wrigley Greenbelt. If you pass under Wardlow Rd or the 405 Freeway, you've gone too far. Ride down the access ramp onto 34th St.
**25.3** Merge onto Wardlow Rd.
**25.6** Arrive back at Metro's Wardlow station. End of ride.

B
*B1* Lakewood Cyclery, 4313 Carson St, Lakewood
*B2* California Cycle Sport
6759 Carson St, Lakewood
*B3* Performance Bicycle
7611 Carson St, Long Beach
*B4* JAX Bicycle Center
3000 Bellflower Blvd, Long Beach
*B5* Sports Authority
6346 Pacific Coast Hwy, Long Beach
*B6* Jones Bicycles
5332 East 2nd St, Belmont Shores
*B7* City Grounds, 435 1st St, Long Beach
*B8* Bikestation Long Beach
222 East 1st St, Long Beach
*B9* The Hub Community Bike Center
1730 Long Beach Blvd, Long Beach
R
*R1* Wheel Fun Rentals
419 Shoreline Village Dr, Long Beach
*R2* Wheel Fun Rentals
RMS Queen Mary, Long Beach
*R3* Alfredo's Beach Club, 700 Shoreline Dr
(Alamitos Beach), Long Beach

**Long Beach Bicycle Periferico: The Perimeter Route**

Altitude ft: 100, 0
Distance miles: 0, 4, 8, 12, 16, 20, 24, 25.6

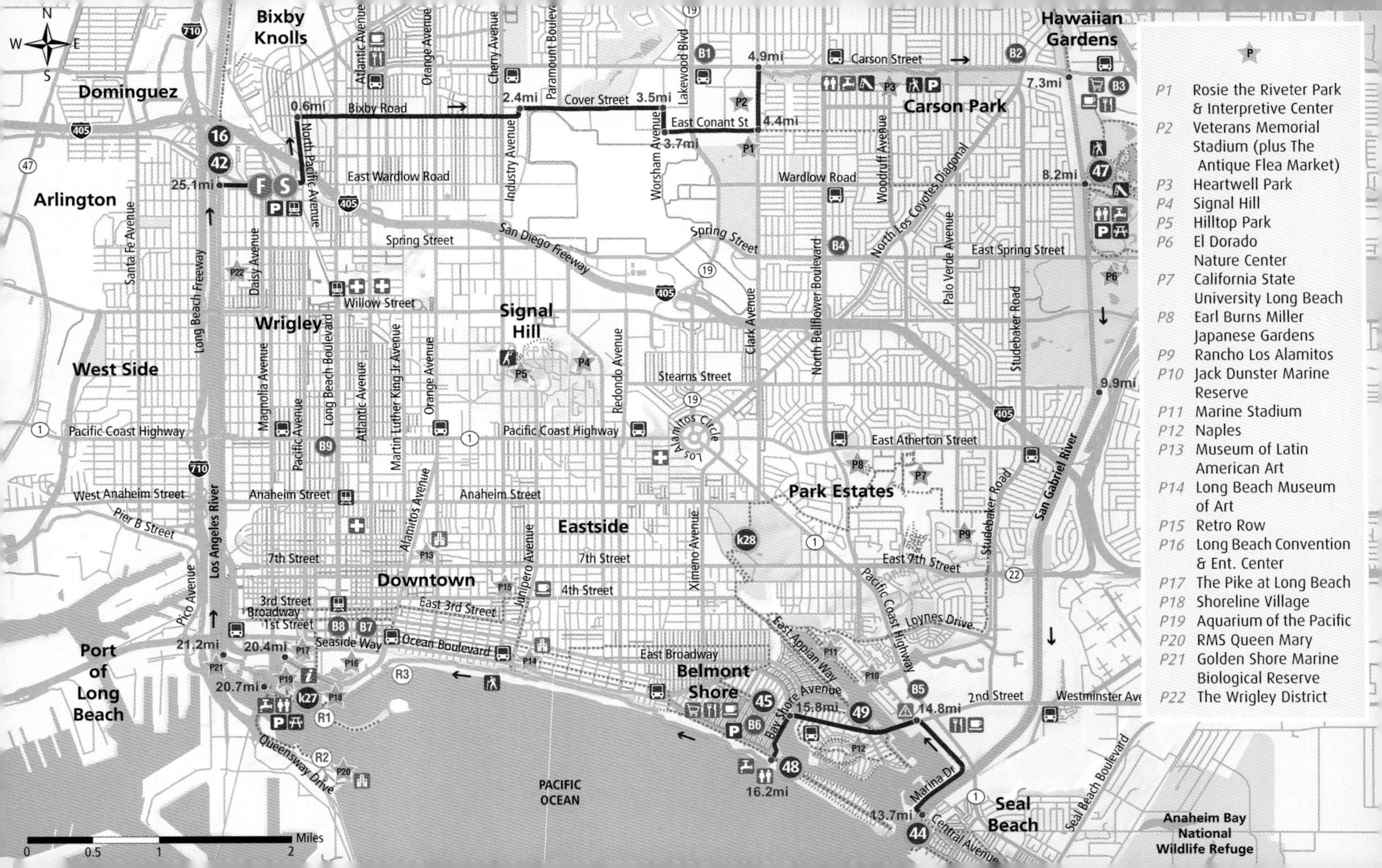

Bixby Knolls
Dominguez
Arlington
West Side
Wrigley
Signal Hill
Downtown
Eastside
Park Estates
Carson Park
Hawaiian Gardens
Belmont Shore
Seal Beach
Port of Long Beach
PACIFIC OCEAN
Anaheim Bay National Wildlife Refuge
Bixby Road
Cover Street
East Conant St
Carson Street
East Wardlow Road
Wardlow Road
Spring Street
San Diego Freeway
East Spring Street
Willow Street
Stearns Street
Pacific Coast Highway
East Atherton Street
West Anaheim Street
Anaheim Street
Pier B Street
7th Street
East 7th Street
4th Street
3rd Street
Broadway
1st Street
East 3rd Street
Seaside Way
Ocean Boulevard
East Broadway
East Appian Way
Bay Shore Avenue
Loynes Drive
2nd Street
Westminster Ave
Marina Dr
Central Avenue
Seal Beach Boulevard
Queensway Drive
Long Beach Freeway
Los Angeles River
San Gabriel River
Pico Avenue
Santa Fe Avenue
Daisy Avenue
Magnolia Avenue
Pacific Avenue
Long Beach Boulevard
Atlantic Avenue
Martin Luther King Jr Avenue
Orange Avenue
Alamitos Avenue
Junipero Avenue
Redondo Avenue
Cherry Avenue
Paramount Boulevard
Industry Avenue
Lakewood Blvd
Worsham Avenue
Clark Avenue
Ximeno Avenue
Los Alamitos Circle
North Bellflower Boulevard
Woodruff Avenue
North Los Coyotes Diagonal
Palo Verde Avenue
Studebaker Road
North Pacific Avenue
0.6mi
2.4mi
3.5mi
3.7mi
4.4mi
4.9mi
7.3mi
8.2mi
9.9mi
13.7mi
14.8mi
15.8mi
16.2mi
20.4mi
20.7mi
21.2mi
25.1mi
Miles
0
0.5
1
2
P1 Rosie the Riveter Park & Interpretive Center
P2 Veterans Memorial Stadium (plus The Antique Flea Market)
P3 Heartwell Park
P4 Signal Hill
P5 Hilltop Park
P6 El Dorado Nature Center
P7 California State University Long Beach
P8 Earl Burns Miller Japanese Gardens
P9 Rancho Los Alamitos
P10 Jack Dunster Marine Reserve
P11 Marine Stadium
P12 Naples
P13 Museum of Latin American Art
P14 Long Beach Museum of Art
P15 Retro Row
P16 Long Beach Convention & Ent. Center
P17 The Pike at Long Beach
P18 Shoreline Village
P19 Aquarium of the Pacific
P20 RMS Queen Mary
P21 Golden Shore Marine Biological Reserve
P22 The Wrigley District

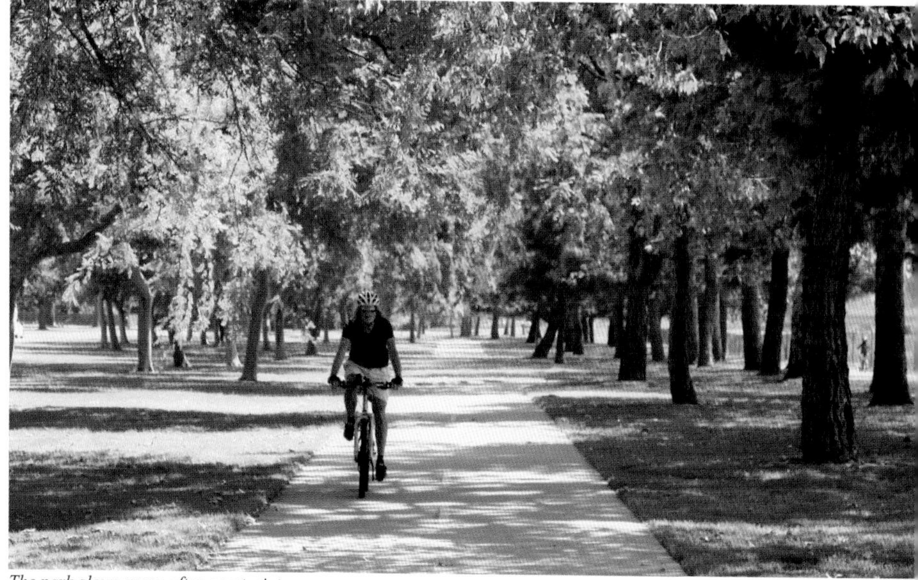

*The park glows green after a wet winter.*

## At a Glance

**Distance** 3.9 miles **Elevation Gain** 100 feet

### Terrain

A pair of flat, easy loops with a couple of minor inclines form this route. The loop south of Wardlow Road is a concrete bike path, while its counterpart to the north is an asphalt road.

### Traffic

Walkers, joggers and skaters share the bike path, so watch out for them. Automobile traffic within the park tends to be courteous and slow moving.

### How to Get There

Exit the 605 Freeway at Spring Street or at Willow/Katella, then drive west a short distance to the park's entrance. All-day vehicle entry fees are modest: $5 on weekdays, $7 on the weekends and $8 on holidays.

### Food and Drink

Long Beach Towne Center, just north of the park and accessible via a short ride on the San Gabriel River Bike Path, has a Walmart, restaurants, a Starbucks and Ben & Jerry's ice cream.

### Side Trip

The San Gabriel River Bike Path (see Rides 16 and 46) runs along the park's western edge with entry points at Wardlow or Spring Street. You can venture as far south as the beach at Naples (six miles) or as far north as the San Gabriel Mountains (32 miles) on this vehicle-free bikeway.

**Links to** 16 46

**Where to Bike Rating** 

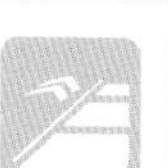
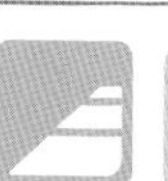
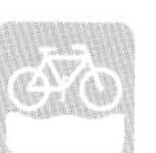

## About...

El Dorado East Regional Park is the biggest urban park in the Long Beach area. Within its 400 acres, ducks and geese flock, anglers cast their lines (there are three lakes), archers draw their bows, model glider planes soar overhead and families picnic beneath shady trees. That's just a sampling of the diverse activities that co-exist peacefully in this grassy park.

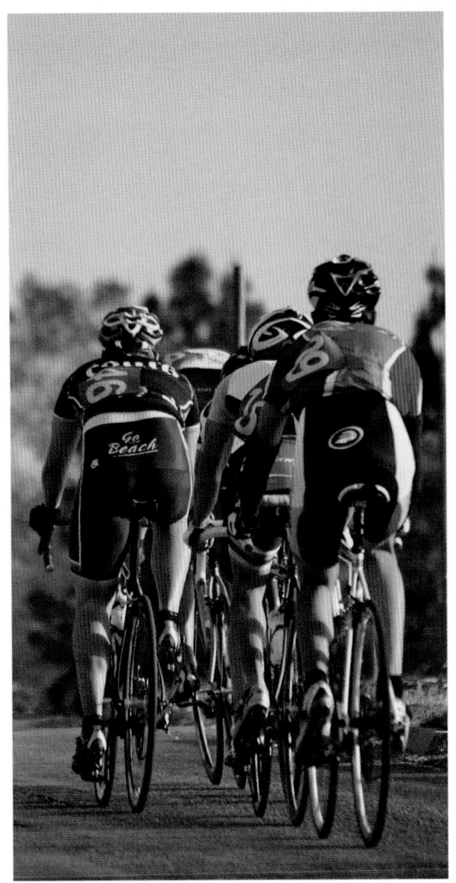


*Tuesday evenings, from March through August, El Dorado hosts criterium races.*

This is a dual-loop ride, with one circuit in the park's northern section and the other ringing its southern tract. A short passageway under Wardlow Road (the city street that cleaves El Dorado Park) connects these loops. We begin our ride from the parking area near El Dorado's entrance, off Spring Street, but you can actually pedal from any of the seven different car lots throughout the park.

From the archery range, the bike path follows the park's outer edges, passing first through a meadow with shade trees. Low hills separate this flat field from the rest of the park, so it's easy to imagine yourself riding through a great, secluded landscape (though traffic buzz from the nearby freeway may occasionally trespass on that idyllic daydream). After coasting by plenty of picnic spots and BBQ pits, you'll pass through the short tunnel to the park's northern side. For the next couple of miles, you'll be riding among cars—so be attentive. El Dorado's two lakes north of Wardlow Road attract abundant birdlife, including herons, egrets, ducks and geese.

On this side of the park, the loop becomes the track for weekly criterium races, "The Tuesday Twilight Racing Series," held from March to August. This series has been integral to Southern California's grassroots racing culture for more than 25 years. On race evenings, consider a late-afternoon spin around the park before you dismount to watch the aspiring champions chase each other around the 1.75-mile circuit as the sun sets.

In broad daylight, the El Dorado Park ride has an outstandingly kid-friendly southern loop. You'll also find more than five miles of ride extensions, some on the access roads that wind through the park's southern terrain.

*While Ride 47 has not been deemed kid-friendly in its entirety, it does include substantial sections which are entirely safe for family use.*

# Ride Log

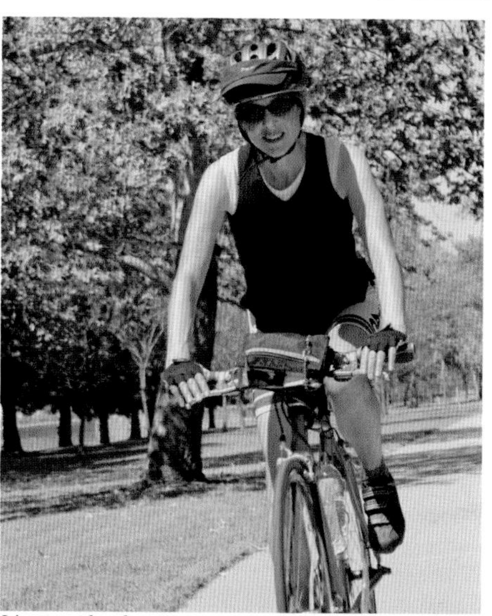
*It's easy riding here.*

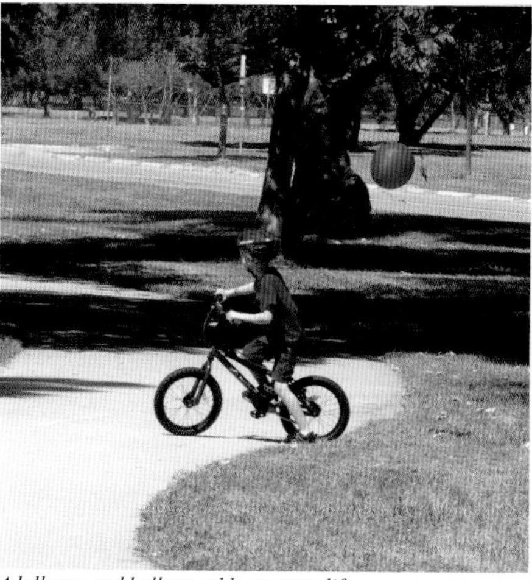
*A lollypop-red balloon adds an extra lift.*

**0.0** From the archery range's parking lot, cross the access road, join the bike path and then ride east toward the Spring St entrance road.

**0.9** Cross the old, unused access road (which is gated barring vehicles) and resume riding on the bike path.

**1.2** Turn right and follow the paved roadway as it passes under Wardlow Rd.

**1.3** Stay to the right at the Y, following the sign to Arbor Day Grove.

**1.7** Pass Arbor Day Grove.

**1.8** Pass El Dorado Express train ride (Saturday and Sunday 10:30 a.m. to 4:00 p.m., $2.00 per person) at Caboose Corners.

**2.6** Stay to the left at the Y—there's a big, open meadow for model airplane flying on the left.

**3.0** Stay to the right at the Y and ride towards the San Gabriel River.

**3.1** Cross under Wardlow Rd.

**3.2** Rejoin the bike path on the right.

**3.7** Stay to the left at the Y, turning away from the river, and cross an access road.

**3.9** Return to the archery range parking area. End of loop.

*P1* Tuesday Twilight Criterium Races (March through August)
*P2* El Dorado Nature Center
*P3* Pedal Boat Dock and snack bar (summer weekends)

B
*B1* JAX Bicycle Center
3000 Bellflower Blvd, Long Beach
*B2* California Cycle Sport
6759 Carson St, Lakewood
*B3* Performace Cycles
7611 E. Carson Blvd, Long Beach

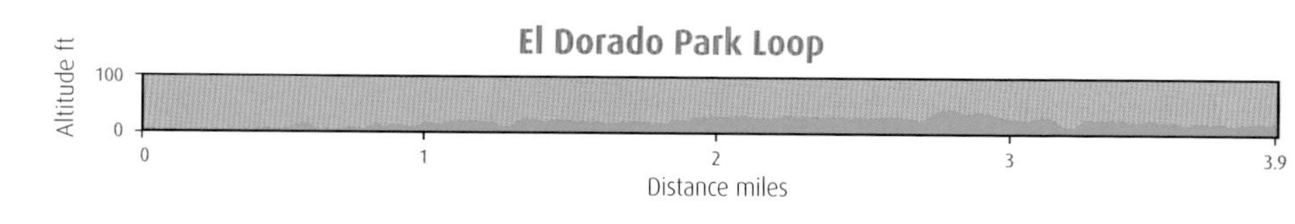

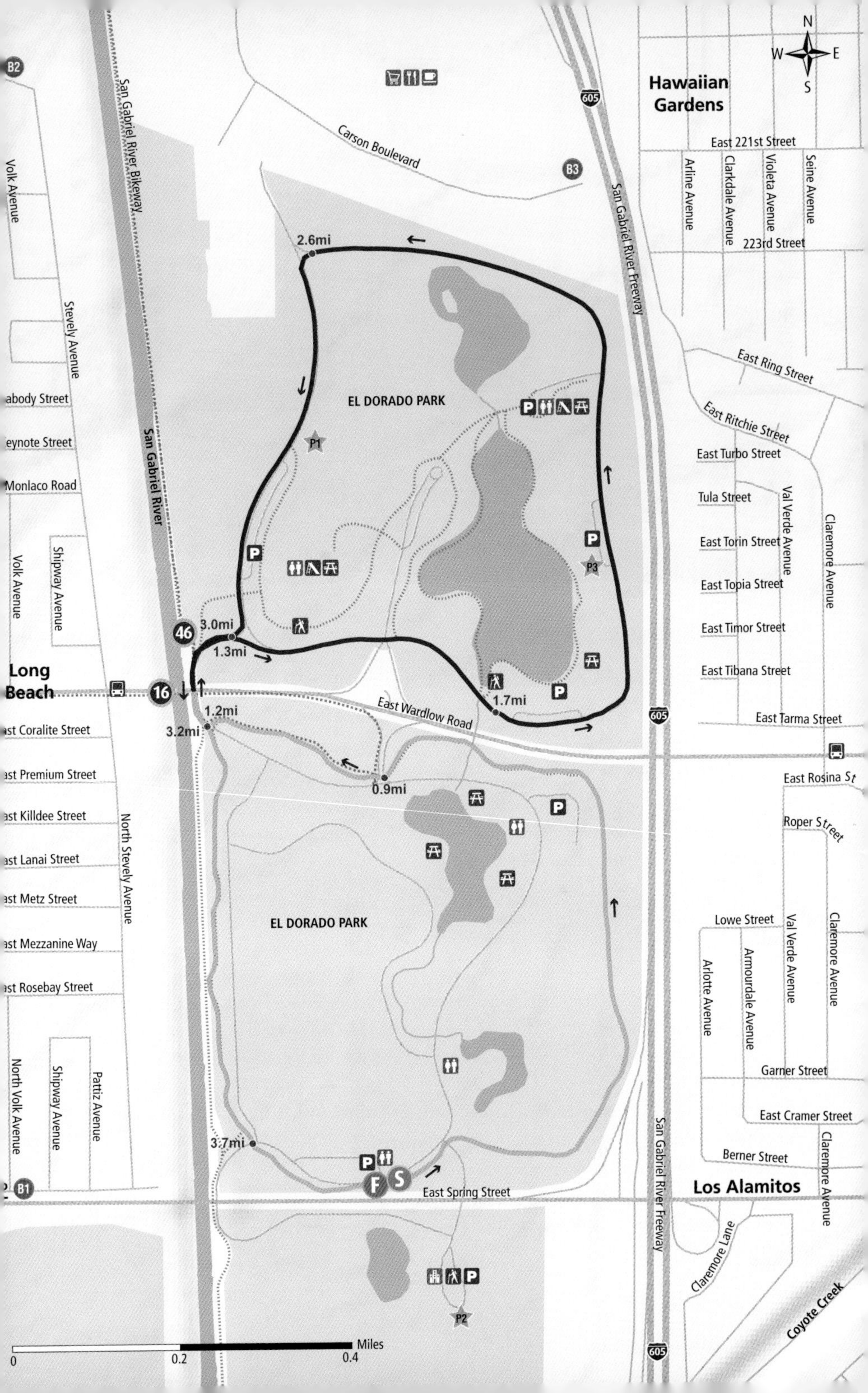

N
W
E
S
Hawaiian Gardens
Carson Boulevard
San Gabriel River Bikeway
San Gabriel River Freeway
605
B2
B3
East 221st Street
Arline Avenue
Clarkdale Avenue
Violeta Avenue
Seine Avenue
223rd Street
Volk Avenue
Stevely Avenue
2.6mi
EL DORADO PARK
P1
East Ring Street
East Ritchie Street
East Turbo Street
Tula Street
Val Verde Avenue
East Torin Street
Claremore Avenue
East Topia Street
East Timor Street
East Tibana Street
East Tarma Street
abody Street
eynote Street
Monlaco Road
San Gabriel River
Shipway Avenue
Volk Avenue
P3
46
3.0mi
1.3mi
Long Beach
16
1.7mi
East Wardlow Road
1.2mi
3.2mi
ast Coralite Street
ast Premium Street
ast Killdee Street
ast Lanai Street
ast Metz Street
ast Mezzanine Way
ast Rosebay Street
North Stevely Avenue
0.9mi
East Rosina St
Roper Street
EL DORADO PARK
Lowe Street
Val Verde Avenue
Claremore Avenue
Arlotte Avenue
Armourdale Avenue
Garner Street
East Cramer Street
Berner Street
North Volk Avenue
Shipway Avenue
Pattiz Avenue
3.7mi
F
S
B1
East Spring Street
Los Alamitos
Claremore Avenue
Claremore Lane
P2
Coyote Creek
Miles
0
0.2
0.4

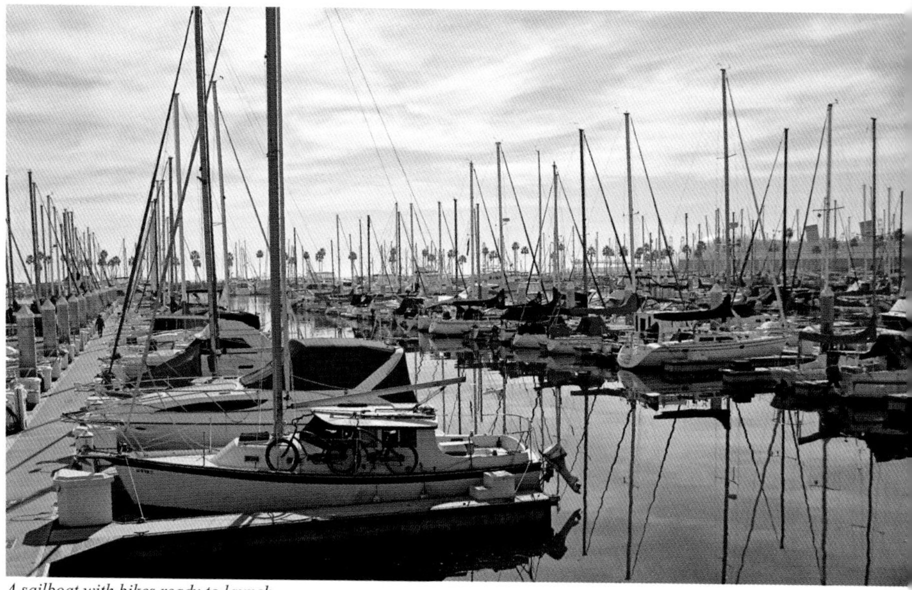

*A sailboat with bikes ready to launch.*

## At a Glance

**Distance** 15.0 miles **Elevation Gain** 500 feet

### Terrain

The mostly concrete and asphalt shoreline bike path has two short climbs, one over the Queensway Bridge and the other, at the ride's end, up to Bixby and Bluff parks.

### Traffic

This ride is on bike paths, except for a short stretch of fairly quiet street riding on Ocean Boulevard between 54th Place and Alamitos Park.

### How to Get There

From the 710 Freeway, take Broadway into downtown Long Beach. Continue east about two miles to Bixby Park. You can park there or on adjacent streets. Alternatively, take Metro Blue Line south to the Long Beach Transit Mall, then bicycle east on Broadway and First Street to the park.

### Food and Drink

Second Street in Belmont Shores has plenty of options espresso joints, ice cream stands and restaurants. Take 54th Place north to Bay Shore Avenue. Continue on Bay Shore for a couple of blocks, then left onto Second Street

### Side Trip

Take a shipboard tour of *RMS Queen Mary*, the retired 1936 ocean liner, now a museum and hotel-dining complex permanently moored in Long Beach. Tours include engine rooms and deluxe Art Deco interiors Anchored beside it is *The Scorpion*, a decommissioned Soviet-era attack submarine, also open for visits.

**Links to** 42 44 45 46 49 k27

**Where to Bike Rating** 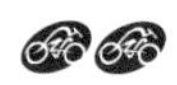

 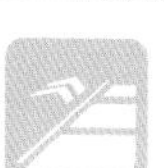  

## About...

This is a laid-back, beach cruiser-style tour of the Long Beach shoreline. Near its western end, the route borders The Pike, a small amusement park, and the Aquarium of the Pacific. After crossing the Queensway Bridge and looping around to the majestic *Queen Mary,* the vintage ocean liner, you'll proceed east on four-plus miles of bicycle-and-pedestrian path along the city's main beach. The ride turnaround is Alamitos Park. The long, car-free stretch from Shoreline Village to 54th Place is great for families with kids.

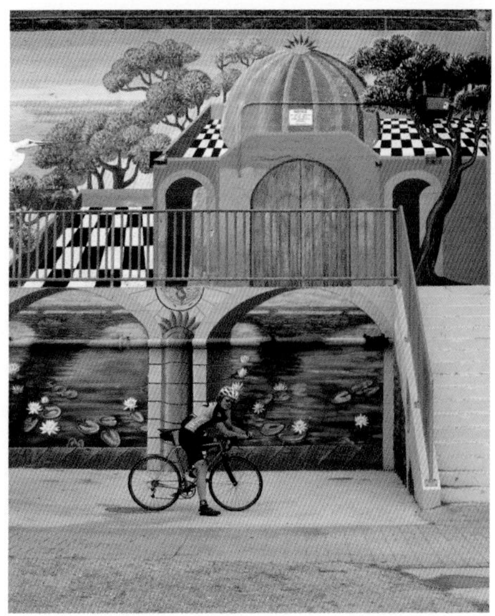

*You'll pass this mural (maybe once part of a restaurant?) along the beach path.*

Like many Southern California ocean-side cities, Long Beach was once famous for its popular amusement zone, known here as The Pike. Its wooden amusement pier, a teeming tourist attraction packed with eclectic and tacky delights, is long gone, but the spirit of fun by the sea lives on in Long Beach's modern (more low-key and cleaned-up) incarnation of The Pike: a smaller entertainment area with a Ferris wheel and rollercoaster-shaped pedestrian bridge. Neighboring tourist magnets include the Aquarium of the Pacific, focused on local marine life; and Shoreline Village, a cluster of eateries and rides in a faux-New England fishing port. Just as cycling was the transportation of choice in the old days, it still fits the setting. So, pedal on....

The next destination is *RMS Queen Mary*, a retired 1936 ocean liner, permanently moored here, now a museum and hotel-dining complex peacefully co-existing beside a vintage attack submarine. (See: Side Trip).

As you ride back over the Queensway Bridge, be sure to stop mid-span at the road deck's highpoint for views of the entire Long Beach shoreline, all the way east to Alamitos Bay. You can see Terminal Island, a vast shipping container-processing compound, serving the ports of Long Beach and Los Angeles (the island also houses a Federal prison).

From the bridge, the ride turns south, alongside a small-craft marina, bristling with masts. After breezing out onto the breakwater, past fishermen and sailboats, you'll continue on the Shoreline Pedestrian/Bicycle Path along a sheltered beach extending more than four miles, from downtown Long Beach to the San Gabriel River's outlet at Alamitos Bay. When the wind's strong, this stretch attracts flocks of kite boarders: surfers pulled along by colorful, billowy kites. The palm-studded islands you'll see offshore are actually oil rigs, masquerading as balmy tropical retreats. The city's fame as an oil town dates back to the 1920s, when bubbling crude was first discovered in the area. In those days, the Long Beach Oil Field, with its Alamitos No. 1 gusher, was considered one of the most productive in the world.

Burning snack energy instead of petroleum fuel, you'll finally arrive at the end of the ocean-side bike path. Here, at 54th Place, the route turns onto Ocean Boulevard, where you'll pass between ocean and bay, as you coast toward the turnaround, near the marina at Alamitos Park.

*While Ride 48 has not been deemed kid-friendly in its entirety, it does include substantial sections which are entirely safe for family use.*

# Ride Log

**0.0** Begin the ride at the southeast corner of Bixby Park, at the intersection of Ocean Blvd and Junipero Ave. Cross Ocean and descend to the beach.

**0.2** Turn right onto Long Beach Bikeway 2.

**1.3** Just past the Alfredo's Beach Club concessions stand, turn left and then right, continuing on Bikeway 2 parallel to the marina.

**1.8** Turn right onto Long Beach Bikeway 17 running parallel to Shoreline Village Dr.

**1.9** Cross Shoreline Dr and continue on Bikeway 17 past Rainbow Lagoon Park.

**2.1** Cross Pine Ave.

**2.4** Turn left at Queens Way, crossing Shoreline Dr. Continue on Bikeway 17.

**2.5** Cross Aquarium Way, then angle to right on the bike path towards *RMS Queen Mary*.

**2.8** Cross Queensway Bridge.

**3.1** Join Queensway Dr where the bikeway ends. Watch for cross traffic.

**3.3** Enter Harry Bridges Park, follow the path/sidewalk along the harbor's edge.

**3.5** Leave the park and continue straight along the edge of the Catalina Express parking lot to the *Queen Mary* and the Russian submarine *Scorpion*. After visiting those two landmarks, ride back through the parking lot and Harry Bridges Park onto Queensway Dr.

**4.2** Join Bikeway 17, watch for cross traffic.

**4.5** Cross Queensway Bridge.

**4.9** Merge with Bikeway 2.

**5.0** Cross Shoreline Dr, turn right onto Bikeway 17.

**5.2** Cross Pine Ave and pass by Rainbow Lagoon Park.

**5.5** Cross Shoreline Dr at the signal and continue on Bikeway 17 parallel to Shoreline Village Dr.

**5.6** Turn right on Bikeway 2. Continue along the breakwater past Shoreline Village.

**6.3** Arrive at the end of the breakwater. Return by the same route.

**6.8** Turn right at Shoreline Village and continue straight along the marina on Bikeway 2.

**7.4** Make a left, then a right turn, continue along the beach.

**9.7** Cross Belmont Pier.

**10.7** Turn right onto Ocean Blvd.

**11.7** Arrive at Alamitos Park. After enjoying this park and beach area, return along Ocean Blvd.

**12.8** Turn left and rejoin Bikeway 2 at 54th Pl.

**13.9** Cross Belmont Pier.

**14.7** Turn right onto Junipero Ave and ascend the short hill.

**15.0** Cross Ocean Blvd to Bixby Park. End of ride.

B
*B1* City Grounds Long Beach
435 E First St, Long Beach
*B2* The Hub Community Bike Center
1730 Long Beach Blvd, Long Beach
*B3* Bike Station
222 E Broadway, Long Beach
*B4* Jones Bicycles & Skateboards
5332 E Second St, Long Beach
*B5* Sports Authority
6346 Pacific Coast Hwy, Long Beach

R
*R1* Wheel Fun Rentals
419 Shoreline Village Dr, Long Beach
*R2* Wheel Fun Rentals
RMS Queen Mary, Long Beach
*R3* Alfredo's Beach Club
700 Shoreline Dr (Alamitos Bch), Long Beach

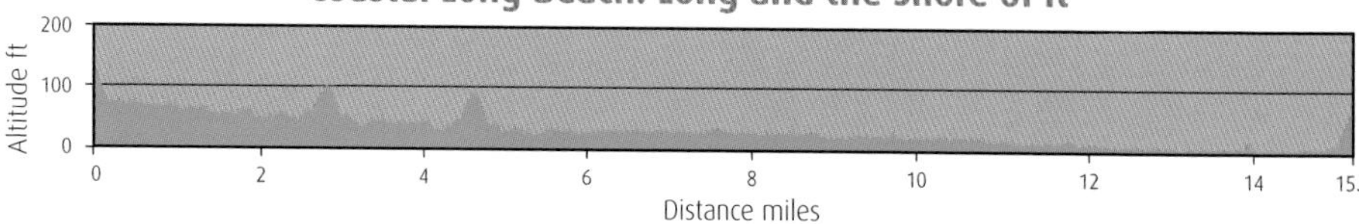

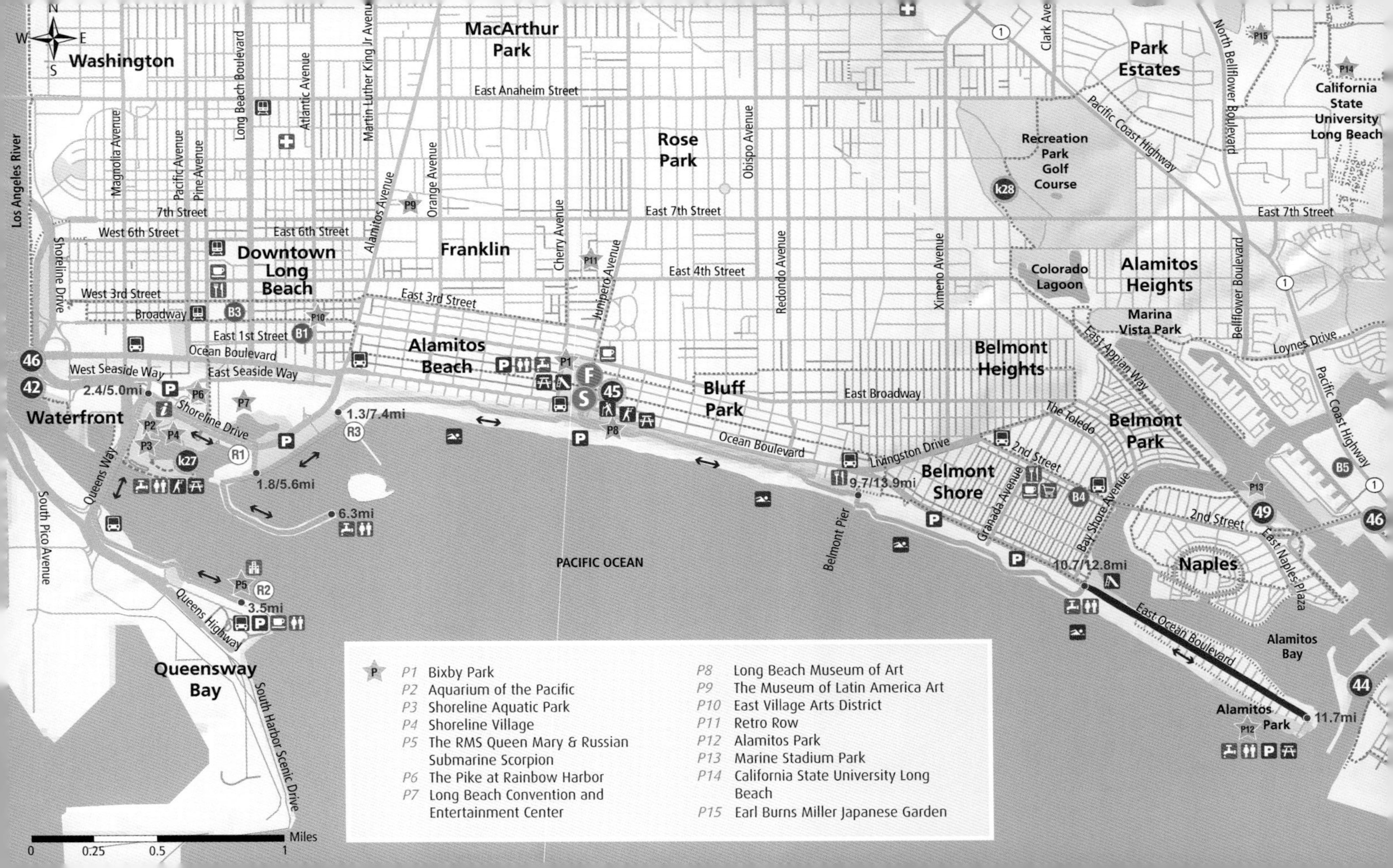

Washington
MacArthur Park
Rose Park
Park Estates
California State University Long Beach
Recreation Park Golf Course
Franklin
Downtown Long Beach
Alamitos Heights
Colorado Lagoon
Marina Vista Park
Alamitos Beach
Bluff Park
Belmont Heights
Belmont Park
Belmont Shore
Naples
Alamitos Bay
Alamitos Park
Waterfront
Queensway Bay
PACIFIC OCEAN
Los Angeles River
Shoreline Drive
Magnolia Avenue
Pacific Avenue
Pine Avenue
Long Beach Boulevard
Atlantic Avenue
Martin Luther King Jr Avenue
Alamitos Avenue
Orange Avenue
Cherry Avenue
Junipero Avenue
Obispo Avenue
Redondo Avenue
Ximeno Avenue
Clark Ave
North Bellflower Boulevard
Bellflower Boulevard
Pacific Coast Highway
East Anaheim Street
7th Street
East 7th Street
West 6th Street
East 6th Street
West 3rd Street
East 3rd Street
East 4th Street
Broadway
East 1st Street
Ocean Boulevard
West Seaside Way
East Seaside Way
East Broadway
East Appian Way
Loynes Drive
The Toledo
Livingston Drive
2nd Street
Granada Avenue
Bay Shore Avenue
East Naples Plaza
East Ocean Boulevard
Belmont Pier
Queens Way
South Pico Avenue
Queens Highway
South Harbor Scenic Drive
2.4/5.0mi
1.3/7.4mi
1.8/5.6mi
6.3mi
3.5mi
9.7/13.9mi
10.7/12.8mi
11.7mi
P1 Bixby Park
P2 Aquarium of the Pacific
P3 Shoreline Aquatic Park
P4 Shoreline Village
P5 The RMS Queen Mary & Russian Submarine Scorpion
P6 The Pike at Rainbow Harbor
P7 Long Beach Convention and Entertainment Center
P8 Long Beach Museum of Art
P9 The Museum of Latin America Art
P10 East Village Arts District
P11 Retro Row
P12 Alamitos Park
P13 Marine Stadium Park
P14 California State University Long Beach
P15 Earl Burns Miller Japanese Garden
Miles
0
0.25
0.5
1

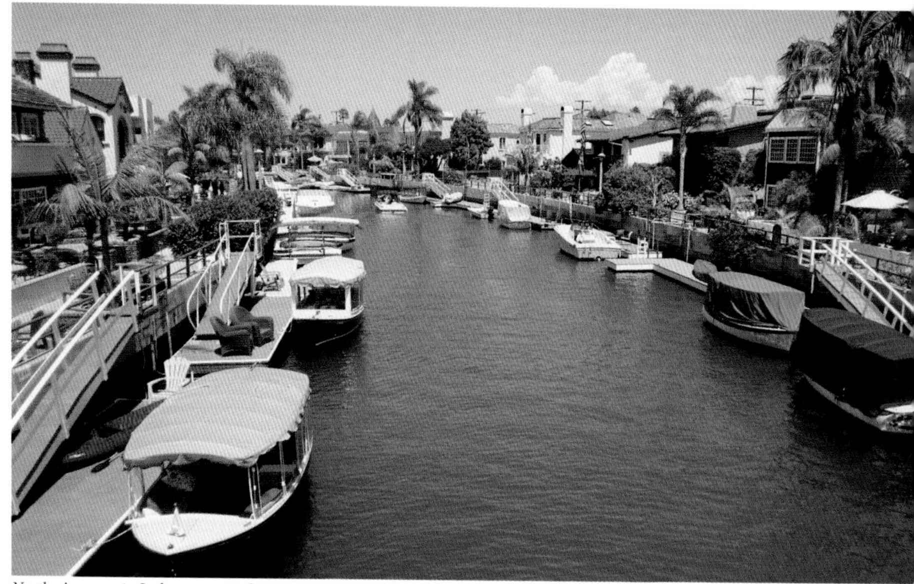

*Naples' romantic Italianate canals were fashioned from swamps around 1903.*

## At a Glance

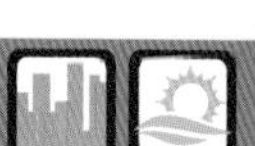

**Distance** 12.4 miles **Elevation Gain** 400 feet

### Terrain

This mostly flat ride is on city streets and paved bike paths.

### Traffic

Traffic tends to be light in residential Naples, Bixby Hill, Bixby Village and Alamitos Heights, as well as the Cal State Long Beach campus. Elsewhere, expect moderate traffic, increasing around Marine Park on weekends.

### How to Get There

Drive south on the 405 Freeway to southeast Long Beach. Exit at Seal Beach Boulevard and go south. Turn right onto Westminster Avenue (becomes Second Street). Cross Pacific Coast Highway, then turn right onto Appian Way and park street-side or in one of the lots near Mother's Beach at Marine Park.

### Food and Drink

Eateries are plentiful on Second Street in Belmont Shores and in the shopping centers on Westminster Avenue and Pacific Coast Highway. There's a Starbuck at Seventh Street across from Recreation Park.

### Side Trip

Rancho Los Alamitos is a National Register site once occupied by native Tongva people, then Spaniards and, later, Mexicans. Visit the adobe ranch house (ca. 1800) and historic gardens (Wednesdays through Sundays, 1:00 p.m. to 5:00 p.m.; free of charge). The historic barnyard will reopen in 2012. (6400 Bixby Hill Road—enter through security gate at Anaheim and Palo Verde; tel. 562-431-3541).

**Links to** 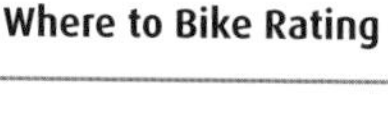


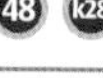

**Where to Bike Rating** 

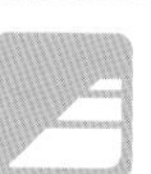

# About...

Long Beach derives its name from a great stretch of oceanfront, but—don't be fooled—there's plenty to explore inland, as well. This ride takes you on a whirl from a 1932 Olympics venue to an Italian-styled neighborhood of quaint canals and bridges, followed by the campus of California State University Long Beach, with its Japanese garden and huge, blue pyramid, before you loop back, coasting along a couple of waterways en route.

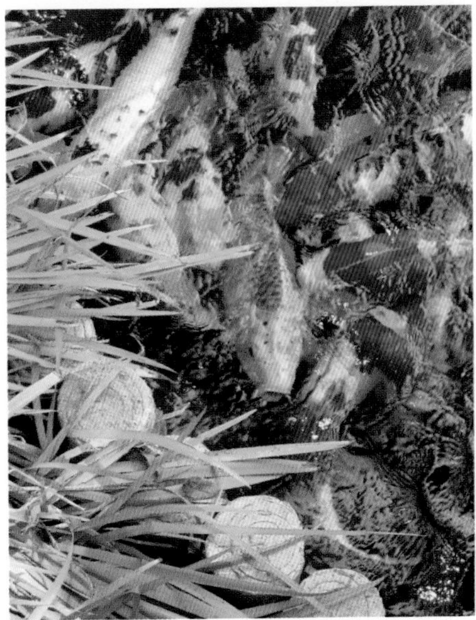

*At the Earl Burns Miller Japanese Garden, the koi are big, colorful and abundant.*

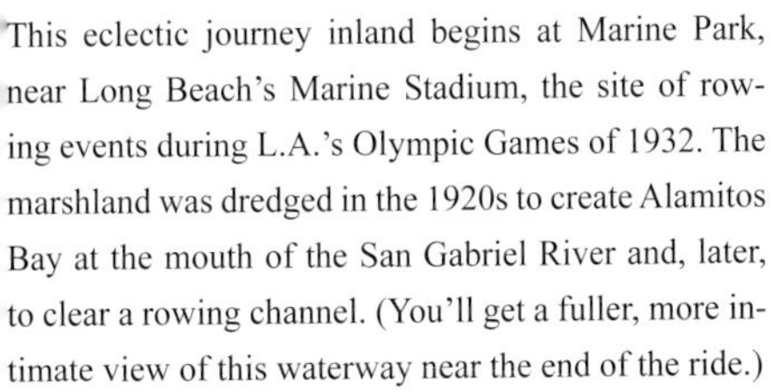

This eclectic journey inland begins at Marine Park, near Long Beach's Marine Stadium, the site of rowing events during L.A.'s Olympic Games of 1932. The marshland was dredged in the 1920s to create Alamitos Bay at the mouth of the San Gabriel River and, later, to clear a rowing channel. (You'll get a fuller, more intimate view of this waterway near the end of the ride.)

Next stop: Naples, a manmade island, dubbed "Dreamland of Southern California" by its original promoters who bought up swampy real estate around 1903 to create, and cash in on, a romanticized enclave with canals, gondolas and high-arching bridges. Inspired by the Italian-styled "Venice of America" (now Venice, California), this project was completed in the 1920s, only to be rebuilt after the 1933 Long Beach earthquake. Early on, Naples was featured in Pacific Electric's Triangle Trolley Trip, an excursion from L.A. Unlike Venice's canals today, which ban motorized boats, these wider waterways, connecting directly to the ocean, see everything from yachts to gondolas and inflatable rafts. Except during Naples Island's Christmas Boat Parade (usually the second Saturday of December), its quiet residential streets are ideal for leisurely cycling.

From Naples, continue down Appian Way, along Marine Stadium, past Colorado Lagoon, a wetlands habitat with a lifeguarded swimming beach (an area poised for revitalization). Soon you'll ride through Recreation Park on bike path and then, on a lightly traveled way past the golf clubhouse.

After crossing Pacific Coast Highway (at the crosswalk, with the light!) and winding through a residential neighborhood, you'll reach Cal State Long Beach. A campus highlight is the lushly serene Earl Burns Miller Japanese Garden, a meditative oasis with a pond of colorful koi. Free to visitors: It's open Tuesdays through Fridays, and Sundays (closed Mondays and on Saturdays—see **www.csulb.edu/**).

Once you've emerged from this transcendent "foray to Japan," you may be startled to come upon the campus' nod to Egypt: the Walter Pyramid, an 18-story-high stadium, clad in blue corrugated aluminum. Go figure.

On the ride back to the start, near "Naples, Italy," you'll coast along waterside bike paths in Channel View Park and, later, Marine Stadium, skirting past rowers or water skiers as you approach the "international finish line" of this one-time Olympic venue.

# Ride Log

**0.0** From Marine Park, turn left onto Appian Way.

**0.5** Make a U-turn at the end of Appian Way.

**0.7** Turn left onto The Toledo.

**1.2** Continue past the Naples fountain.

**1.7** Cross Second St. Continue on Sorrento Dr.

**2.1** Turn left onto Appian Way.

**3.4** Turn right onto Park Ave.

**3.5** Turn right onto Sixth St.

**3.6** Turn left onto the bike path into Recreation Park. If you reach Federation Dr you've gone too far.

**3.7** Cross Seventh St.

**3.9** Turn right, continuing on the bike path.

**4.0** Turn left onto Federation Dr.

**4.1** Turn right into the Recreation Park Municipal Golf Course.

**4.3** Pass the golf course clubhouse.

**4.4** Pass around the security gate and then, turn right onto the bike path. Merge with Anaheim St for a short distance. Be in the rightmost straight-through lane.

**4.6** Cross Pacific Coast Hwy, continuing on El Parque St.

**4.7** Turn right onto Anaheim Rd.

**5.3** Turn left onto Bellflower Blvd.

**5.4** Enter the Cal State Long Beach campus on Beach Dr.

**5.5** Turn left onto Earl Warren Dr.

**5.9** Turn right onto the unnamed street bisecting two parking areas.

**6.0** Turn left onto Merriam Way.

**6.1** Turn right onto the access street north of the parking structure.

**6.2** Turn right onto the bike path and pass the Walter Pyramid.

**6.4** Turn left at the "Beach" quad and continue on the bike path. Pass swimming pools and tennis courts.

**6.7** Turn right onto Deukmejian Way.

**6.8** Turn left onto State University Dr/Anaheim Rd.

**7.2** Turn right, joining Long Beach Bikeway 10 at the gate.

**7.8** Enter Channel View Park.

**8.3** Turn right onto Vista St.

**8.6** Turn left onto Bikeway 10 across from Margo Ave. The bike path runs along the sidewalk west of Bixby Village Dr.

**9.0** Cross Pacific Coast Hwy and Loynes Dr at the signal. The bikeway parallels the sidewalk on the south side of Loynes.

**9.3** Cross Bellflower Blvd.

**9.6** Merge onto the sidewalk bike path at Eliot St.

**9.7** Turn left onto Boathouse Ln.

**10.3** Make at U-turn at the Pete Archer Rowing Center.

**10.9** Turn left and rejoin the bike path.

**11.2** Turn left onto Colorado St, left onto Nieto Ave, and then left onto Appian Way.

**12.4** Arrive back at Mother's Beach.

P

*P1* Marine Park—Mother's Beach
*P2* Naples Fountain
*P3* Marine Stadium Park
*P4* Colorado Lagoon
*P5* California State University Long Beach
*P6* Earl Burns Miller Japanese Gardens
*P7* Rancho Los Alamitos
*P8* Jack Dunster Marine Reserve

B

*B1* Jones Bicycles and Skateboards
5332 E Second St, Belmont Shores
*B2* Sports Authority
6346 Pacific Coast Hwy, Long Beach
*B3* Kings Bike Store
1190 Pacific Coast Hwy, Seal Beach
*B4* Main Street Cyclery
317 Main St, Seal Bach

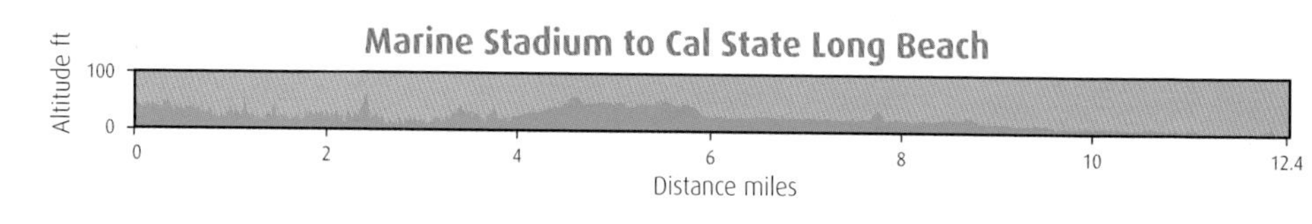

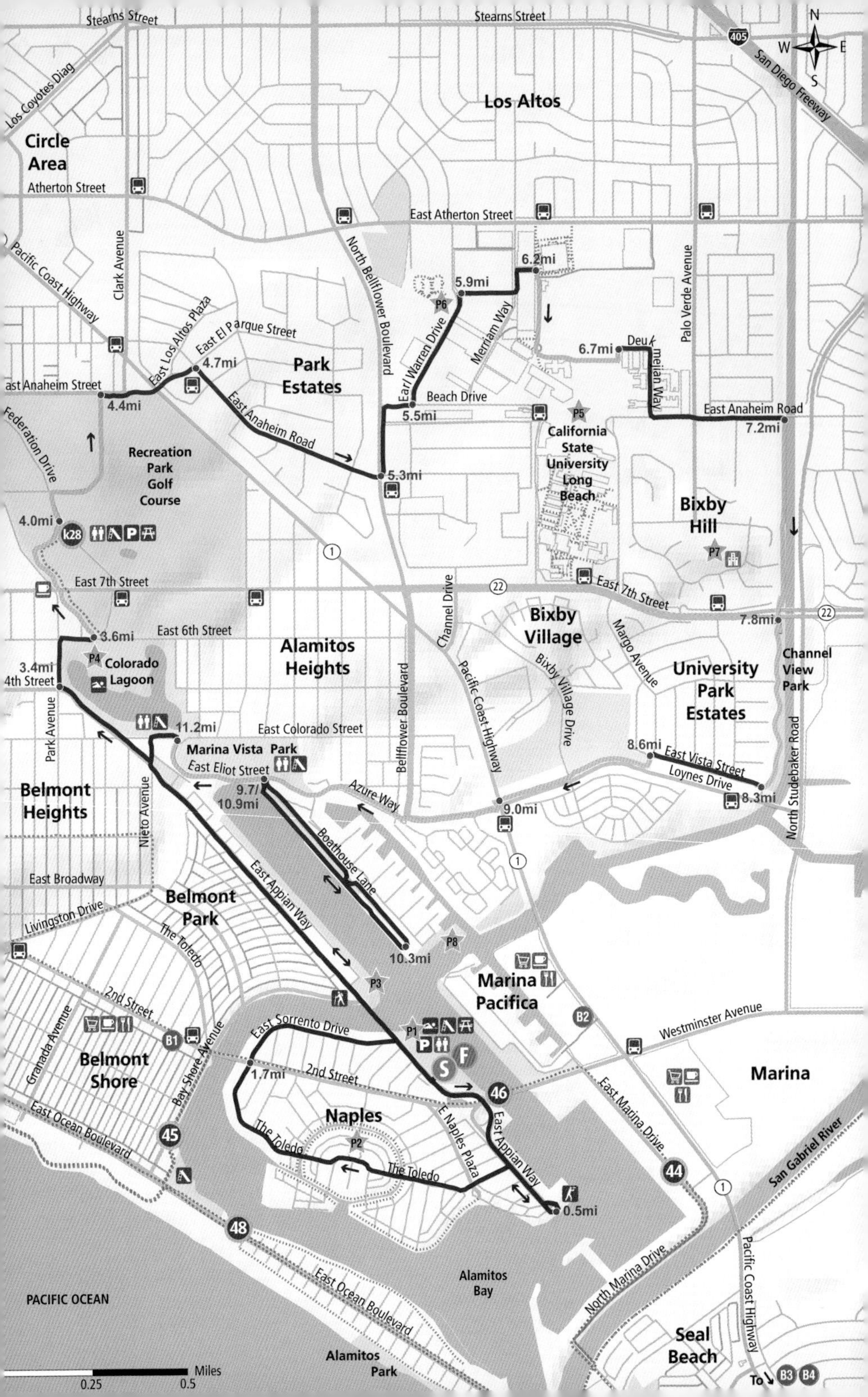

Stearns Street
Los Coyotes Diag
Circle Area
Atherton Street
Los Altos
San Diego Freeway
405
East Atherton Street
Clark Avenue
Pacific Coast Highway
North Bellflower Boulevard
6.2mi
5.9mi
P6
Earl Warren Drive
Merriam Way
Palo Verde Avenue
East El Parque Street
East Los Altos Plaza
4.7mi
Park Estates
6.7mi
Deukmejian Way
East Anaheim Street
4.4mi
East Anaheim Road
Beach Drive
5.5mi
P5
California State University Long Beach
East Anaheim Road
7.2mi
Federation Drive
Recreation Park Golf Course
5.3mi
Bixby Hill
P7
4.0mi
K28
East 7th Street
Channel Drive
22
East 7th Street
7.8mi
3.6mi
East 6th Street
Alamitos Heights
Bixby Village
Margo Avenue
Channel View Park
P4
Colorado Lagoon
3.4mi
4th Street
Bixby Village Drive
University Park Estates
Park Avenue
11.2mi
East Colorado Street
Bellflower Boulevard
Pacific Coast Highway
Marina Vista Park
East Eliot Street
8.6mi
East Vista Street
Loynes Drive
North Studebaker Road
Belmont Heights
9.7/ 10.9mi
Azure Way
9.0mi
8.3mi
Nieto Avenue
Boathouse Lane
East Broadway
Belmont Park
East Appian Way
Livingston Drive
The Toledo
P8
10.3mi
Marina Pacifica
P3
2nd Street
Granada Avenue
East Sorrento Drive
P1
B2
Westminster Avenue
B1
Bay Shore Avenue
Belmont Shore
1.7mi
2nd Street
S
F
46
Marina
Naples
E Naples Plaza
East Appian Way
East Marina Drive
East Ocean Boulevard
45
The Toledo
P2
The Toledo
San Gabriel River
44
0.5mi
48
North Marina Drive
Pacific Coast Highway
Alamitos Bay
PACIFIC OCEAN
East Ocean Boulevard
Seal Beach
Alamitos Park
Miles
0.25
0.5
To B3 B4

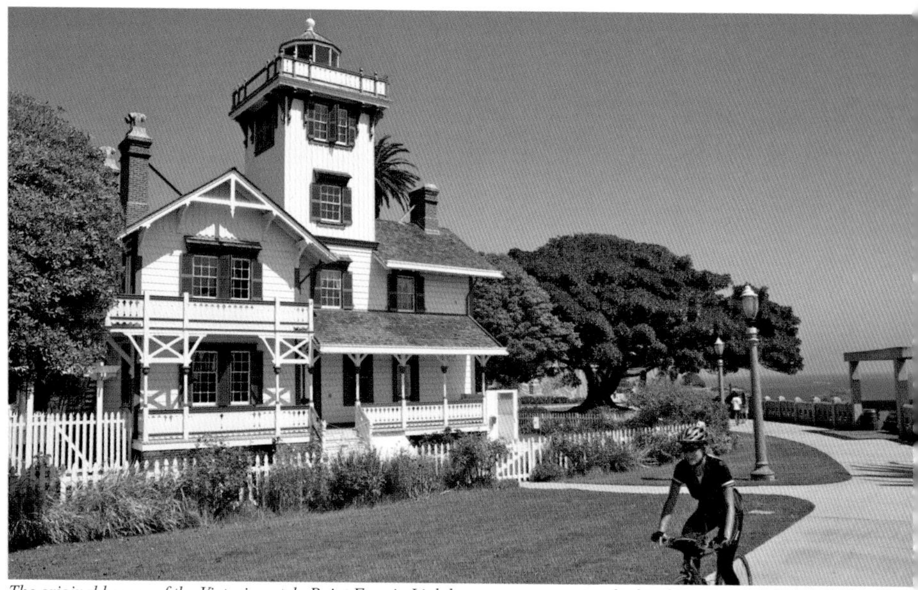

*The original keeper of the Victorian-style Point Fermin Lighthouse was a woman, who lived here with her sister.*

## At a Glance

**Distance** 11.0 miles **Elevation Gain** 700 feet

### Terrain

From a flat, leisurely harborside bike path, the route ascends briefly through hilly residential streets and then continues two miles on level bike lanes atop cliffs overlooking the ocean.

### Traffic

The ride features bike paths and lanes in roughly equal proportions (except for short stretches on ordinary, but quiet, streets). Traffic is generally light.

### How to Get There

To reach the ride start, near the *S. S. Lane Victory*, take the 110 Freeway south to Highway 47, then toward the Vincent Thomas Bridge and Terminal Island. Exit at Harbor Boulevard. From the center lane, continue straight through the intersection to parking ($1.00 per hour).

### Food and Drink

Lighthouse Deli & Café, on 39th Street, and Walker's Café, across Paseo Del Mar from Point Fermin Lighthouse, offer diner fare in vintage ambience. Near the ride's end, Sacred Grounds, on Sixth Street, serves excellent coffees, teas and treats in a laid-back atmosphere.

### Side Trip

Quite a sight, the huge Korean Bell of Friendship, on a hilltop above the coast, was a gift to L.A. from the Republic of Korea, commemorating the American bicentennial and the friendship between the two nations. Turn right on Gaffey Street, up the hill to the "Peace Park."

**Links to** 

**Where to Bike Rating** 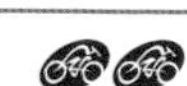

## About...

Times have certainly changed since 1840, when Richard Henry Dana, in his classic seafaring account, *Two Years Before the Mast*, described San Pedro as "the hell of California." These days we consistently find ourselves refreshed by rides along this harbor and rugged but beautiful coastline. Beginning with the Fanfare fountain, our route links eclectic waterfront landmarks, landscapes and curiosities—from the Vincent Thomas Bridge to Point Fermin Park—along the bluffs, all the way west to tidal pools and white sand shores of Royal Palms State Beach.

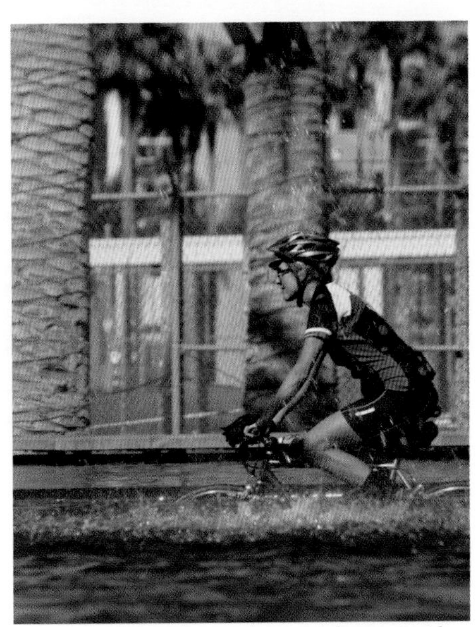

*The Fanfare fountain's waters have parted—you can ride or walk between them.*

The ride begins along San Pedro's working waterfront, where mantis-like cranes shuttle steel containers of goods between massive containerships and the shore. This thriving shipping port sees a flurry of other maritime departures and arrivals, as well, including Catalina Island's ferry, cruise ships and the *S. S. Lane Victory*, a World War II-era freighter, now an itinerant floating museum.

San Pedro emerged as a major deepwater shipping and fishing port at least as far back as its "discovery," in 1542, by Juan Rodriguez Cabrillo, who claimed it for Spain. Beginning around 1903, the area also developed the world's greatest concentration of albacore tuna canneries—a booming local industry that all but vanished by the mid-1980s.

For views of the harbor before modern-day megaships and uniform cargo containers, stop by the Los Angeles Maritime Museum, just down the path from the start. Or ride past Ports O' Call village, along the Miner and Signal Street quays, to see vintage warehouses and grain silos, where longshoremen once muscled crates and barrels on and off ships via gangplanks.

From San Pedro's working waterfront, the ride makes a short climb through a hilly enclave of clapboard cottages (now coveted real estate) that once housed fishermen and dockworkers. The route continues from there on a bike lane atop bluffs overlooking the ocean. This is Point Fermin, L.A.'s southernmost point—its own *finisterra*, or land's end—with superb views of Catalina Island and the harbor. We recommend exploring Point Fermin's 1874 lighthouse with its small museum, strolling along its park promenade, picnicking here or grabing a bite across the road at Walker's Café.

The cliffs you'll ride along are rich in history. The lighthouse protected vessels from the rugged coastline, and nearby Fort MacArthur used giant shore batteries and, later, Nike missiles to defend the harbor from invasion. Nowadays, the lighthouse and its park host weddings, summertime Shakespeare productions and model glider flyers. And this end of Fort MacArthur, now decommissioned, has become a park, a small museum and, further west at its White Point Park section, a nature preserve.

As the ride returns to the harborside bike path, stop at the Fanfare fountain, a remarkable dynamic water display set to music, sometimes evoking the sails that first reached this port two centuries ago.

*While Ride 50 has not been deemed kid-friendly in its entirety, it does include substantial sections which are entirely safe for family use.*

# Ride Log

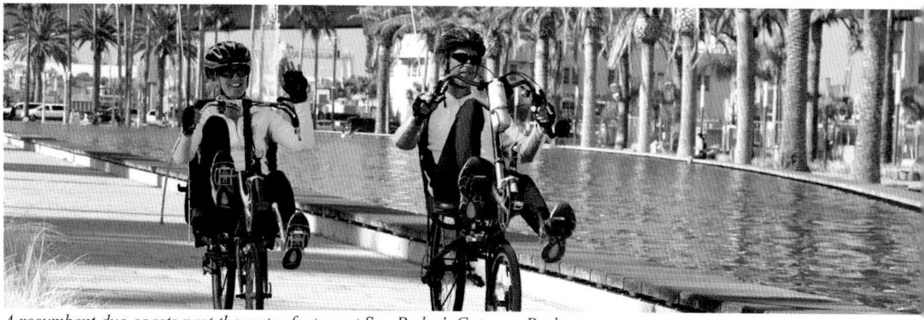

*A recumbent duo coasts past the water feature at San Pedro's Gateway Park.*

**0.0** From the Fanfare fountain at the corner of Front St/ Swinford St and Harbor Blvd, begin riding south along the waterfront bike path.

**0.7** Turn right onto Sixth St, then left onto Harbor Blvd, joining the bike lane.

**1.4** Cross Crescent Ave, then turn right to the bike path.

**1.9** Cross 22nd St. The bike path continues along the sidewalk on the west side of Via Cabrillo-Marina.

**2.2** Turn right and uphill, continuing on the bike path.

**2.4** Turn right onto Shoshonean Rd where the bike path ends.

**2.6** Continue into Cabrillo Beach Park (which has restrooms, drinking fountains and picnic spots).

**2.9** Pass the Cabrillo Marine Aquarium.

**3.0** Exit Cabrillo Beach Park on Oliver Vickery Circle Way.

**3.1** Turn right onto Stephen M. White Dr.

**3.2** Turn left onto Pacific Ave.

**3.5** Turn right onto Shepard St.

**3.9** Pass Point Fermin Park and lighthouse. Shepard becomes Paseo Del Mar.

**5.5** Turn left into the entrance to Royal Palms State Beach (which has restrooms, a picnic area and drinking fountain). Return toward San Pedro on Paseo Del Mar.

**7.4** Turn right onto Pacific Ave, then left onto Bluff Pl. Exercise caution on this short, but steep downhill.

**7.7** Continue straight onto Stephen M. White Dr.

**7.8** Turn right onto Oliver Vickery Circle Way.

**7.9** Continue into Cabrillo Beach Park (which has restrooms, a picnic area and drinking fountain).

**8.0** Pass the Cabrillo Marine Aquarium.

**8.2** Exit Cabrillo Beach Park on Shoshonean Rd.

**8.4** Join the bike path on the left where Shoshonean Rd meets Via Cabrillo-Marina.

**8.7** Turn left onto the sidewalk bike lane on the west side of Via Cabrillo-Marina.

**9.0** Cross 22nd St.

**9.5** Cross Harbor Blvd at the end of the bike path. Continue north.

**10.2** Turn right at Sixth St, join the bike path.

**11.0** Arrive back at Fanfare fountain. End of ride.

## San Pedro's Waterfront

Altitude ft: 0, 100, 200

Distance miles: 0, 2, 4, 6, 8, 10, 11.0

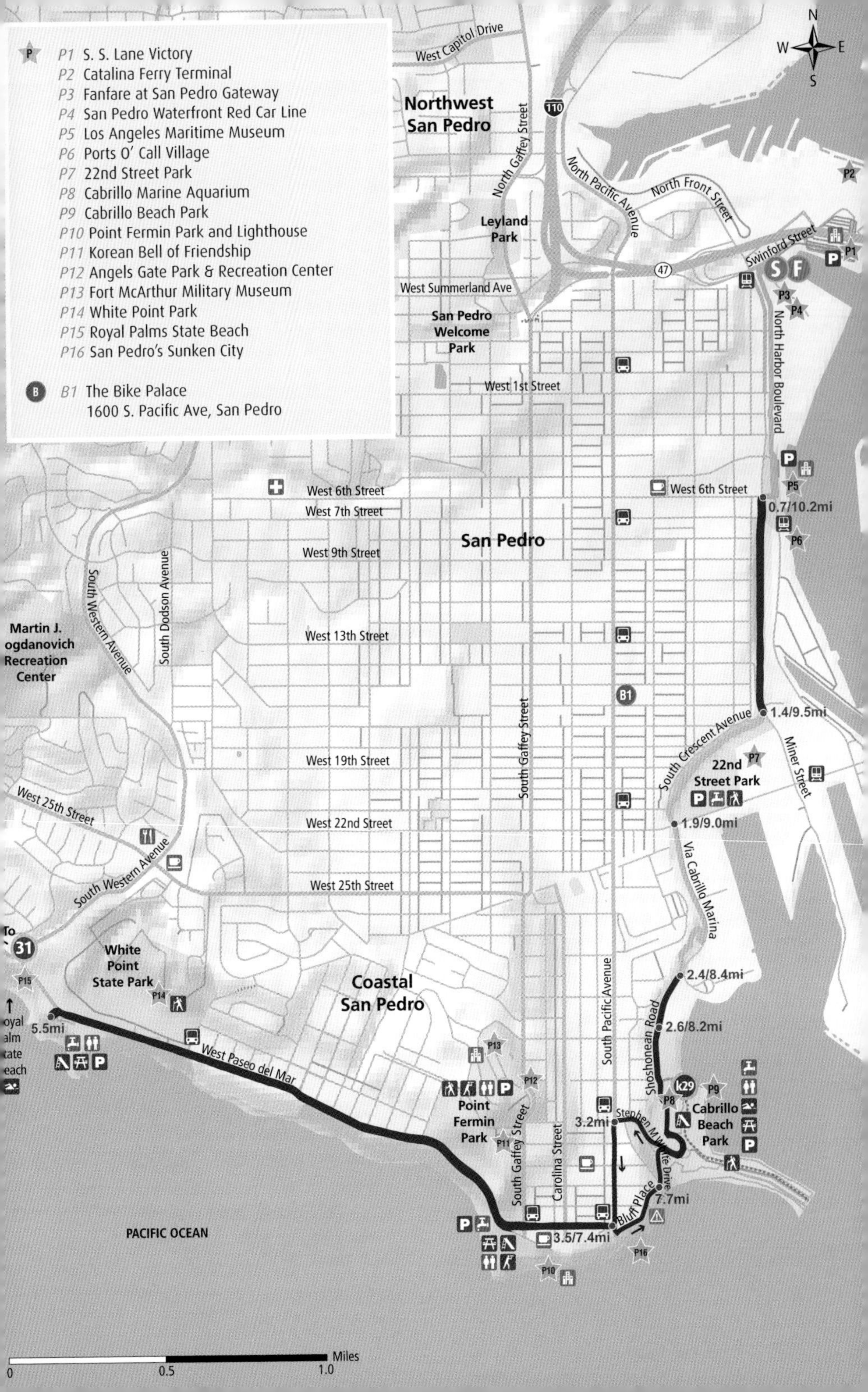

P1 S. S. Lane Victory
P2 Catalina Ferry Terminal
P3 Fanfare at San Pedro Gateway
P4 San Pedro Waterfront Red Car Line
P5 Los Angeles Maritime Museum
P6 Ports O' Call Village
P7 22nd Street Park
P8 Cabrillo Marine Aquarium
P9 Cabrillo Beach Park
P10 Point Fermin Park and Lighthouse
P11 Korean Bell of Friendship
P12 Angels Gate Park & Recreation Center
P13 Fort McArthur Military Museum
P14 White Point Park
P15 Royal Palms State Beach
P16 San Pedro's Sunken City
B1 The Bike Palace
1600 S. Pacific Ave, San Pedro
Northwest San Pedro
San Pedro
Coastal San Pedro
Leyland Park
San Pedro Welcome Park
22nd Street Park
White Point State Park
Point Fermin Park
Cabrillo Beach Park
Martin J. Bogdanovich Recreation Center
To Royal Palm State Beach
PACIFIC OCEAN
West Capitol Drive
North Gaffey Street
North Pacific Avenue
North Front Street
Swinford Street
West Summerland Ave
West 1st Street
North Harbor Boulevard
West 6th Street
West 7th Street
West 9th Street
West 13th Street
West 19th Street
West 22nd Street
West 25th Street
South Western Avenue
South Dodson Avenue
South Gaffey Street
South Pacific Avenue
South Crescent Avenue
Miner Street
Via Cabrillo Marina
Shoshonean Road
Stephen M White Drive
Bluff Place
Carolina Street
West Paseo del Mar
0.7/10.2mi
1.4/9.5mi
1.9/9.0mi
2.4/8.4mi
2.6/8.2mi
3.2mi
3.5/7.4mi
5.5mi
7.7mi
Miles
0
0.5
1.0

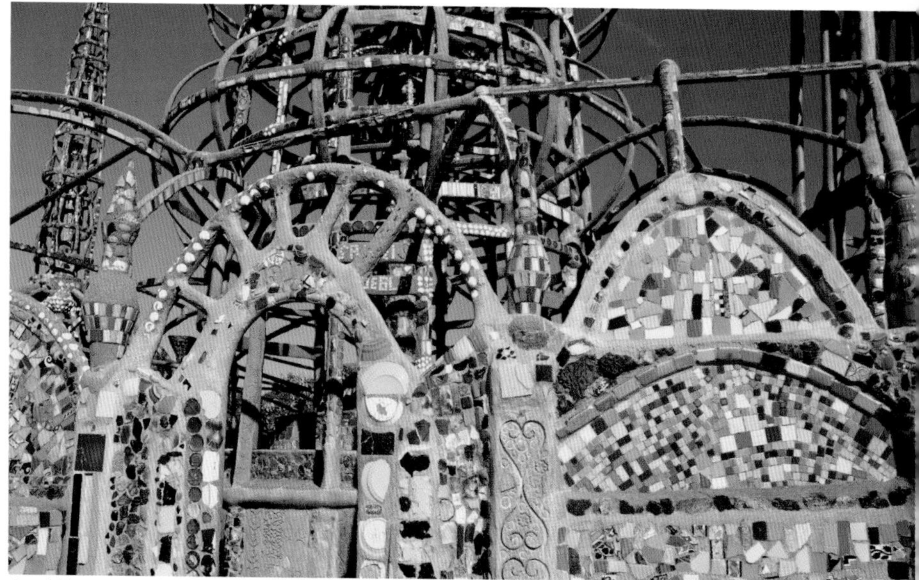

*Jewel-like ceramic shards, broken bottles and many other found objects encrust Simon Rodia's "Nuestro Pueblo," or Watts Towers.*

## At a Glance

**Distance** 15.0 miles **Elevation Gain** 650 feet

### Terrain

This ride begins with a short stretch on the lower Compton Creek Bike Path and continues onto flat city streets. Pavement is good throughout.

### Traffic

The industrial areas north of the start, all the way to El Segundo Boulevard, have very little traffic on weekends. Beyond El Segundo, traffic levels increase moderately.

### How to Get There

From the 710 Freeway, exit onto Del Amo Boulevard westbound. After about three blocks, turn right into the Metro Blue Line's Del Amo station parking lot (free). Or, by train, reach the station via Blue Line from downtown or Long Beach.

### Food and Drink

The Martin Luther King Jr. shopping center, at the intersection of 103rd Street and the Blue Line, has a supermarket and a couple of restaurants.

### Side Trip

For a green diversion from this ride's urban landscape, go west from the Watts Towers along 103rd Street to Ted Watkins Memorial Park. Recently renovated, its 27 acres are newly landscaped, with lawns, shade trees, and picnic areas.

**Links to** 16 42 46

**Where to Bike Rating** 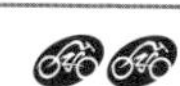

  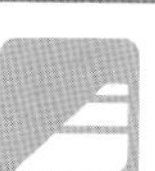 

## About...

Carving a prudent path to an extraordinary destination, this ride offers a sensible route from northern Long Beach through a gritty swath of South Central Los Angeles. Then, from behind a weedy vacant lot, the 99-foot-tall spires of Watts Towers suddenly come into view. This grass-roots masterpiece—one man's vision, built with his own hands—presents dynamic, filigreed forms, ornamented with gem-like bottle pieces, ceramic shards and myriad seashells. For 34 years, from 1921, Simon Rodia worked in relative obscurity on his towers: today, an iconic L.A. landmark.

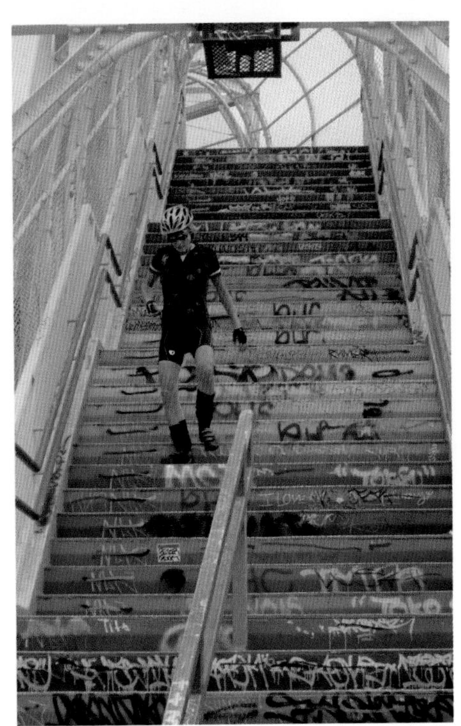

*A block from Watts Towers, rainbow stairs ascend to the pedestrian bridge over Metro's light rail tracks.*

Moderate in vehicular traffic yet high in visibility, much of this route borders the Metro Blue Line (making it easy to hop the train for a stretch). After the journey from northern Long Beach to Watts, it's a dazzling moment when you finally turn onto a forlorn side street, and there they are: the phenomenal Towers of Simon Rodia!

Their creator, Sabato ("Simon" or "Sam") Rodia, was an Italian immigrant, who, in 1921, purchased the triangular site in Watts—then and now a relatively impoverished part of L.A. For the next three decades, while he held day jobs as a handy man, tile layer and construction worker, he toiled single-handedly in his spare time to build what he called "Nuestro Pueblo" (our town), a tribute to the nation that had taken him in.

Though his assemblage crescendos in three towers, two of which rise nearly 100 feet, the work is actually composed of 17 interconnected elements, including sculptural walls, a fountain, bird baths, a ship named Marco Polo and a gazebo. Virtually all the materials were cast-offs—found objects and scraps—that Rodia collected from the neighborhood and as far away as Long Beach. Using only rudimentary hand tools, he first built metal armatures of pipe and rods, then wrapped the frames with wire mesh, coated them with mortar and embedded decorative bits of glass, ceramic shards, pebbles and seashells. Rodia worked solo, made no drawings and, rather than use scaffolding, he simply scampered up the towers, carting materials in buckets and hanging on with a window-washer's belt while he worked.

In 1955, with the project complete, he walked away, deeding the land to a neighbor and moving to Northern California. Apparently, he did not see the towers again before he died, in 1965. Though the city made serious attempts to demolish the structures, local opposition galvanized to save his extraordinary creation—now designated a city, state and national landmark.

When returning to Long Beach, bicycle south along the same route. Or, you can catch a Blue Line at the 103$^{rd}$ Street station, two blocks northwest of Watts Towers, and ride it south a few stops to the Del Amo station.

# Ride Log

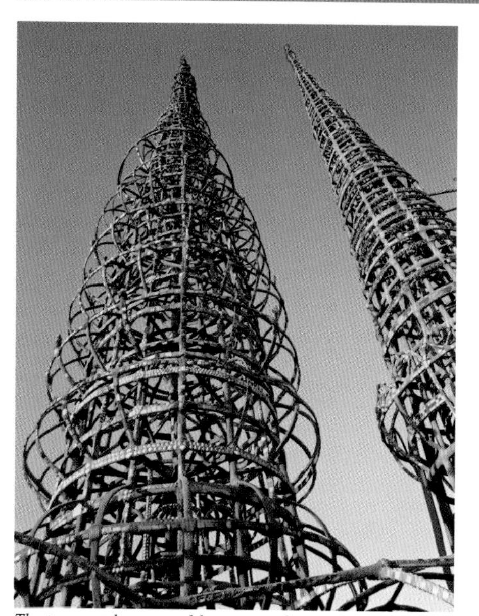

*The towers take on a golden cast as the sun descends.*

- P1 California State University Dominguez Hills
- P2 Rancho Dominguez Adoba Museum
- P3 DeForest Park
- P4 Earvin "Magic" Johnson Recreation Area
- P5 Ralph C Dills Park
- P6 Watts Towers of Simon Rodia
- P7 Ted Watkins Memorial Park
- P8 South Gate Park

- B1 Manny's Bike Shop
  400 Rosecrans Ave, Compton
- B2 Watts Cyclery
  11202 Wilmington Ave, Watts

**0.0** Start at Metro Blue Line's Del Amo station and ride east on the sidewalk a short distance, then turn left onto the Lower Compton Creek Bike Path.

**1.0** Exit the bike path and turn north onto Santa Fe Ave.

**2.0** Cross under the 91 Freeway and Artesia Blvd to join the bike lane along Santa Fe.

**5.0** Turn left onto El Segundo Blvd.

**5.8** Turn right onto Willowbrook Ave just before the Blue Line.

**6.7** When you reach Willowbrook's dead end, ride along the sidewalk beneath the elevated Blue Line tracks for about one block, then cross Willowbrook to the east using the crosswalk.

**6.9** Turn right onto Wilmington Ave.

**7.5** Turn left onto Santa Ana Blvd and arrive at Watts Towers. After experiencing Watts Towers, begin the return trip by turning right onto Wilmington Ave.

**8.2** Angle to the left onto Willowbrook Ave toward the Metro Blue Line station. Continue along the sidewalk beneath the elevated Blue Line tracks for about one block and then, rejoin Willowbrook Ave.

**9.3** Turn left onto El Segundo Blvd.

**10.0** Turn right onto Santa Fe Ave and onto the bike lane south of Pine St.

**13.1** Cross under the 91 Freeway and Artesia Blvd.

**14.0** Cross Santa Fe Ave using the crosswalk and then onto the Lower Compton Creek Bike Path.

**15.0** Arrive back at Del Amo Blvd. End of ride. Turn right and ride along the sidewalk to the Metro station's parking area.

**Experiencing Watts Towers**

Altitude ft: 100, 0
Distance miles: 0, 3, 6, 9, 12, 15.0

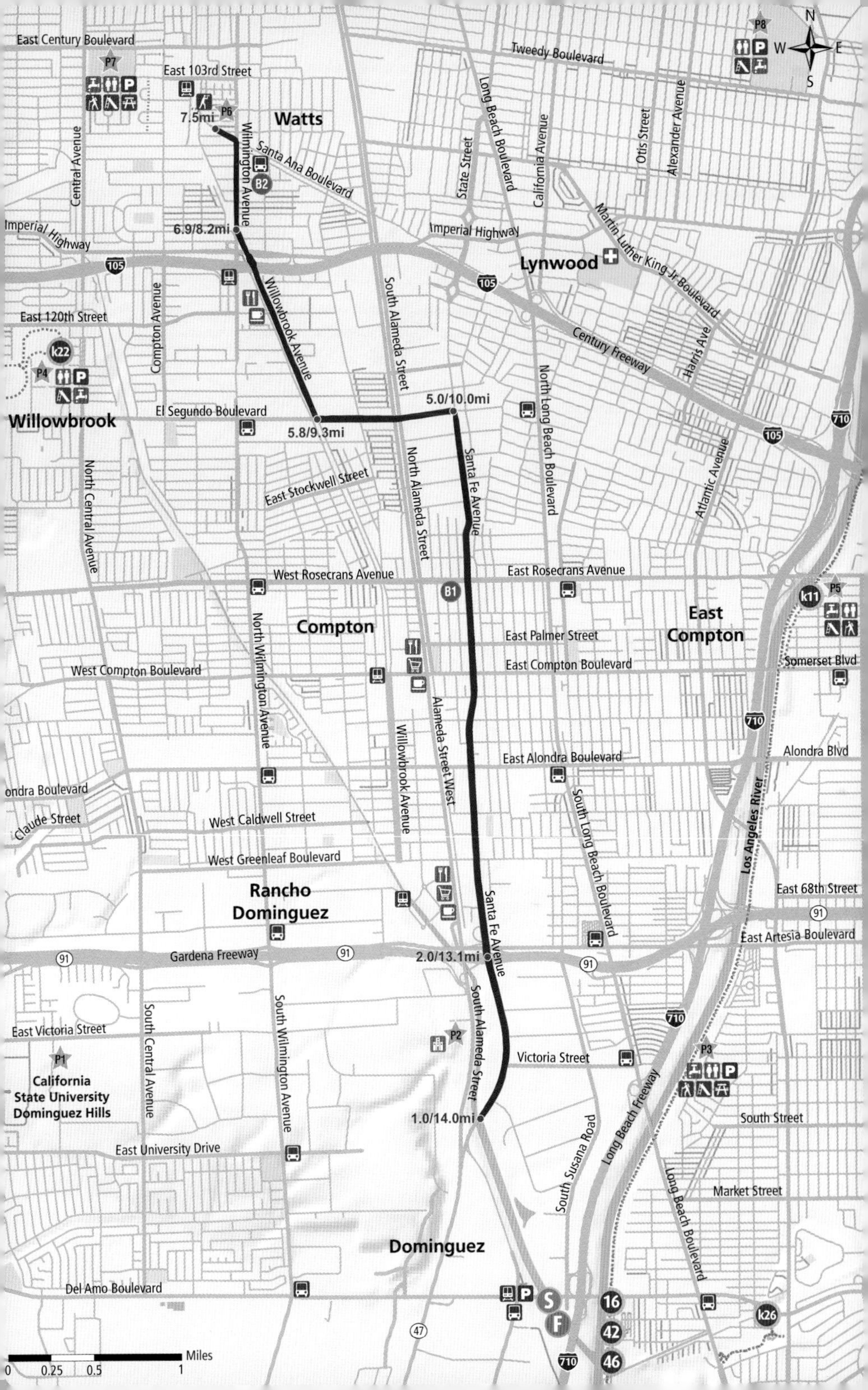

East Century Boulevard
P7
East 103rd Street
7.5mi
P6
Watts
Tweedy Boulevard
P8
N
W
E
S
Long Beach Boulevard
Otis Street
Alexander Avenue
California Avenue
State Street
Wilmington Avenue
Santa Ana Boulevard
B2
Central Avenue
6.9/8.2mi
Imperial Highway
Imperial Highway
Martin Luther King Jr Boulevard
Lynwood
105
105
South Alameda Street
Willowbrook Avenue
Compton Avenue
East 120th Street
Century Freeway
Harris Ave
k22
P4
North Long Beach Boulevard
5.0/10.0mi
El Segundo Boulevard
Willowbrook
5.8/9.3mi
710
105
Atlantic Avenue
North Central Avenue
North Alameda Street
Santa Fe Avenue
East Stockwell Street
West Rosecrans Avenue
East Rosecrans Avenue
B1
k11
P5
Compton
East Compton
North Wilmington Avenue
East Palmer Street
West Compton Boulevard
East Compton Boulevard
Somerset Blvd
710
Alameda Street West
Willowbrook Avenue
East Alondra Boulevard
Alondra Blvd
ondra Boulevard
South Long Beach Boulevard
Claude Street
West Caldwell Street
Los Angeles River
West Greenleaf Boulevard
Santa Fe Avenue
Rancho Dominguez
East 68th Street
91
East Artesia Boulevard
91
Gardena Freeway
91
2.0/13.1mi
91
South Alameda Street
710
East Victoria Street
P2
South Central Avenue
South Wilmington Avenue
P1
California State University Dominguez Hills
Victoria Street
P3
South Street
1.0/14.0mi
East University Drive
South Susana Road
Long Beach Freeway
Long Beach Boulevard
Market Street
Dominguez
Del Amo Boulevard
S
F
16
42
46
k26
47
710
Miles
0
0.25
0.5
1

# Kids' Rides

Learning to ride a two-wheel bicycle is a childhood rite of passage, about finding balance and overcoming fear and doubt—often leading to an exhilarating, wind-in-your-hair sense of independence and freedom.

But in Los Angeles, it can be challenging to find safe and enjoyable training grounds. With hundreds of city parks, the choices would seem endless—except that many are officially off limits to cyclists of any age. (Who knows if those rules would actually be enforced against tykes, but best not risk it.) However we earned our own "wheels and wings" long ago, parking lots and driveways are hardly optimal for our precious little ones. But fear not—we have compiled the following list of 30 essential kids' rides, across L.A. County. All are car free, with nice, flat stretches (suitable for tricycles and others without climbing gears) and high-quality amenities, such as playgrounds, lawns, shaded picnic areas, restrooms, drinking fountains and maybe even summertime water features and ice cream vendors.

Among the highlights are: Wilmington Waterfront Park, a brand new, long and colorful park with bridges and ramps, water jets and free stationary binoculars for views of San Pedro's commercial docks; El Cariso Park, a verdant, mountain-view hub of community activity with kids' rides of three lengths (and swimming pools); Lacy Park, a quiet European-style park, with gracious shade trees, lush lawns, a rose garden and a long bike loop; the Cornfield, a network of trails within a historic, urban landscape near downtown; and near the Santa Monica Pier, where junior cyclists will find no shortage of ocean-side riding.

As your young ones develop into full-fledged cyclists, the gates open to some of the adult rides—those labeled "Kid Friendly" in the Ride Overview—featuring longer bike paths, some with varied terrain and others shared by rollerbladers, joggers and experienced bicyclists. The Marvin Braude Bike Trail on the beach—north of the Venice Fishing Pier to Will Rogers State Beach and south of Playa del Rey to Manhattan Beach—is just the ticket. Ditto for Long Beach's Shoreline Pedestrian/Bicycle Path and most of the Santa Clarita's Cloverleaf. And let's not forget the flat trail and refreshing wilderness at the West Fork of the San Gabriel River, high in the Angeles National Forest, where kids (and their parents) can enjoy the freedom of riding among tall pines, along a swimmable river.

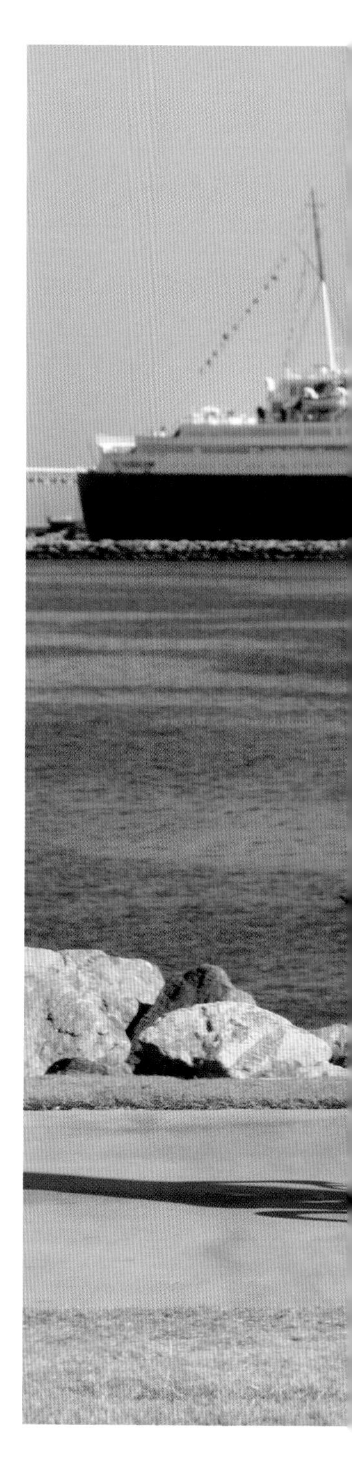

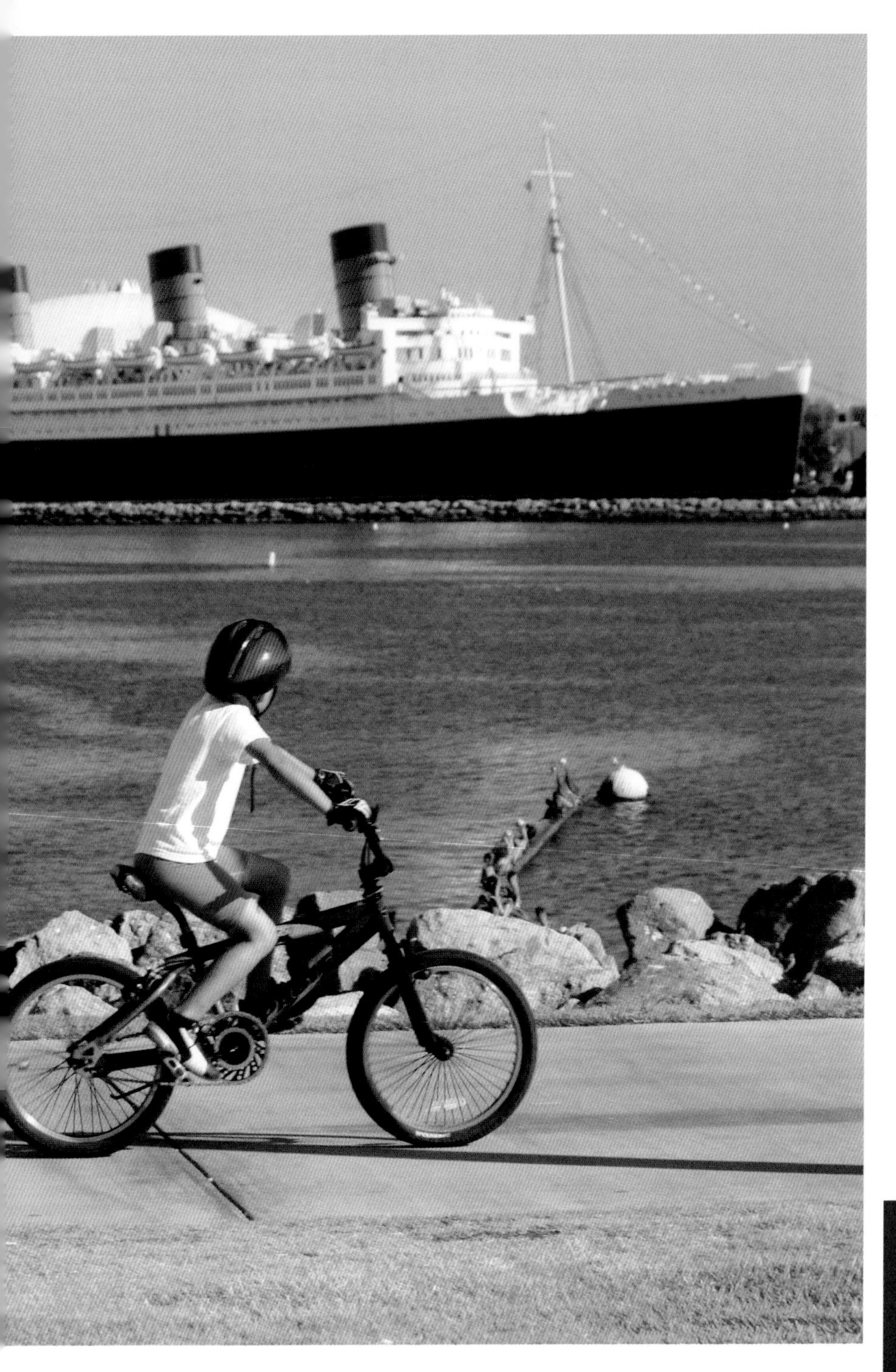

# Ride K1 - The Banks of the Santa Clara River (Santa Clarita)

**Distance** 2.8 miles

## Terrain

An almost level, extremely well paved bike path follows the river banks. Native sagebrush and cottonwoods dot the surrounding hilly landscape. (Usually, this river flows only following a wet winter.)

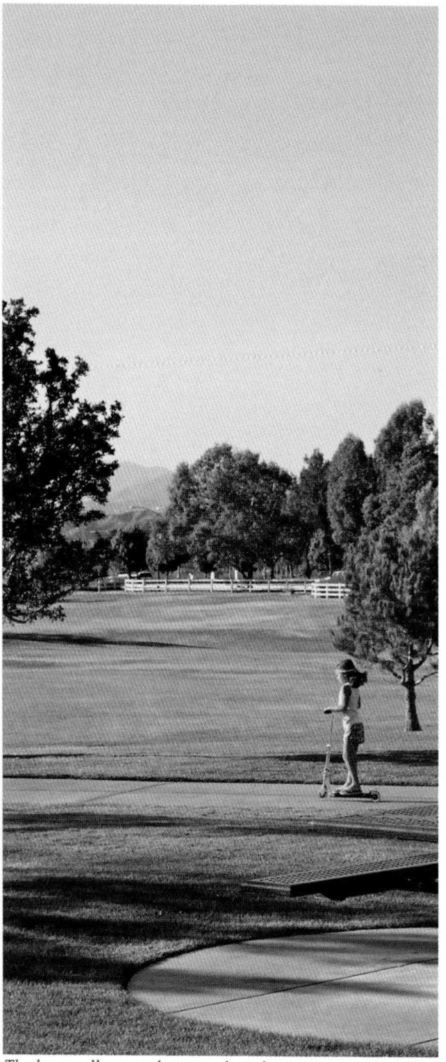

*The lawn rolls on and on—as does this young scooter rider.*

## How to Get There

Exit the 5 Freeway at Magic Mountain Parkwa and drive east. Turn left onto McBean Parkway an right onto Newhall Ranch Road. After Bridgepor Elementary School, make a right on Parkwood Lane at its end, turn right to Bridgeport Park.

## Amenities and Things to Do

You'll find a playground, picnic tables, restrooms drinking fountains and plenty of grassy areas. Thoug riding in the park itself is not officially sanctioned Bridgeport Park—literally touching a neatly define segment of the Santa Clara River bikeways—makes a perfect base for young riders beginning to explore the river routes.

## About

This spin along the north bank of Santa Clara's arroyo, between McBean Parkway and Newhall Ranch Road, offers kids a bite-sized morsel—a taste with amenities and low traffic—of the great network of bike paths weaving through the Santa Clarita Valley. From this "trailhead," it's easy to alter the journey's length. Ambitious young riders can venture further, while those preferring a breather in the playground or in the grass will find it right here.

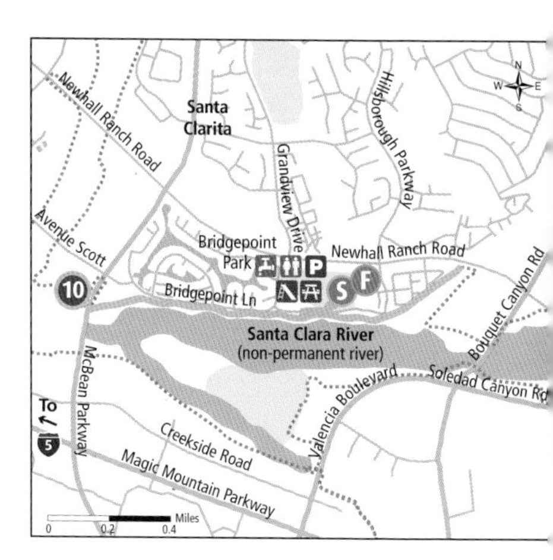

# Ride K2 - Summit Park (Valencia)

**Distance** 1.0 mile

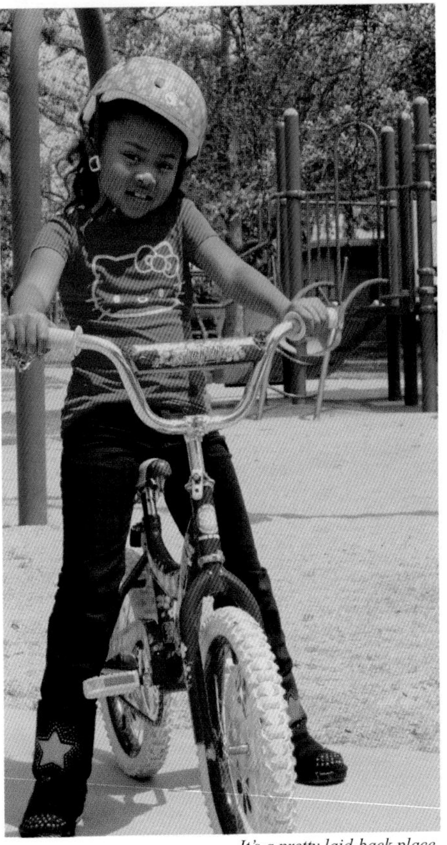

*It's a pretty laid-back place.*

## Terrain

This ride's name may conjure up visions of kids on training wheels scaling high peaks. But in reality, this grassy, tree-shaded park is nearly flat, tucked within a hollow behind the Santa Clarita Family YMCA. The only hill leads to a footbridge over a nearby roadway, connecting the park to pleasant surrounding neighborhoods.

## How to Get There

Exit the 5 Freeway at Valencia Boulevard and drive northeast. Make a right onto McBean Parkway and, after about 0.4 miles, turn into the parking lot for Summit Park and the Santa Clarita Family YMCA.

## Amenities and Things to Do

Summit Park is a quiet, peaceful spot for recreation and family outings. Its offerings include picnic tables, a large gazebo and a playground on a bed of clean river sand. Restrooms are available at the YMCA.

## About

Near the park's center, a roughly oval bike path surrounds a large grassy field. Branching off are three "out-and-back" segments: (a) the longest meanders over the flats to Del Monte Drive; (b) the second crosses a safe, protected footbridge over McBean Parkway; and (c) the final offshoot ventures south along the hollow, past live oaks, cottonwoods and native grasses.

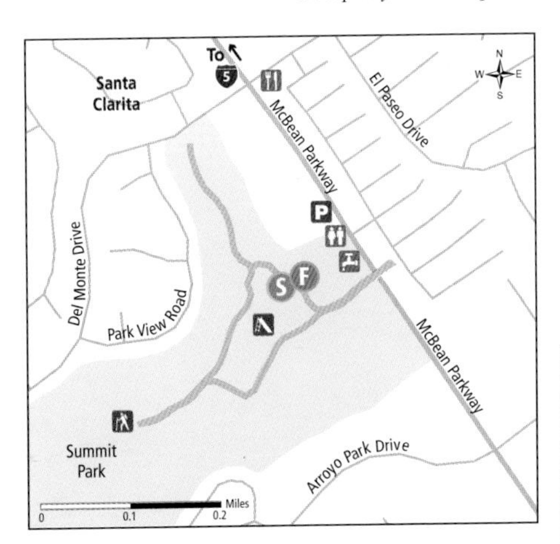

# Ride K3 - Lake Balboa (Van Nuys)

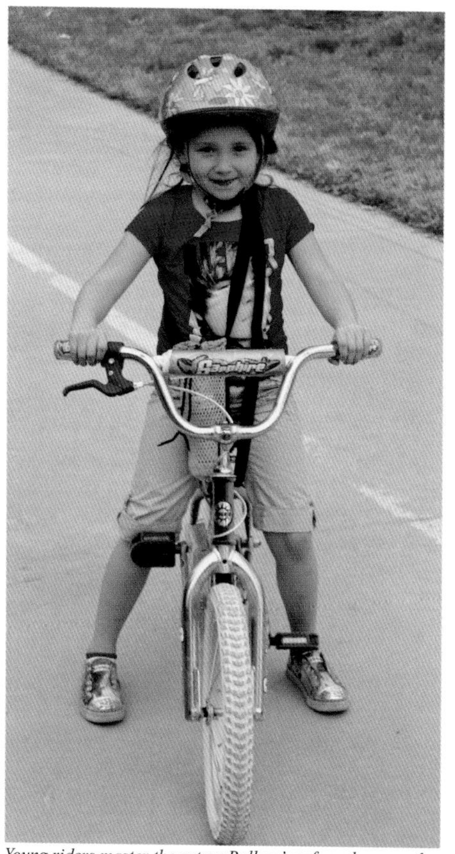

*Young riders master the art on Balboa's safe and easy paths.*

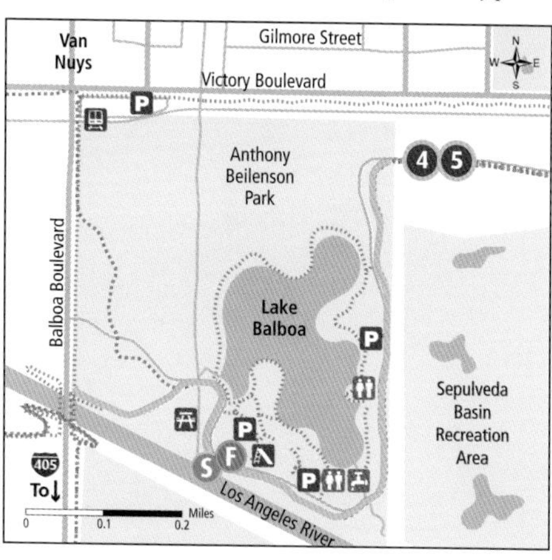


**Distance** 1.1 miles

## Terrain

This crescent-shaped, smooth concrete bike path is mostly flat with a very small hill at one end.

## How to Get There

Lake Balboa, part of Anthony C. Beilenson Park, is just south of Victory Boulevard between Balboa Boulevard and Woodley Avenue. Free parking areas are scattered throughout the park and along the access road.

## Amenities and Things to Do

Beilenson Park offers lots of family attractions, including an elaborate children's play area with swings and plenty of climbing opportunities. A small artificial creek that's suitable for wading runs from the lake to the Los Angeles River. A network of walking paths surrounds the lake, offering places to rest beneath vine-covered arbors and big shade trees. On the lake itself, you can kayak, boat and fish (sorry, no swimming). Pedal cars are available for rent at a kiosk operated by Wheel Fun Rentals.

## About

This kids' ride at Lake Balboa is very pleasant, with lots of safe riding—all with the scenic backdrop of this naturalistic manmade lake. The route offers variations: Cyclists can easily vary the length of this loop or extend it to include other kid-friendly paths in the adjacent Sepulveda Basin Recreation Area (see Adult Ride 5).

# Ride K4 - El Cariso Park (Sylmar)

**Distance** 1.9 miles

## Terrain

El Cariso slopes gradually uphill from south to north. From east to west, the park is mostly flat. The paths are wide, though shared with walkers and joggers.

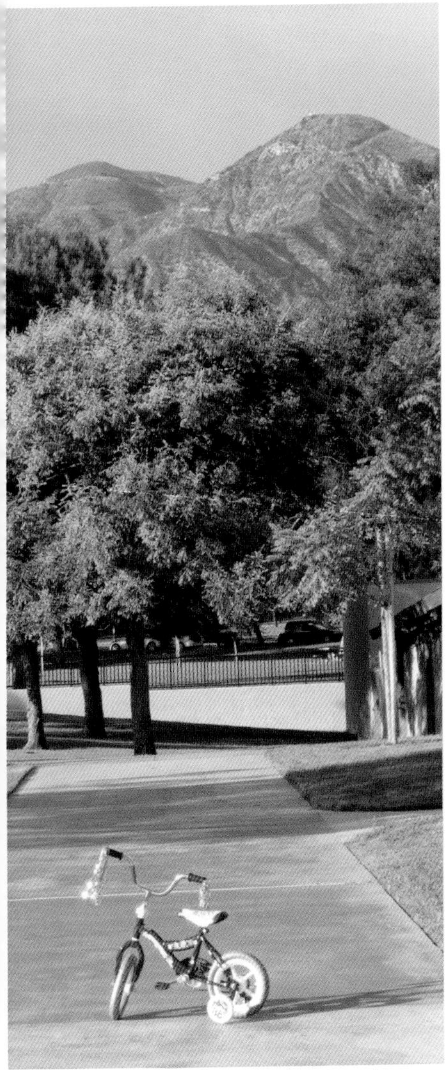

*San Gabriel Mountain peaks appear above the park's lush treetops.*

## How to Get There

From the 201 Freeway to Sylmar, exit onto Hubbard Street and drive northeast, toward the mountains. Along Hubbard, north of Eldridge Avenue, the park has three separate entrances, each connected to a network of free parking lots.

## Amenities and Things to Do

The park's name honors the 12 El Cariso Hotshot firefighters who perished in the 1966 Loop Fire, nearby. A hub of community activity, the park offers junior (and adult) tennis, soccer and swimming, as well as after-school programs. Across its 79 acres, you'll find picnic areas, playgrounds, a basketball court, a baseball diamond, a pair of community pools and tennis courts—all set within mature eucalyptus, pine and oak groves.

## About

Kids on bikes can enjoy the park's three main loops singly or in combination: (a) the "blue path," an easy ring around the tennis courts; (b) the slightly longer "red path," an amoeba-shaped, mostly flat circuit past picnic areas and playgrounds; and (c) the "yellow path," the longest loop, with modest climbing, roughly following the park's periphery.

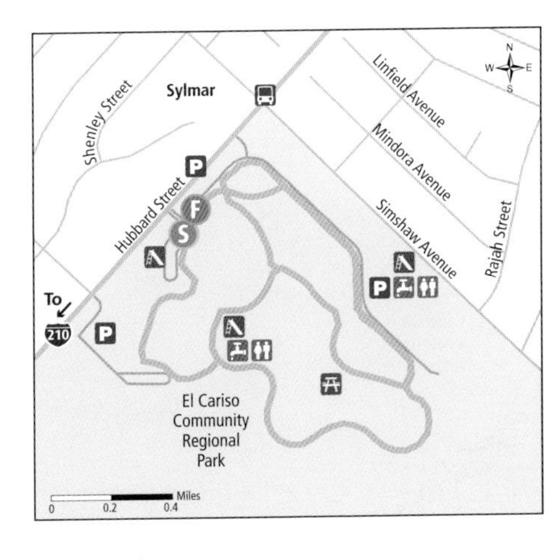

# Ride K5 - Rio de Los Angeles State Park (Cypress Park)

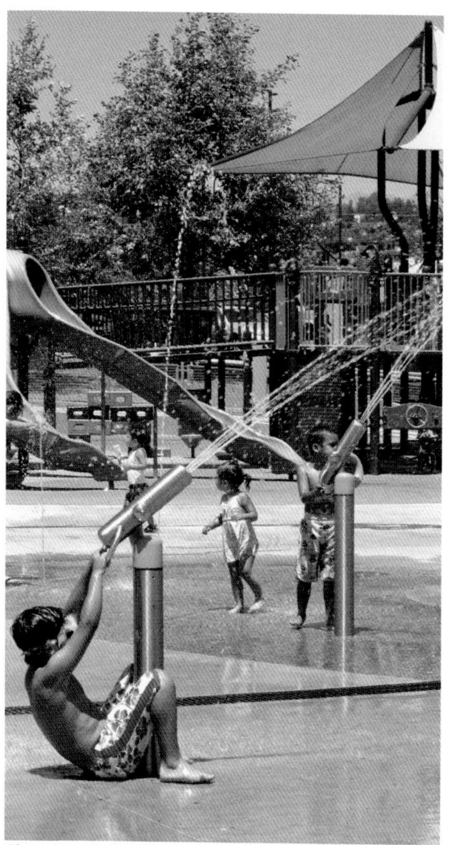

*The splash pad's gentle geysers shoot up alongside mini-water cannons.*

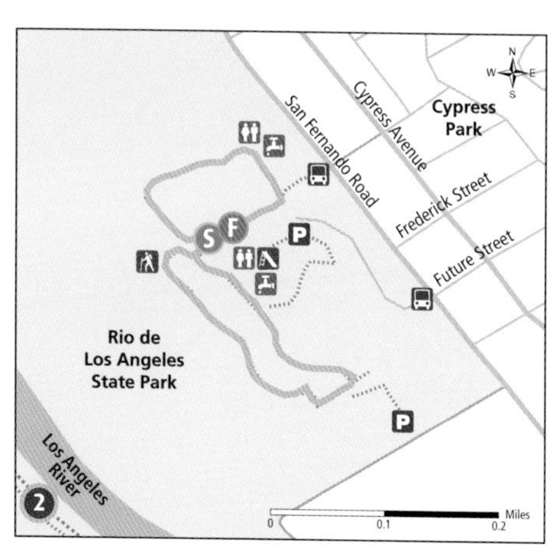


**Distance** 0.9 miles

## Terrain

Flat, hard-packed dirt paths border restored wetlands, athletic fields and picnic areas.

## How to Get There

From the 5 Freeway, take the 2 Freeway a short distance north. Exit onto San Fernando Road and continue south about one mile to Rio de Los Angeles State Park.

## Amenities and Things to Do

Rio de Los Angeles, one of the region's newest state parks, occupies the site of Taylor Yards, a long-abandoned railroad switching facility. Along the park's western side, L.A. River wetlands are gradually re-emerging, laced with walking and biking trails. Athletic fields, including a fully lit soccer pitch, barbecues and picnic areas are among the amenities. The playground has a small summertime water park, or "splash pad." For Cinco de Mayo, the park hosts a three-day carnival with amusement park rides (the Friday, Saturday and Sunday closest to May 5).

## About

The park offers three key bike routes for kids: [a] a relatively big loop, amid young willows, cottonwoods and other native plants, explores the park's re-emerging natural side, its Oxbow section; [b] a shorter loop winds around baseball fields and past a picnic area, ending at a good playground; and [c] the most ambitious ride combines both loops into a kid-sized Tour del Rio de Los Angeles.

## Ride K6 - Arroyo Seco (Montecito Heights)

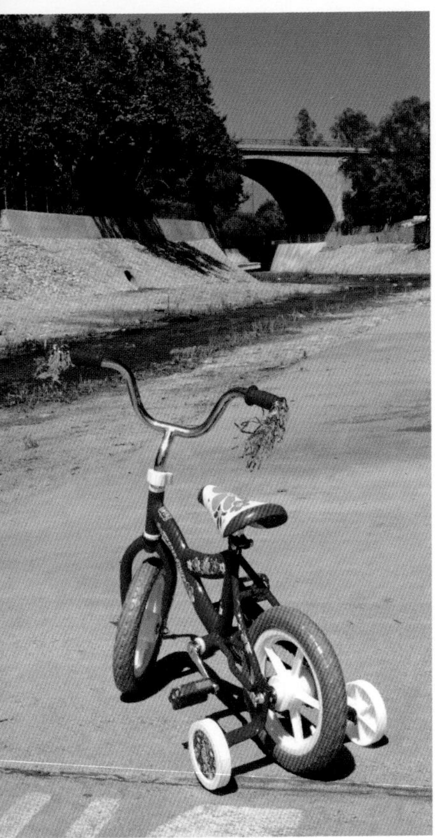

*Completely car-free Arroyo Seco is great for young riders.*

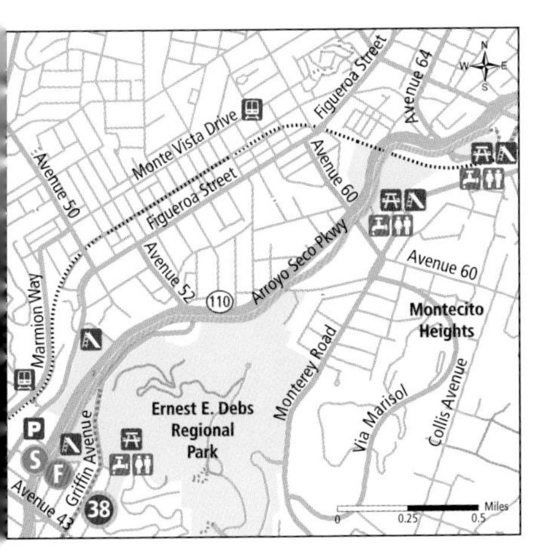


**Distance** 2.1 miles

### Terrain

This concrete bicycle path meanders along the Arroyo Seco Canyon, with a slight uphill grade from beginning to end. The route is occasionally cluttered with sand, leaves, twigs and other creek debris. Avoid this ride on or right after rainy days.

### How to Get There

From the 110 Freeway, exit at East Avenue 43, go east to Homer Street, and then north one block to the Montecito Heights Recreation Center. The Arroyo Seco Bike Path begins at the west end of the center's parking lot.

### Amenities and Things to Do

City parks—Montecito Heights Recreation Center and Hermon Park—line much of the east side of Arroyo Seco. Each one, accessed from the bike path via a short access ramp, offers playgrounds, restrooms and picnic areas beneath hundreds of oaks, sycamores and cottonwoods. A slightly arcing bridge across Arroyo Seco and the freeway, just north of the recreation center, leads to another play area: Sycamore Grove Park. The ride over the bridge to this park is an experience that many kids enjoy.

### About

Ideal for young cyclists, the safe Arroyo Seco ride follows a creek, with the sounds of flowing water, beneath a canopy of trees. Though this once-natural watercourse is contained within a concrete channel, the route along this creek bed of cast-in-place river rocks still suggests adventures worthy of Tom Sawyer and Becky Thatcher.

# Ride K7 - Lacy Park (San Marino)

**Distance** 0.5 miles

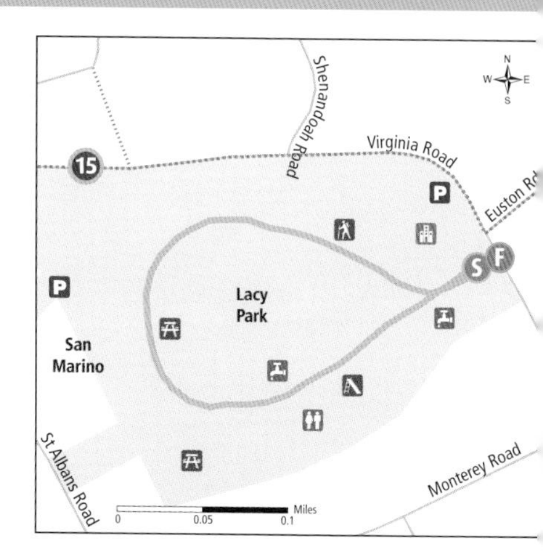


## Terrain

This gem of a ride (in a hidden, verdant park) encircles a great lawn along a wide, level, paved path. The riding conditions are excellent, except for a few small rough spots.

## How to Get There

From Huntington Drive, turn north on Virginia Road toward the mountains. Two small parking lots flank Lacy's entrance. If those lots are full, park on the adjacent streets.

## Amenities and Things to Do

Lacy Park has a playground with swings, slides, and rocking horses, all on a bed of fine woodchips. Around the park perimeter, an extensive network of paths meanders through shady groves, offering great places to stroll and explore. When making the grand tour with the kids, don't miss the rose arbor at the park's west entrance, off St. Albans Road. Picnic tables and drinking fountains are perched across the grounds.

## About

San Marino is an upscale enclave, with stately homes surrounded by immaculate lawns and landscaping. The city apparently borrowed that template in creating this amenity, reminiscent of a quiet European park, with gracious shade trees, rose bushes and lush lawns, ringed by dense hedges and wrought-iron fences. Children will surely enjoy riding in this picturesque and relaxed setting. Note: Bicycles are allowed only on the inner circle, not on the outer walking paths. Lacy Park has a certain undeniable exclusivity: On weekends, San Marino charges non-neighborhood residents a $4.00 entrance fee.

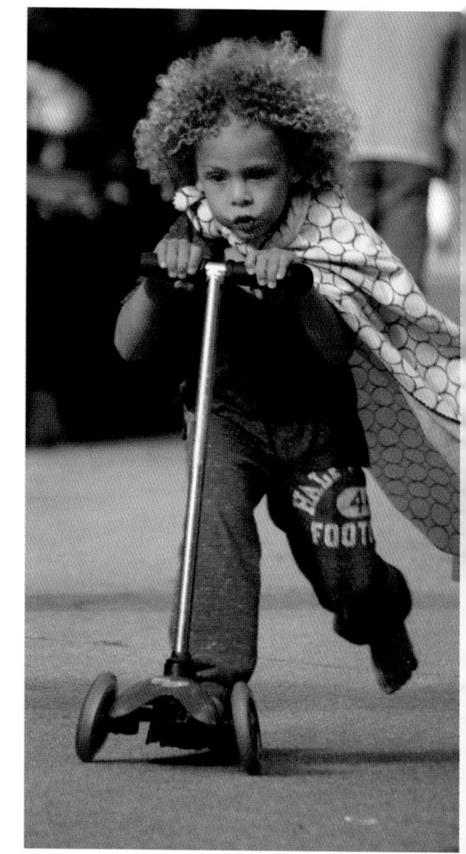

*A caped boy flies on his scooter.*

## Ride K8 - Belvedere Park (East Los Angeles)

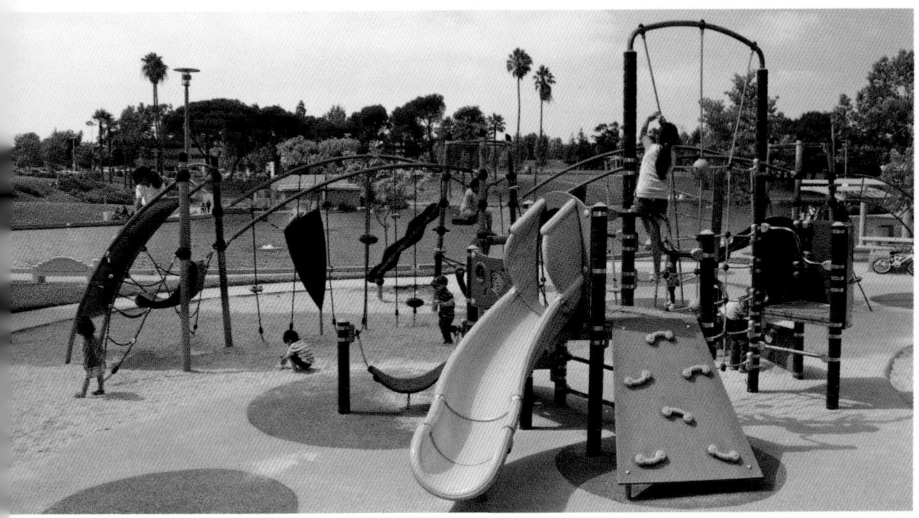
*This apparatus is a kid magnet.*

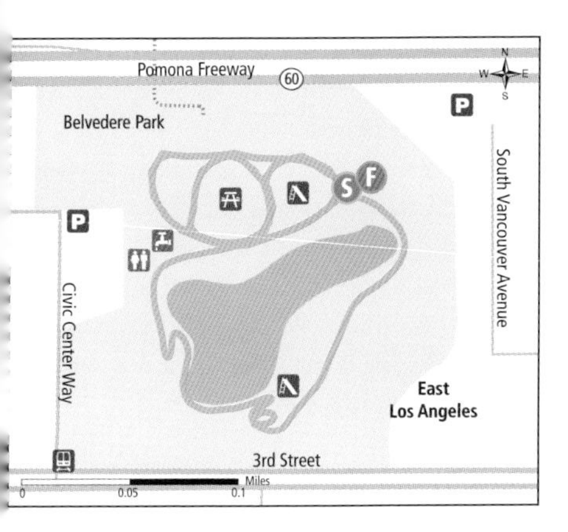


**Distance** 1.0 mile

### Terrain

All the paths are smooth concrete (only narrow in a couple of areas). An easy switchback links the park's upper network of paths to the lakeside below.

### How to Get There

From the 60 Freeway, exit onto Atlantic Boulevard heading south. A block later, make a right onto Pomona Boulevard and then, a right on Civic Center Way to Belevedere Park's free parking lot. Or take the Metro Gold line to the Atlantic station, across the street from the park.

### Amenities and Things to Do

Right at the civic core of East Los Angeles, Belvedere Park is also its recreation hub. Lawns, flowers, shade trees, an amphitheater, two playgrounds and canopied picnic tables surround a serene lake with fountains. Ducks and other waterfowl, including exotic species, populate the lake—enlivened each spring by newly hatched ducklings and goslings, which you can watch at close range.

### About

Belvedere Park offers many options for young riders. At the upper level, the path circles a shady lawn, swinging by a play area overlooking the lake. Short cross-paths add variety. This route joins a second loop, gradually descending to the water and another playground. A gentle switchback ramps back up to higher ground, returning to the starting point.

## Ride K9 - Legg Lake (South El Monte)

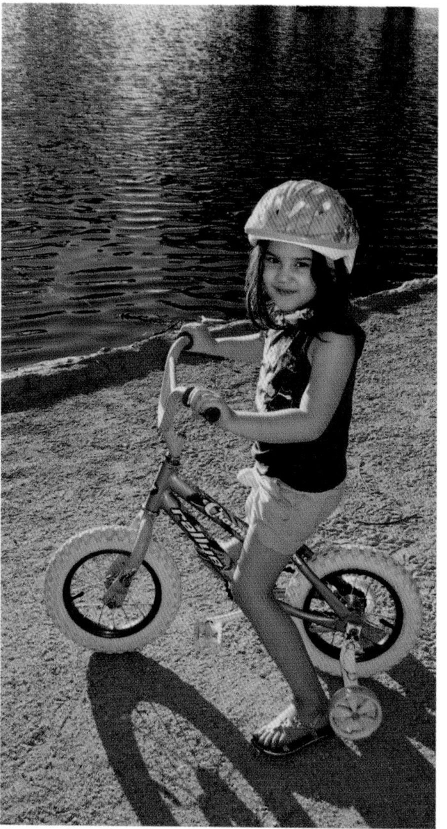
*A great place for a first ride.*

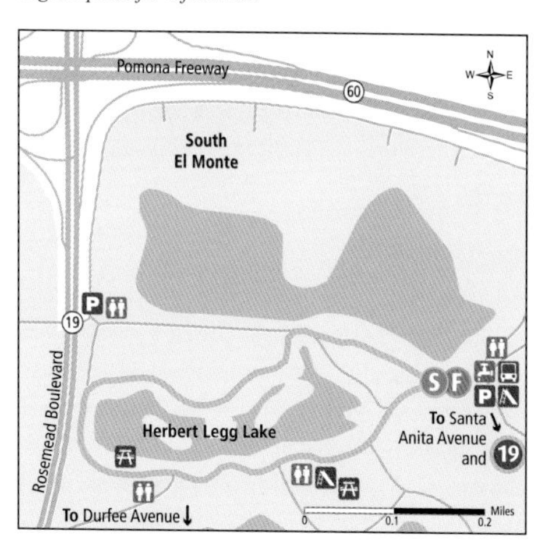


**Distance** 1.0 mile

### Terrain

A smooth, virtually flat, hard-packed dirt bike path rings one of the park's three lakes. The area is rarely crowded with bike traffic, even on busy weekends.

### How to Get There

Exit the 60 Freeway at Rosemead Boulevard, travel south and follow the signs to Legg Lake. You'll find paid parking areas on Rosemead Boulevard and, south of the lakes, on Durfee Avenue, as well as one free lot off Santa Anita Avenue, on the park's east side.

### Amenities and Things to Do

A jovial, blue, two-headed dragon, dancing octopuses, and oversize turtles are among the whimsical, cast-concrete "inhabitants" of the park—all welcoming climbing and imaginative play. The park also offers a wading pool for a light dip (though swimming is not permitted in any of the three lakes), plus playgrounds, covered picnic areas and great spots under shady trees or along lakeshores for stringing up a hammock or unfurling a beach blanket. Pedal cars and pedal boats are both available for rental. On Saturdays and Sundays, you'll find a mobile hot dog cart at the Rosemead Boulevard parking lot.

### About

The park's three lakes line up roughly on a north-south axis. Bike paths around Legg, Center and North lakes meander through meadows, lush with mature shade trees. A couple of footbridges invite cyclists across the narrow streams that link this trio of lakes. On the stretch around the middle lake, the path connects at several points to a larger web of bike routes, offering options for extended riding adventures.

# Ride K10 - Santa Fe Dam Recreation Area (Irwindale)

**Distance** 1.2 miles

### Terrain

Tracing a lazy figure-eight along a lake's shores, this flat, paved bike path wends its way through tree-shaded picnic and play areas.

### How to Get There

Santa Fe Dam Recreation Area is near the junction of the 605 and 210 freeways. If you're arriving on the 605, exit at Arrow Highway. Alternatively, from the 210, get off at North Irwindale Avenue and proceed south to Arrow Highway. From Arrow Highway, take Azusa Canyon Road north up over the dam to parking areas near the lake.

### Amenities and Things to Do

Santa Fe Dam Recreation Area makes it easy to combine diverse family activities with cycling excursions. The amenities include a lifeguarded swimming area with a white-sand beach (summers Thursday through Sunday) and the "Little Squirt Water Play Area" (open summer weekends), a splashy playground set in a shallow pool, complete with two water slides and an array of nozzles and fountains fed by kid-controlled valves. Throughout the park, you'll find plenty of picnic and BBQ spots. Wheel Fun rents pedal cars, pedal boats and kayaks. It also has a snack bar, with cold drinks, ice cream and other goodies.

### About

This "best of" ride begins near Parking Lot 3, leading the little ones by the park's playgrounds, past the creek that feeds the lake, all the way back to the swim beach. The recreation area's extensive network of low-key bicycle paths offers an enticing menu of additional rides—safe, varied, fun and relaxing—for kids and young families.

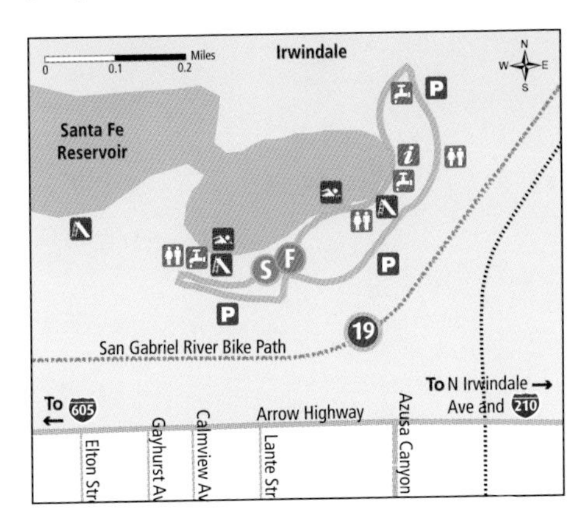


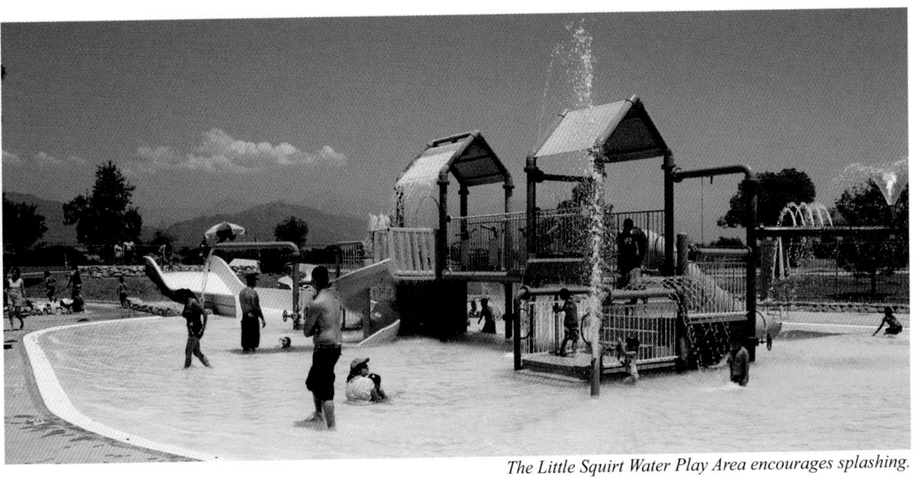

*The Little Squirt Water Play Area encourages splashing.*

# Ride 11 - Ralph C. Dills Park (Paramount)

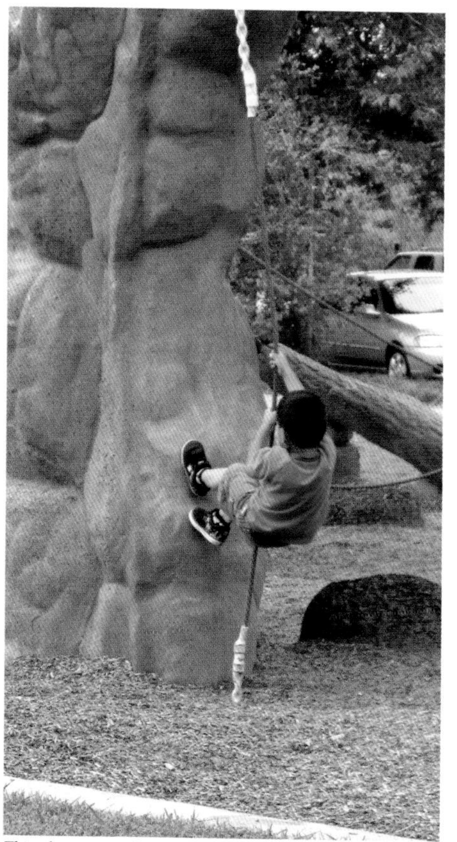

*This play area rocks—with manmade boulders rigged for young climbers.*

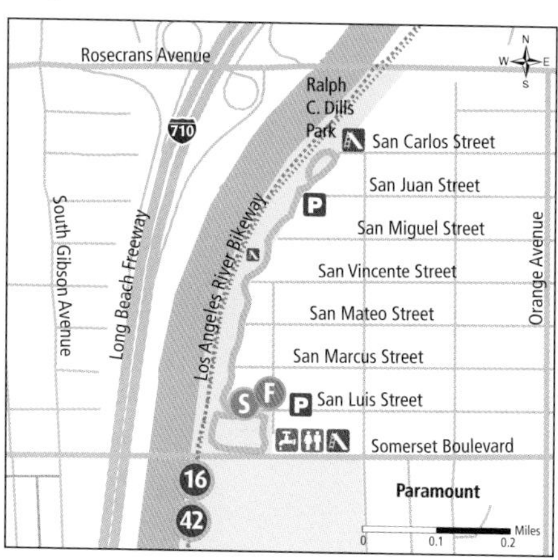


**Distance** 0.7 miles

### Terrain

The park's wide, level jogging and nature trail, surfaced in hard-packed dirt doubles as a bike path.

### How to Get There

From the 710 Freeway, exit at Rosecrans Avenue and drive east, crossing the L.A. River. Turn right on Orange Avenue, followed by a left on San Marcus Street, and then, a right onto San Antonio Street to the park's south end.

### Amenities and Things to Do

Dills Park—formerly named "Banana Park" for its long, curved shape—is a half-mile-long green belt adjacent to the L.A. River. Nestled in the park's wildflower-speckled landscaping are inventive playgrounds, including Rocks and Ropes, a young climbers' paradise with rope-rigged faux rock formations; and Fallen Tree, a slide and jungle gym, sculpted to resemble hollow tree trunks.

### About

Dills' ride options include the small, circular path around an athletic field/lawn at the park's south end. From there, you can pick up the main path, snaking north through aromatic and seemingly untamed landscapes of coastal sage scrub, live oak and native flowers favored by butterflies. To extend these rides, ramps at either end of the park onto the L.A. River Bike Trail, offering miles of protected, kid-friendly pathways.

# Ride K12 - Wilderness Park (Downey)

**Distance** 0.8 miles

## Terrain

Within this 26-acre park, a flat, smooth, wide concrete path weaves around three small lakes, expanses of lawn and a good-sized playground.

## How to Get There

From the 5 or the 605 Freeway, exit at Florence Avenue and take Little Lake Road to the park. (From the southbound 5, the Florence exit leads straight onto Little Lake Road.) You can park in Wilderness's lot or along the access road.

## Amenities and Things to Do

Despite the park's proximity to two major freeways, its atmosphere is remarkably tranquil, thanks to a tree canopy and fountains springing from its lakes. This otherwise typical neighborhood green space offers plenty of play areas, including a playground equipped with climbing and swinging apparatus, plus "Jeeps" for imaginary driving. Picnickers will also find tables and BBQ grills.

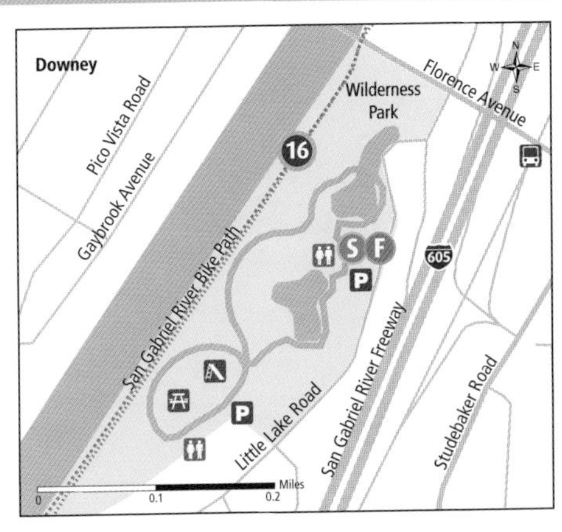


## About

Young cyclists can simply follow the park's main pathway, a loose figure-eight—or extend the journey into three or four smaller interconnected loops. Another great option is to continue onto the San Gabriel River Bike Trail via the modest ramp facing the community building. Along this trail, one recommended destination is Santa Fe Springs Park, about three-quarters of a mile north, offering another playground, plus a summer wading pool.

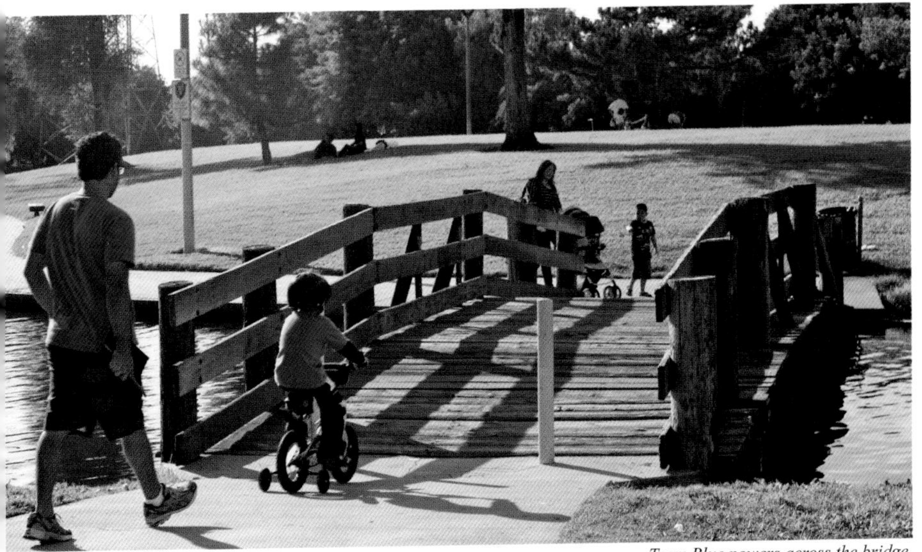

*Team Blue powers across the bridge.*

# Ride K13 - Santa Monica Pier (Santa Monica)

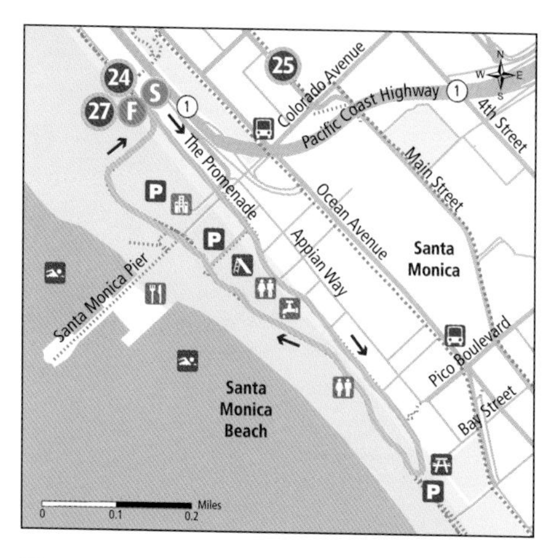


**Distance** 1.3 miles

## Terrain

Two connecting loops—combining a leisurely promenade with a flat, smooth-paved concrete bike path—form this route. Popular with walkers, skaters and cyclists, it's particularly well traveled on weekends.

## How to Get There

From the 10 Freeway, exit at Fourth/Fifth Street, make a left onto Fourth and a right onto Pico Boulevard. At Neilson Way, turn left and two blocks later, a right on Bicknell Avenue. Continue into the paid parking lot west of Crescent Bay Park. Or you might get lucky and find free or metered parking on nearby streets.

## Amenities and Things to Do

Even for fledgling cyclists, there's no shortage of ocean-side fun here within a few turns of the pedal. Pacific Park, atop the Santa Monica Pier, is the last glimmer of Southern California's classic amusement piers, with a Ferris wheel, rollercoaster, game arcade and vintage carousel. Tucked beneath the pier, you'll find the small Santa Monica Pier Aquarium. At beach level, entertainment options range from ocean swimming and sandcastle building to swinging and climbing in the playground. Snack venues abound, on the pier and near the aquarium.

## About

This adventure offers young riders a pint-sized whirl on the Marvin Braude Bike Trail, right near the Santa Monica Pier. The return trip can follow either the bike path or the promenade bordering hotels, bicycle rental stalls and snack stands. More ambitious riders can continue further north or south on the bike path, extending the trip, as desired.

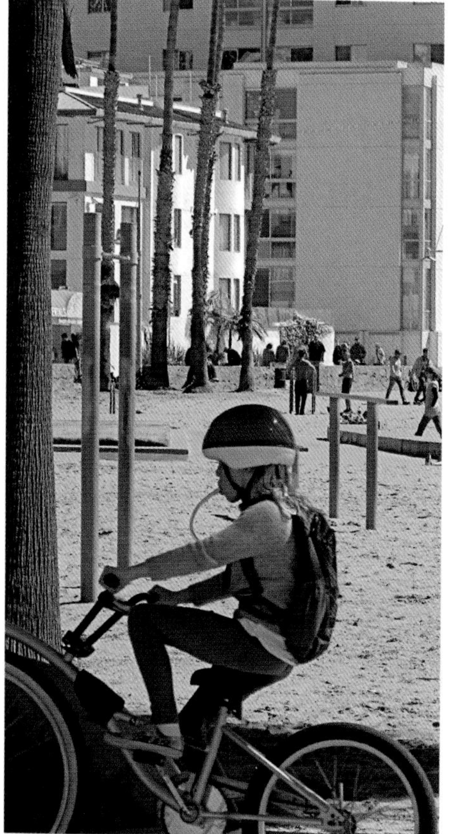

*Staying hydrated: highly recommended, especially on sunny beachside rides.*

# Ride K14 - Burton W. Chase Park (Marina del Rey)

**Distance** 0.5 miles

## Terrain

Set along a marina, with sailboats and other small craft, this is a flat, paved bike path.

## How to Get There

Burton W. Chase Park is at the end of Mindanao Way. It can be accessed from Lincoln Boulevard or Admiralty Way. Parking with coin-operated meters is available adjacent to the park and in parking areas on Mindanao Way.

## Amenities and Things to Do

This park's amenities include generous shade trees, low grassy hills, picnic tables, BBQs and an indoor gathering space (which you can reserve for events, such as meetings or family reunions, by calling 310-305-9595). This is also the summertime site of a concert series, as well as "Marina Movie Nights," free outdoor screenings of feature-length family films. Food sources are near at hand: The shopping center at the corner of Admiralty and Mindanao Ways has plenty of restaurants, many with take-out menus, several snack and coffee shops, plus a Ralph's supermarket.

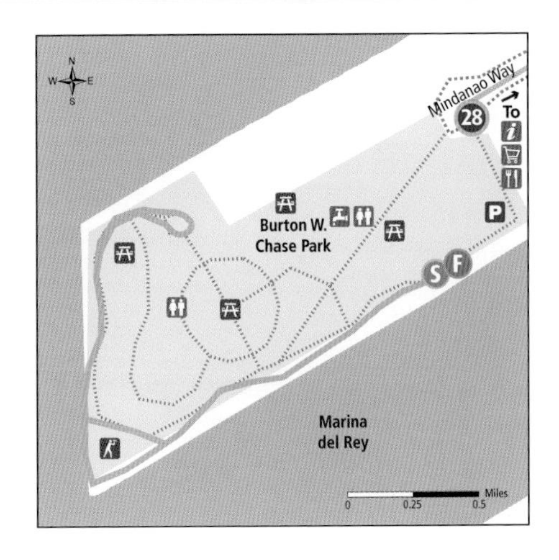


## About

The park is at the tip of a quay extending into the small-craft harbor of Marina del Rey. The nautical activity provides a spectacular backdrop. While cycling, kids and their adult companions can watch sailboats catching the wind out to sea or returning to port from Santa Monica Bay. You might spot dolphins swimming in the navigation channels or harbor seals sunning on nearby buoys and docks. This park is a relaxing family destination.

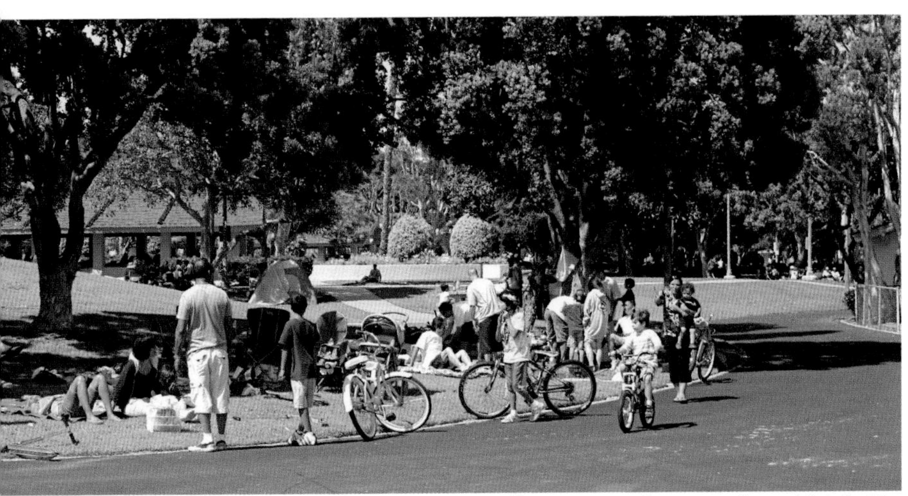

*Sunday in the Park with George: Burton Chase is a magnet for young cyclists and their families.*

# Ride K15 - Clover Park (Santa Monica)

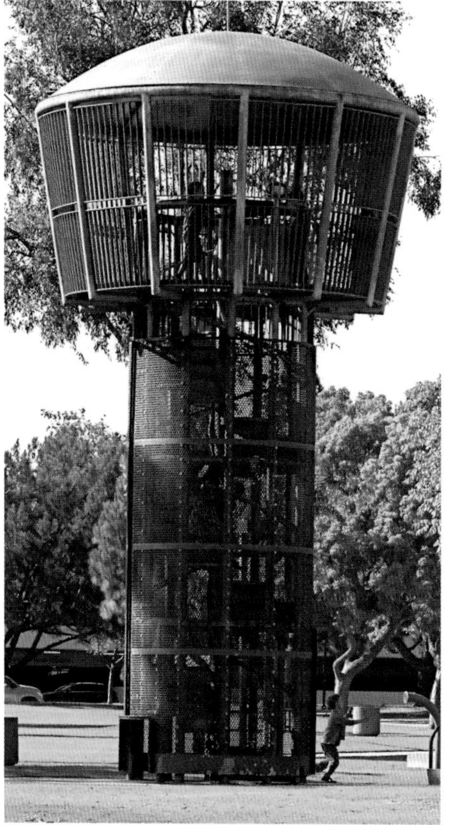

*A kids' climbing apparatus masquerades as a junior "air-traffic control tower."*

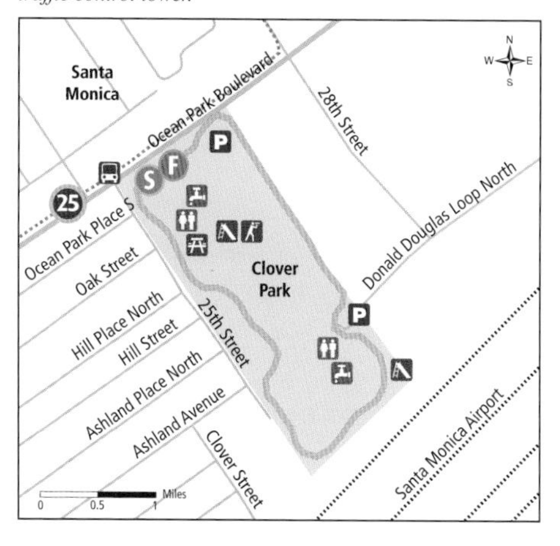


**Distance** 0.8 miles

## Terrain

This almost entirely flat ride follows a paved oblong path around the periphery of Clover Park.

## How to Get There

Clover Park is on Ocean Park Boulevard, between 25th and 28th streets, adjacent to the Santa Monica airport. Parking is available along any of the streets bordering the park and in two free parking lots: one off Ocean Park and the other off 28th Street.

## Amenities and Things to Do

Along the wide bike path, which doubles as a walking and jogging route, there are two terrific children's play areas, one featuring the park's whimsical centerpiece: a gray-and-lavender steel tower, reminiscent of an airport's control tower. This unusual play structure has a cage-like shell, allowing kids to safely ascend a spiral stair within it, rising more than 20 feet for protected views of the airport and surrounding neighborhoods. The park has picnic tables, BBQ grills, athletic fields and tennis courts, as well as many tree-shaded areas where adults can kick back while the tots cycle along.

## About

Although Clover Park is on a major thoroughfare running between a business district and the Santa Monica airport, the park is a surprisingly spacious and pleasant urban amenity. Topping its list of attractions is the fully visible airport runway where small aircraft frequently land and take off: a fascinating sight for many kids in the park. A micro velo-track—a flat paved oval no more that a couple hundred feet long—runs from the kiddy control tower to the adjacent playground (perfect for the plastic-tricycle set). The park can get crowded on summer weekends.

# Ride K16 - Westwood Park (Los Angeles/Westwood)

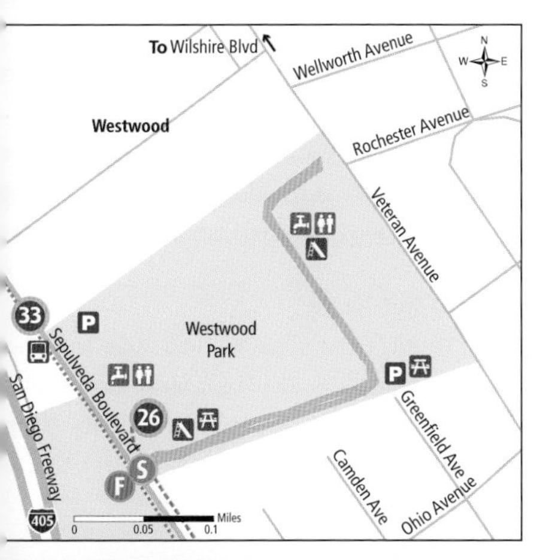


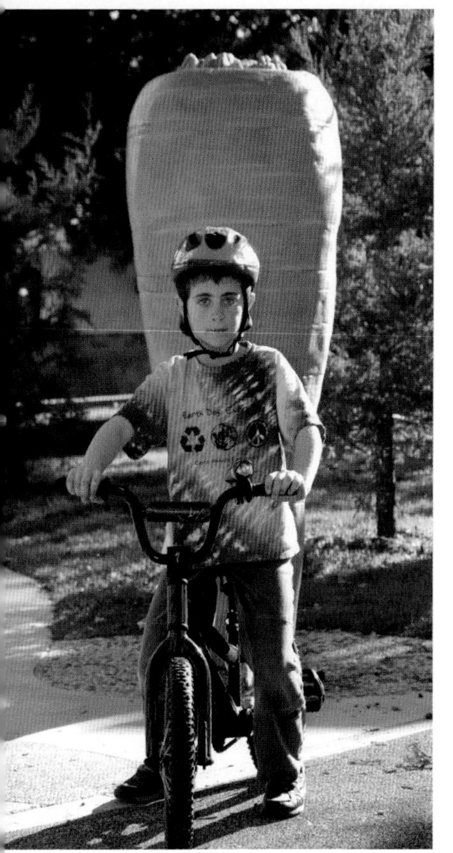

*Sprouting up among the children, giant carrots set the tone for this playground.*

**Distance** 0.7 miles

## Terrain

This flat asphalt path within a modest-sized urban park has zero vehicular traffic.

## How to Get There

From the 405 Freeway: Either exit at Wilshire Boulevard, take Wilshire east and then, Veteran Avenue south; or exit at Santa Monica Boulevard, head east on Santa Monica and north on Sepulveda Boulevard. On the park's north, south and west sides, you'll find parking lots.

## Amenities and Things to Do

Westwood Recreation Center, on the park's Sepulveda side, is a public facility with a 25-meter indoor swimming pool and two gyms. The outdoor Westwood Tennis Center, within the park, offers classes for kids as young as four years old. Its pro shop sells refreshments: bottled water, ice cream and sodas (8:00 a.m. to 9:00 p.m. weekdays; 8:00 a.m. to 5:00 p.m. weekends).

## About

This short bike ride traces a lazy Z through athletic fields and stands of trees, among tennis and basketball courts, soccer fields and picnic areas. A playground punctuates either end of the journey. Aidan's Place was the second universally accessible playground in the U.S. For kids of all abilities, it offers an airplane, a castle, water play, slides and bouncy surfaces. Giant root veggies mark the Carrot Seed Sensory Nook, a place for storytelling or quiet time. Its curved, tactile wall, clad in colorful, ceramic tiles, donated by Michelle Griffoul Studios, illustrates the tale of a growing carrot seed. Big red, pushable buttons invite kids to activate the wall's sound components. The park's open green space encourages running around, picnicking or even celebrating birthdays. This family-friendly park, near Westwood Village and UCLA, buzzes with activity on weekends.

# Ride K17 - Hermosa Beach Strand (Hermosa Beach)

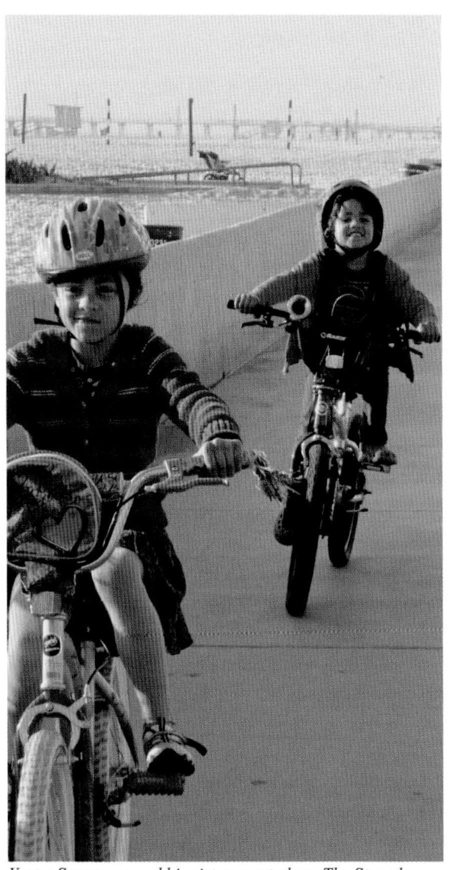

*Young Superman and his sister coast along The Strand.*

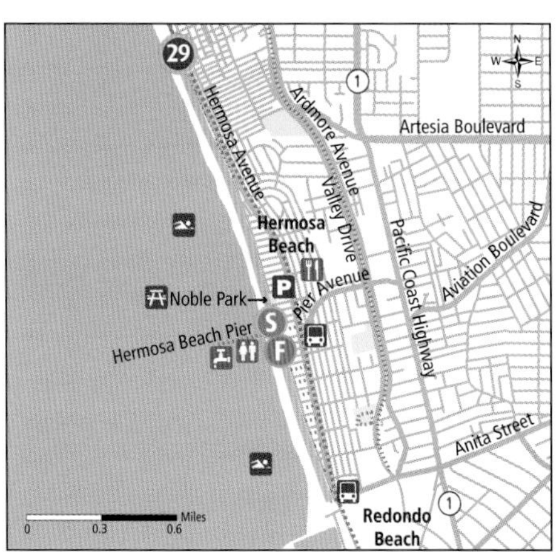


**Distance** 1.8 miles

## Terrain

This flat and generously wide path is essentially smooth ribbon of concrete along the length of Hermos Beach. The posted speed limit is eight miles per hour!

## How to Get There

From Pacific Coast Highway, turn west onto Pie Avenue toward the beach. At 13th Street and Hermos Avenue, just north of Pier Avenue, you'll find a pai parking structure. Also, many of the surrounding cit streets offer metered parking.

## Amenities and Things to Do

Hermosa Beach, with its broad, clean swath of san and abundance of lifeguard stations, is a great spot fo swimming and playing. During prime time, especiall on weekends, the scene is populated by beachcomber in bikinis and surfer shorts, volleyball players, pedaler on colorful beach cruisers, picnicking families unde brightly striped beach umbrellas and kids enjoyin surfside swing sets. The adjacent, relatively smal Noble Park, at 14th Street and The Strand, offers shor walking paths through grassy hillocks and a few youn shade trees. For snacks: The many restaurants near th pier include a Coldstone Creamery ice cream shop an a Starbucks on Hermosa near 13th Street.

## About

This is a leisurely route, where parents can strol chatting over a latte, while their children pedal safel alongside them. As junior riders gain confidence (o for more experienced young cyclists), we recommen extending this route to the north from 34th Street, wher The Strand connects with the kid-friendly Marvi Braude Bike Trail. One small caveat: The Stran can be *muy popular* on weekends—this ride is leas crowded (and, for many people, most relaxing) o weekday mornings.

# Ride 18 - Highridge Park (Rolling Hills Estates)

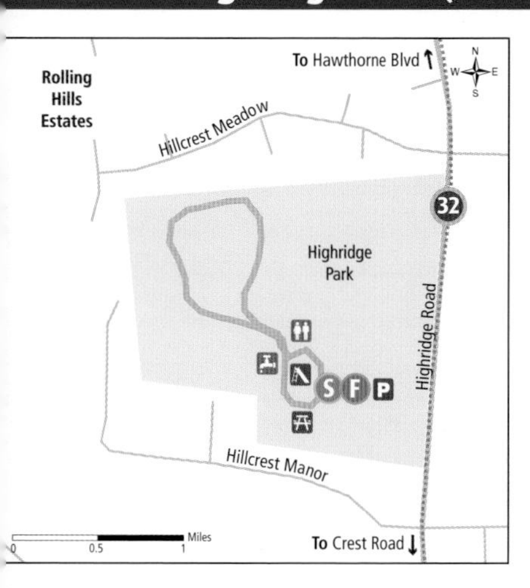


**istance** 0.4 miles

## errain

'his ride follows a fairly smooth, hard-packed dirt path ‚ith a slight grade change from one end to the other.

## low to Get There

ptly named, Highridge Park is near the top of the Palos /erdes Peninsula. From the 110 Freeway, drive west n Pacific Coast Highway, then make a left (south) on Hawthorne Boulevard. Go about 3.4 miles, past the Peninsula Shopping Center, and make a right at the signal onto Highridge Road. Continue straight to the park.

## Amenities and Things to Do

Nestled against an upscale residential neighborhood, Highridge is a peaceful, well-tended park, with long, white "horse farm" fences, a baseball diamond, bridal path and soccer fields. The tree canopy helps shade a playground and picnic area. *Après*-ride refreshments are available a short drive away at the Peninsula Shopping Center.

## About

The Highridge circuit traces a quirky figure-eight. Riders make a small loop around the playground area before picking up a modest downhill connector to the bigger loop, rolling by the baseball diamond and through the park's most wooded corner before returning to the playground. For young cyclists craving a longer ride, you might add the paved bike path that borders the park's front lawn and continues south for about half a mile. (Since this ride extension crosses streets and access roads, however, parents should supervise kids along this segment.)

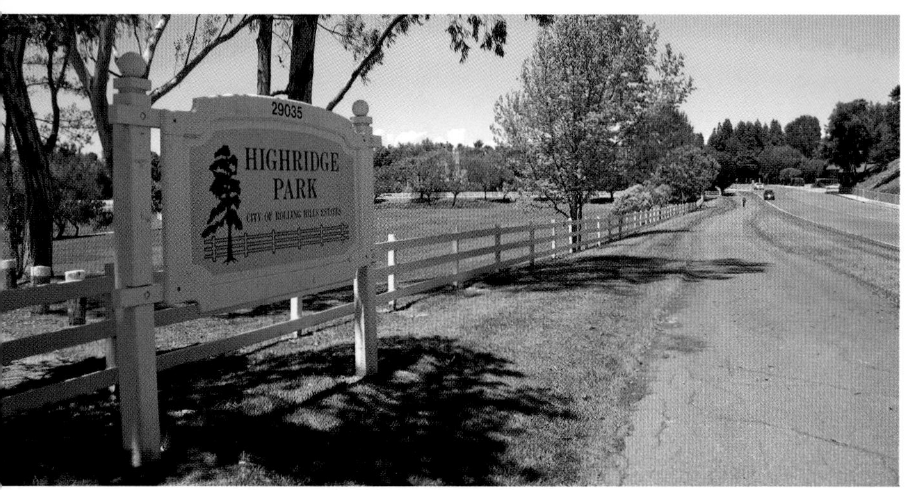


*This part of the Palos Verdes Peninsula is horse country—long rail-and-post fences abound.*

# Ride K19 - The Cornfield (Downtown Los Angeles)

**Distance** 1.5 miles

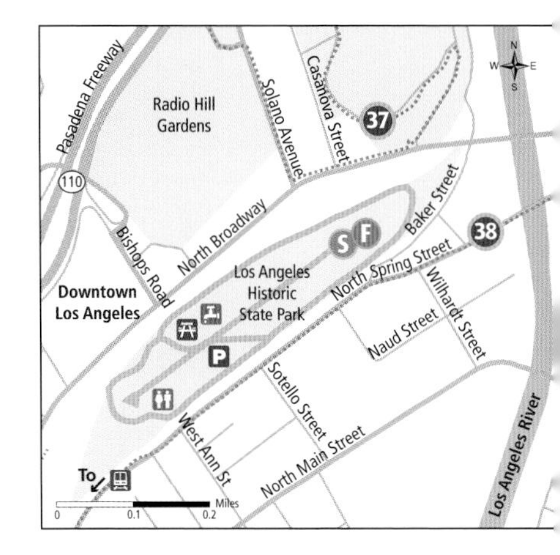


## Terrain

This ride offers flat, smooth, compacted dirt paths.

## How to Get There

Exit the 101 Freeway at Alameda Street (which becomes North Spring Street) and head north to "The Cornfield" (formally the Los Angeles State Historic Park). From the 110 Freeway, exit at Hill Street, turn left at West College, right on North Spring Street and then, north to the park. Metro Gold Line trains stop one block away, at the Chinatown station.

## Amenities and Things to Do

The Cornfield is a unique urban landscape on the riverside site of an abandoned rail yard - the transcontinental railroad's original terminus in the city; the 19th century Pacific Hotel; and, long before that, native Tongva villages. By bicycle, kids can explore vast open meadows, wildflowers, community gardens and the footprints of past buildings, artistically outlined in recycled glass. Metro Gold Line trains zip past, and downtown skyscrapers provide a backdrop. The park hosts many seasonal family events, such as the "Outdoor Cinema Food Fest," with films an a movable feast from scores of ethnic food trucks, ubiquitous treat in L.A. From April to September, par employees and volunteers lead sunset campfire talks.

## About

A network of trails offers a variety of kids' ride including a long perimeter loop (divisible into tw smaller loops) and a separate, central, arrow-straigh path, rising to a mound with views over the entire park

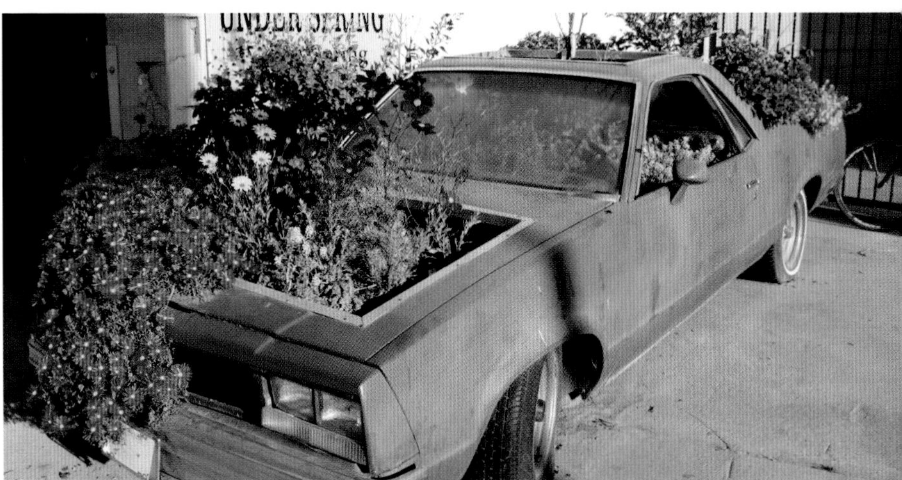

*Relics of the Cornfield's provence as an art project flourish in its immediate surrounding*

## Ride K20 - Kenneth Hahn State Rec. Area (Baldwin Hills)

**Distance** 0.8 miles

### Terrain

This asphalt path is roughly circular, dipping down on the park's north side and climbing slightly near the end of the loop.

### How to Get There

From either direction on the 10 Freeway, exit at Fairfax and drive south about 1.5 miles, merging with La Cienega en route. Follow signs to the recreation area entrance. Drive through the park to the hilltop parking (free on weekdays; $6 on weekends and holidays).

### Amenities and Things to Do

More than seven miles of walking and hiking trails meander through the park's hillsides, ridges, canyons, oak woodlands, grasslands and low-growing coastal sage. The array of activities here nicely complements cycling. The lower area includes three playgrounds, big fields and a Japanese garden. More Japanese landscaping and a pleasant walking path surround Gwen Moore Lake, a picturesque fishing pond fed by a short manmade creek cascading into several low waterfalls. In the upper area, a big purple, smiling dragon "supervises" Jackson's Frontierland, yet another playground. Nearby, you'll find BBQs and shaded tables: ideal for picnics and birthday parties.

### About

A large, bowl-shaped meadow called Janice's Green Valley, in the park's upper area, provides the terrain for this bike loop. Its splendid views offer distant glimpses of the Hollywood Sign, Hollywood Hills, Westside beaches and Downtown L.A. We recommend riding this circuit counter-clockwise to benefit from a more gradual ascent on the south side.

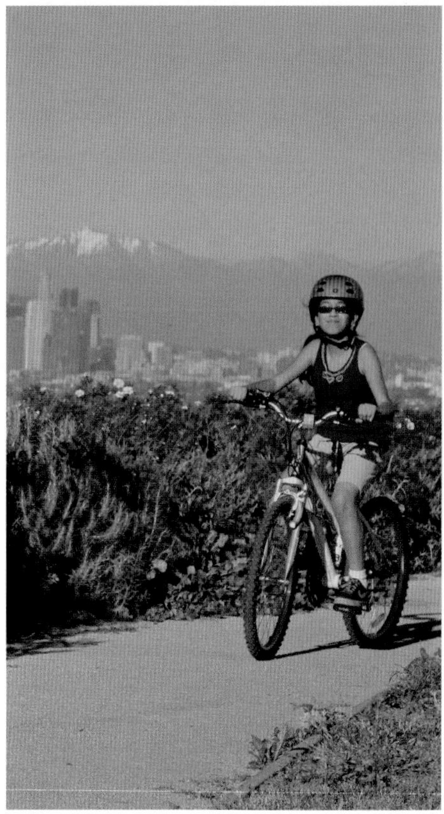

*Beyond the flowering meadows are distant views of Downtown L.A. and the mountains beyond.*

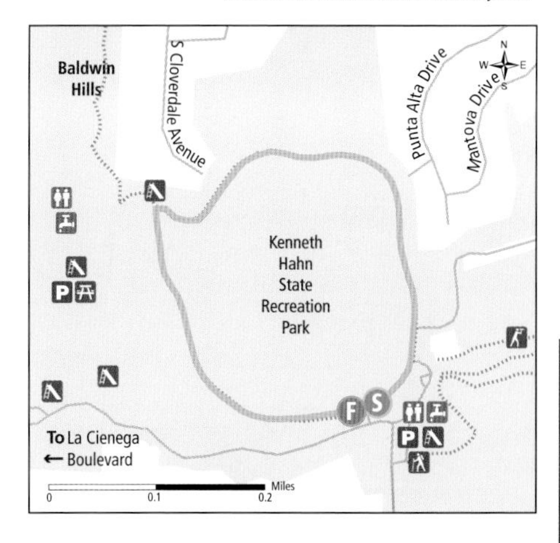

## Ride K21 - Ladera Park (Ladera Heights)

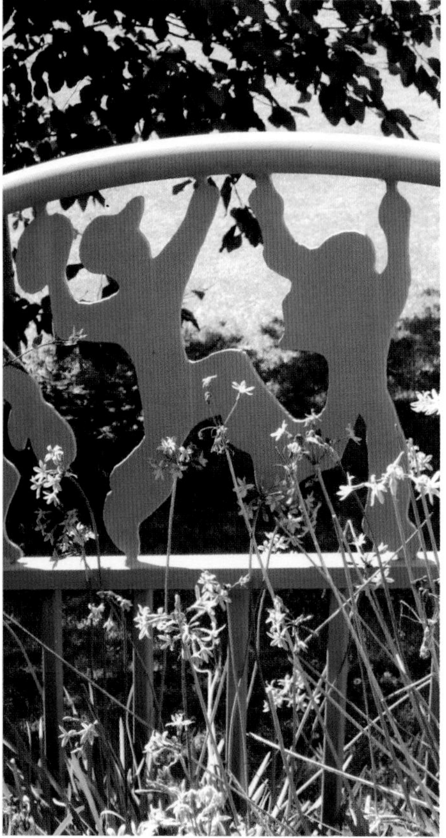

*Fences amid flowers celebrate play in the great outdoors.*

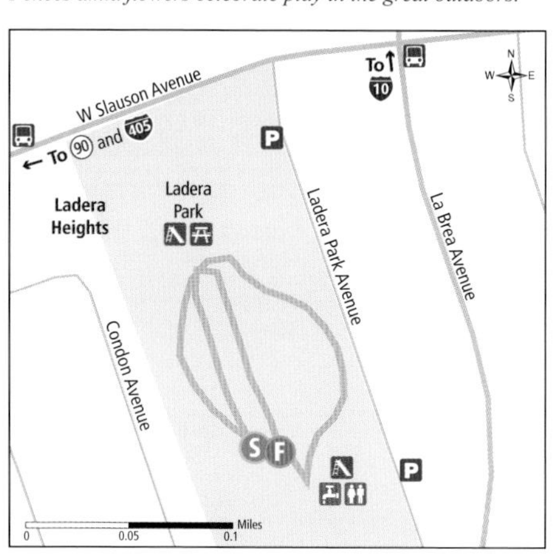


**Distance** 0.5 miles

### Terrain

Paved in smooth concrete, the route is a pair of concentric, interconnected loops: The inner circuit is flat while outer ring includes two small climbs and descents.

### How to Get There

From the Westside and 405 Freeway, exit onto the 90 Freeway toward Slauson Avenue. Continue east on Slauson approximately two miles to the park. From Mid-city and the 10 Freeway, travel south on La Brea Avenue about three miles, make a right onto Slauson and, after a short distance, a left onto Ladera Park Avenue (which has on-street parking).

### Amenities and Things to Do

A playground anchors either end of the park, which also includes a community center, basketball courts, an outdoor amphitheater, a vine-covered arbor and many spots for family picnics and barbecues.

### About

Though only 15.9 acres, Ladera Park is a lush oasis: a long grassy glen, shaded by abundant mature trees. This ride's two loops travel nearly the length of the park. The inner, easier ring surrounds the picnic areas, extending down the valley floor. The outer circuit lets riders look out over the park. Most little legs will be able to make these modest, gently sloped climbs. The downhill runs back to the lower level are also fun and hardly daunting.

# Ride K22 - "Magic" Johnson Recreation Area (Willowbrook)

**Distance** 1.4 miles

## Terrain

The park offers a network of lakeside cycling-and-walking paths with good concrete or asphalt paving.

## How to Get There

Take either the 110, 710 or 405 to the 105 Freeway. Exit at Central Avenue in the Willowbrook neighborhood. Continue south to El Segundo Boulevard or 120th Street and turn right to the access street or one of the parking lots.

## Amenities and Things to Do

Magic Johnson, the man, has become a community leader and philanthropist, following his illustrious basketball career—first, as a star point guard with the Los Angeles Lakers during that team's heyday in the 1980s; and then as a member of the 1992 Olympic gold-medal-winning "Dream Team." Unlike its magical namesake, however, this recreation area is scarce on glitter: just a modest playground, plus a few picnic tables and pergolas across the lawns. But the park definitely engages the community, with locals flocking here to celebrate *Quinceaneras* ("sweet fifteen," for Latinas), photograph weddings, play by the lakes or just hang out.

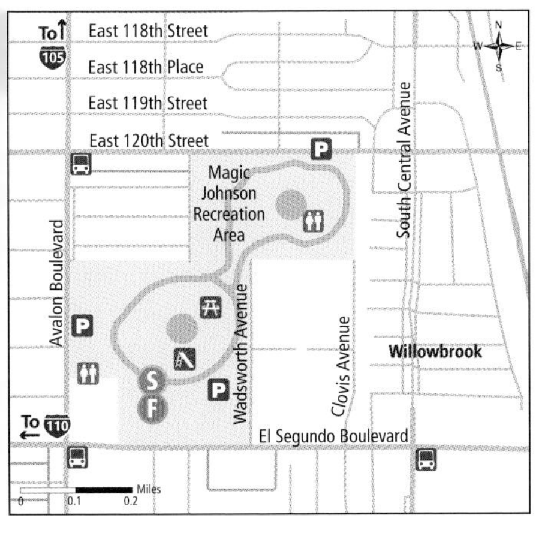


## About

With views of ducks, geese and palm-studded islands, this ride offers roughly a figure eight for cycling (or walking) circuit around two manmade lakes. For shorter spins, you can split the ride into two loops via the wooden bridge between them.

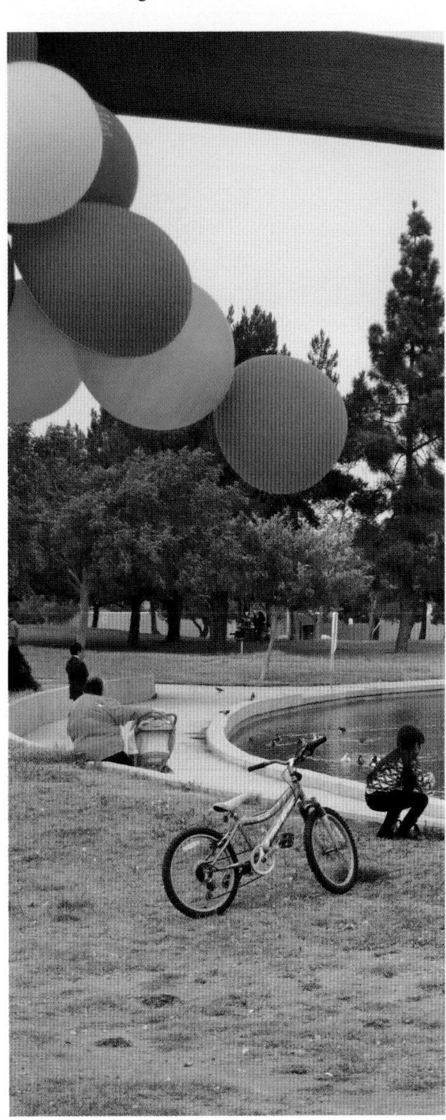

*Cyclists, splashing ducks and birthday picnics.*

# Ride K23 - John Anson Ford Park (Bell Gardens)

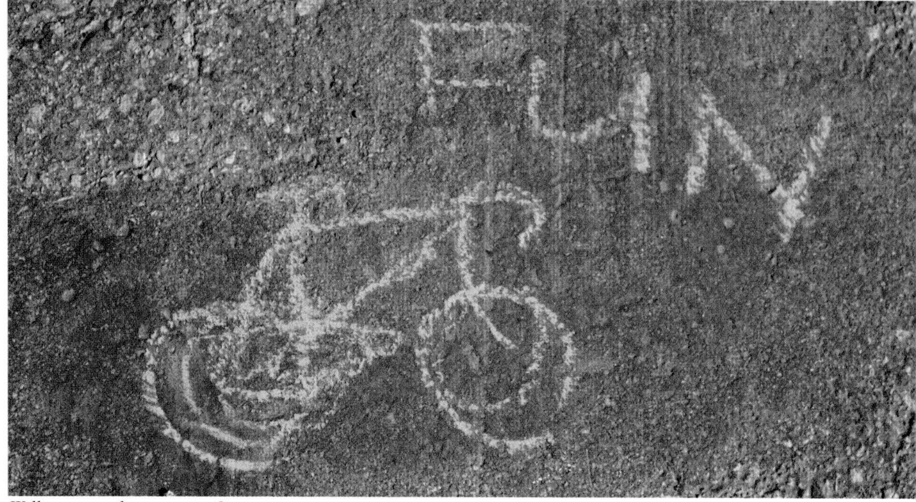


*Well, yes—need we say more?*

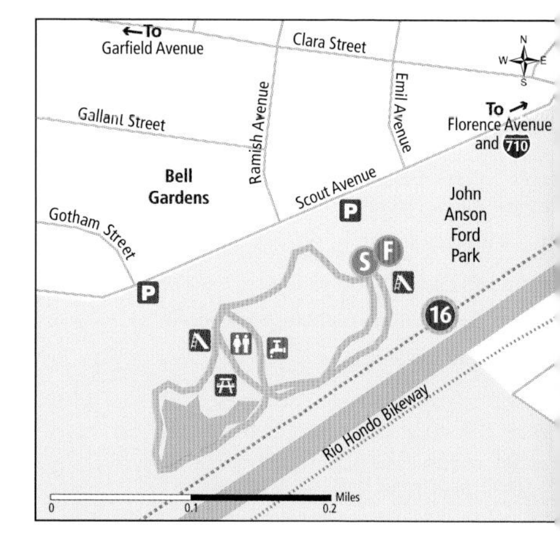


**Distance** 0.8 miles

## Terrain

Fairly smooth, concrete paths, shared by cyclists and pedestrians, suggest several rides through the park.

## How to Get There

Exit the 710 Freeway at Florence Avenue, drive east for about 1.5 miles. Turn right onto Scout Avenue to the park. Scout Avenue and Park Lane usually provide ample parking.

## Amenities and Things to Do

Named for a long-serving county supervisor and champion of the arts, John Anson Ford Park is a nexus of outdoor activity for the community of Bell Gardens, offering both kids' and adults' soccer, baseball, basketball and swimming. There's also a duck pond, a modest playground and shady lawns. Occasional pushcart vendors sell ice cream and cold drinks.

## About

Like many community parks along L.A.'s rivers, this one includes about a mile of cycling-and-pedestrian pathways, a playground and picnic areas, all set amid mature shade trees around a water feature—here a pond that ducks and geese seem to adore. A great plus is the option to extend a kids' ride onto the Rio Hondo Bike Path, bordering the park's south side. Along this river bike path, you'll find Treasure Island Park (well, not exactly an island or a treasure trove, but, hey, it does offer BBQs beneath nice trees), about 1.5 miles north, and Crawford Park, approximately three-quarters of a mile south.

# Ride K24 - Columbia Park (Torrance)

**Distance** 1.5 miles

## Terrain

A wide, level, hard-packed dirt path switches to concrete around the playground and picnic areas.

## How to Get There

Exit the 450 Freeway at Hawthorne Boulevard. Take Hawthorne south and turn left on 190th to Prairie Avenue. The park has a big parking area off 190th, with smaller ones on Prairie and on 186th Street.

## Amenities and Things to Do

Though much of this largely flat, 52-acre park is devoted to soccer and baseball, the eastern third has a playground, gazebos and shady picnic areas. A grove of cherry trees, the gift of Soka Gakkai, a Buddhist group, blossoms here in the spring. (By 2007, the park had received 70 cherry trees, and the donors committed to contributing 30 more each year thereafter.)

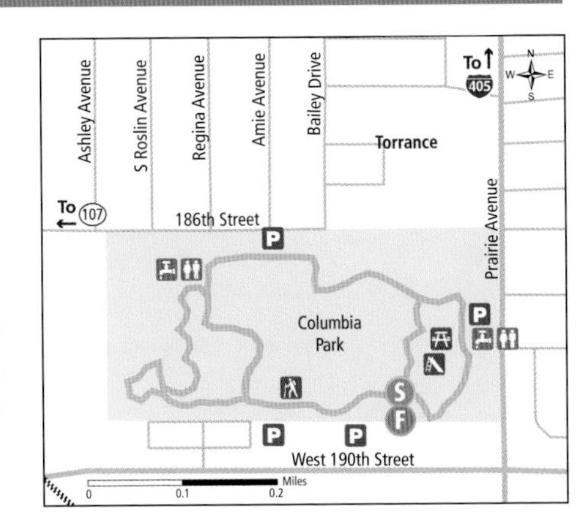


## About

The shared walking/jogging/biking path provides for a safe cycling experience with a variety of routes, from a short circle around the picnic-and-play area to a longer journey that twists around and between soccer fields and a radio broadcast tower, amounting to more than a mile of riding.

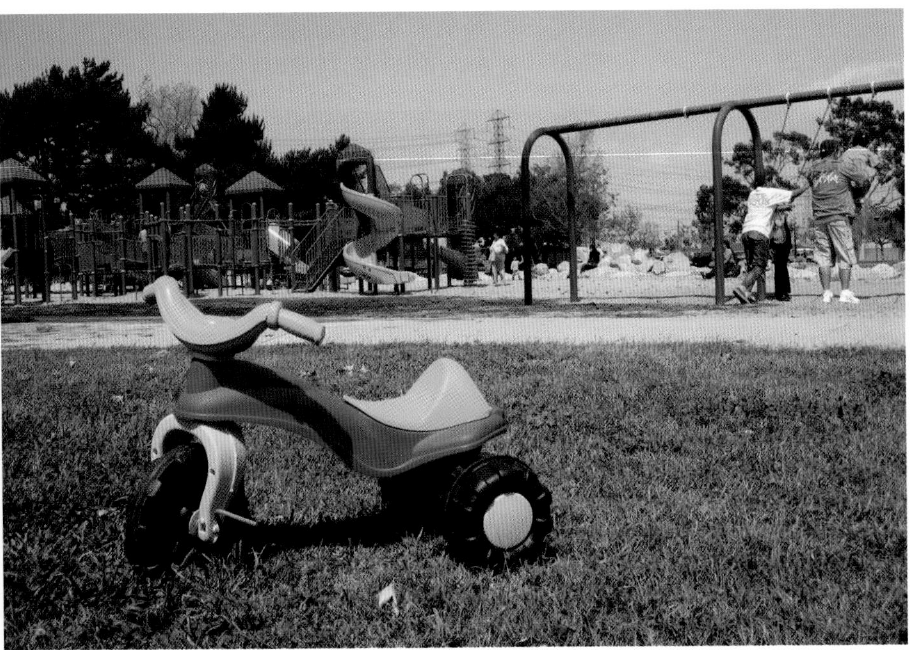

*There's a playful mix of swings, mini-bridges, corkscrew slides—and bikes.*

# Ride K25 - Ken Malloy Harbor Regional Park (Harbor City)

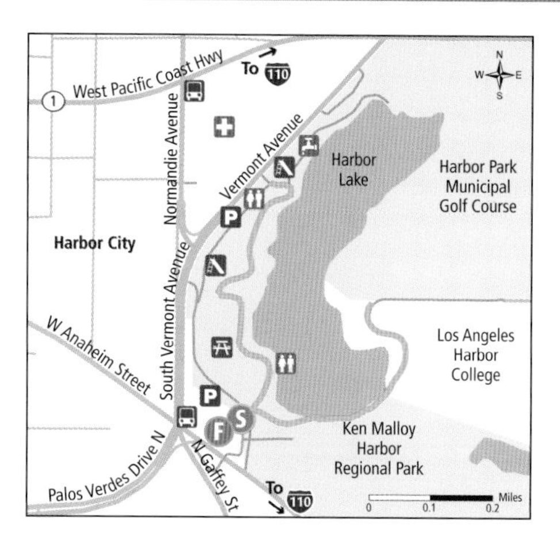


**Distance** 0.9 miles

## Terrain

This lakeside path is flat with one small hill in the middle. The surface needs repaving, but is still bikeable. Just be attentive to bumps, cracks and potholes.

## How to Get There

From the 110 Freeway in the Wilmington and Harbor City area, exit at Pacific Coast Highway and drive west. Turn left onto Vermont Avenue and then, into the parking lot beside the playground.

## Amenities and Things to Do

The centerpiece of the 231-acre park is Machado Lake and surrounding wetlands. Picnic areas and a recently upgraded playground overlook the lake. Harbor Park is excellent for bird watching, with dozens of resident and migrating species, so keep your eyes peeled, especially near the wetlands.

## About

The park has been unloved by the Department of Recreation and Parks and needs a facelift, but until that happens, it's still a good place to cycle. Beginning at the sailboat-themed playground, this excursion proceeds along Machado Lake's shoreline and heads up a short, steep hill before descending to the low-lying path across the lake's dam and spillway. In this "bottom" area, dense rushes, reeds and other plant life thrive, making it a favorite habitat for birds. The journey here begins to feel like a ride into a jungle.

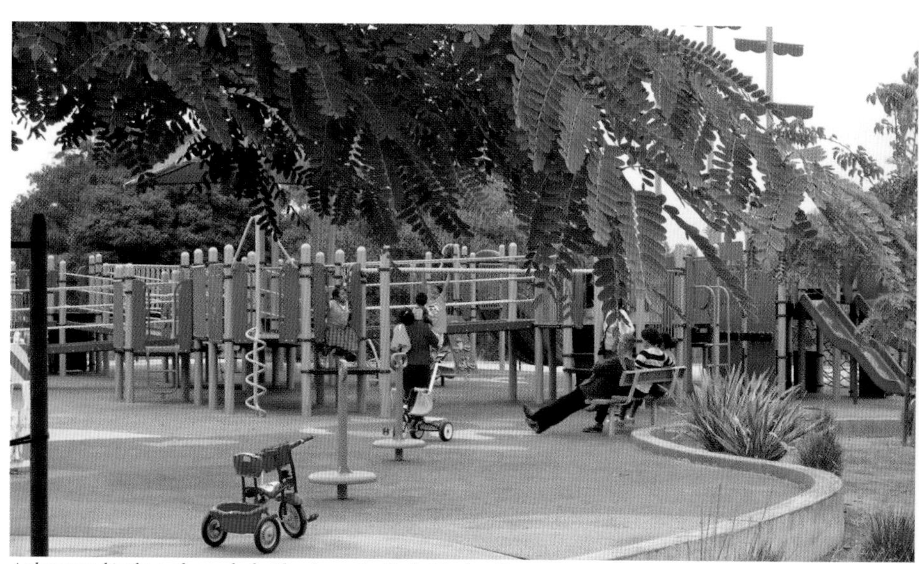

*A playground in the park: sparked with color and spiked with play ship masts.*

# Ride K26 - Scherer Park (Long Beach)

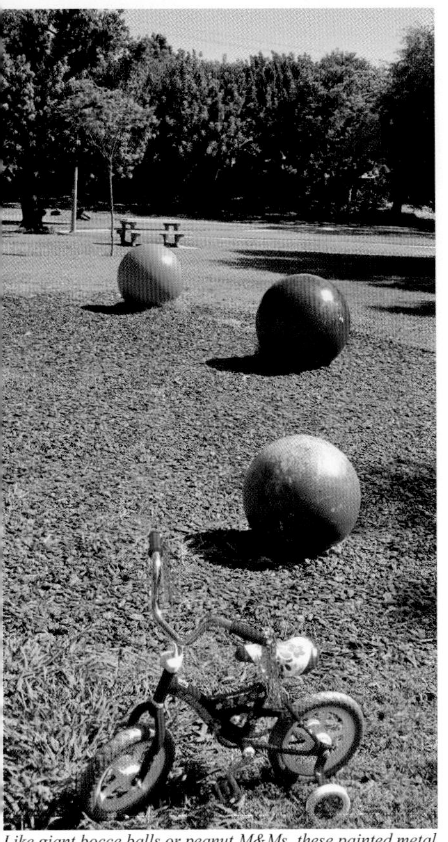

*Like giant bocce balls or peanut M&Ms, these painted metal spheres perform as seats or sculptures.*

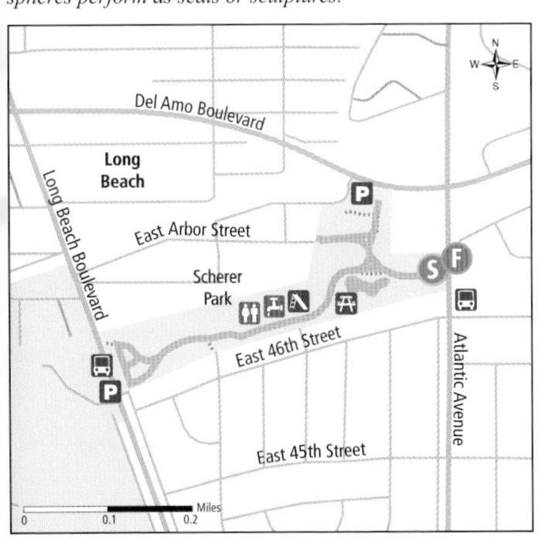


**Distance** 1.0 miles

## Terrain

This gentle, mostly flat concrete path has a short climb at one end.

## How to Get There

Head toward Long Beach on the 710 Freeway, exit at Del Amo Boulevard and drive east about one mile. Look for parking on Del Amo or, just south, on Atlantic Avenue or off Long Beach Boulevard.

## Amenities and Things to Do

Scherer Park is tucked amid quiet residential neighborhoods in northern Long Beach. The hill, sloping down from Atlantic Avenue and ample landscaping shelter the park from street noise. A duck pond and dog park, a playground, tennis and basketball courts, as well as pergolas and other spots for picnics and relaxation make this a popular neighborhood park.

## About

Young cyclists can ride the multi-purpose concrete path that traverses the entire length of the park, passing the community center and a play area with swings and a jungle gym, before eventually ascending the hill to the overlook at Scherer's eastern end. Branches off the main path lead around the duck pond, past the long cascade designed to flow through the park and across a small wooden bridge. Shaded picnic tables and colorful sculptures resembling giant bocce balls (or mega-Peanut M&Ms) are sprinkled across the terrain.

# Ride K27 - Shoreline Aquatic Park (Long Beach)

**Distance** 0.6 miles

## Terrain

This harbor-side path is wide, flat and paved in smooth concrete.

## How to Get There

Follow the 710 Freeway south until its end in Long Beach. Continue on Shoreline Drive to Aquarium Way and through the roundabout onto Golden Shore Street. Go past the aquarium to the parking lot, with views of the Queen Mary.

## Amenities and Things to Do

Set between a small-craft marina and a shipping channel, Shoreline Aquatic Park is modest in size, but expansive in views and nearby activities. The majestic Queen Mary, a 1936 ocean liner which you can tour, is moored permanently across the channel. The park includes a large anchor to climb (beats a jungle gym) and a towering beacon, the Lion's Lighthouse for Sight, atop a grassy hill. Just next door, the Aquarium of The Pacific, offers a shark lagoon, where you can touch the creatures, and the Lorikeet Forest, full of colorful birds. Shoreline Village, with plenty of snacking options, is right nearby, as is The Pike amusement park.

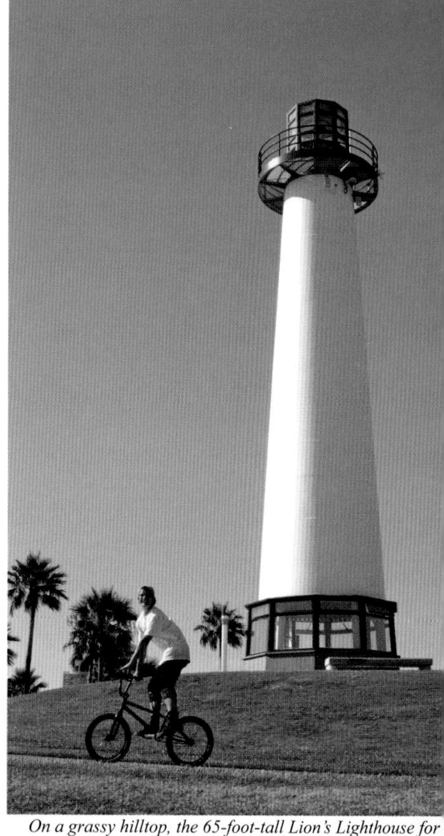

*On a grassy hilltop, the 65-foot-tall Lion's Lighthouse for Sight was built in 2000.*

## About

From a plaza beside sailboat moorings, this ride runs along the park's edge, around its lawns and towering hilltop lighthouse. Views toward the Queen Mary open up as the route swings around a bend and then borders the marine channel all the way to the turnaround at a second, smaller, lighthouse.

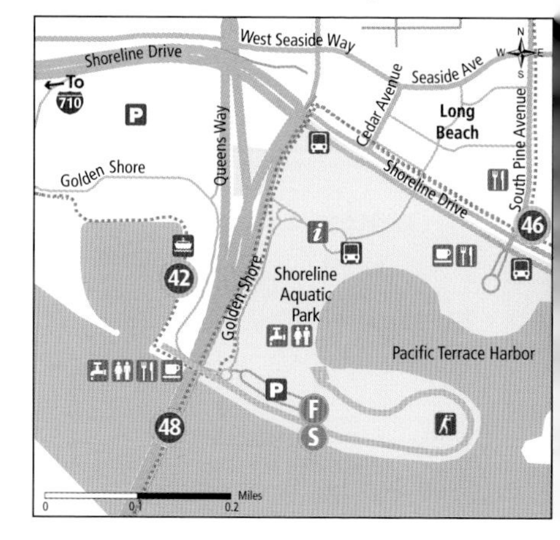

## Ride K28 - Recreation Park (Long Beach)

**istance** 0.8 miles

### 'errain

ecreation Park slopes gently uphill from the start t Sixth Street. (Across the whole ride, it's a rise of only about 50 feet.) The concrete bike path is in good condition, except for occasional cracks.

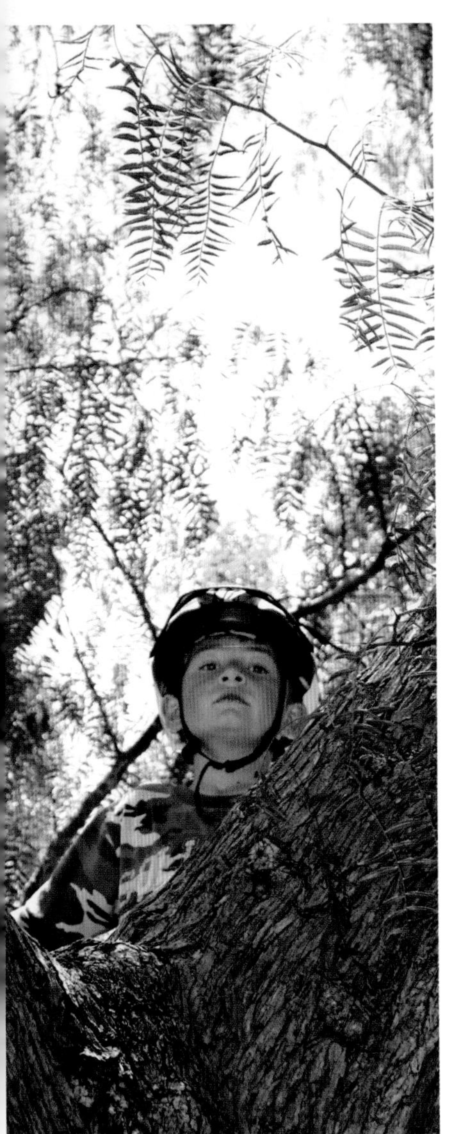

*A young cyclist in camouflage leaves the bike path and scampers up a tree.*

### How to Get There

From the 405 Freeway south, exit onto State Route 22/ Seventh Street. Continue west for about two miles and turn onto Federation Drive, which offers street parking both north and south of Seventh Street.

### Amenities and Things to Do

At 211 acres, Recreation Park is one of Long Beach's bigger parks, though most of its land is given over to a pair of golf courses. The remaining space includes a playground, built anew in 2002, and lots of grassy areas. The city created the park in 1926, so the trees are now big, providing generous shade.

### About

You can enjoy this ride's two segments—one south of Seventh Street and the other north of it—as either: [a] two short, stand-alone jaunts; or [b] a single, longer out-and-back ride of approximately one mile. For the longer option, connecting the north and south legs, be sure to use the crosswalk on Seventh Street east of Park Avenue. Adults should absolutely accompany kids at the crossing.

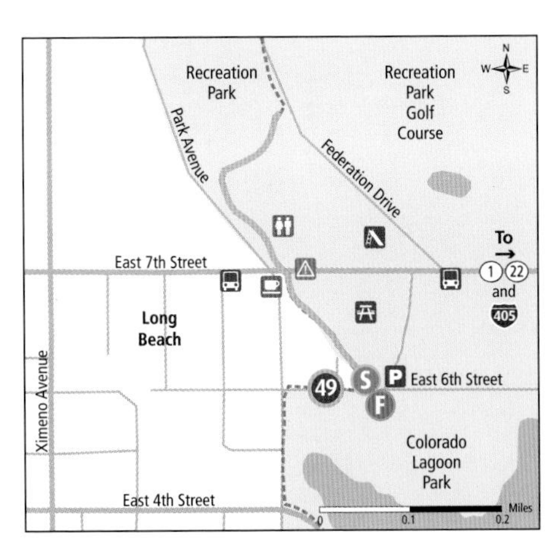

# Ride K29 - Cabrillo Beach (San Pedro)

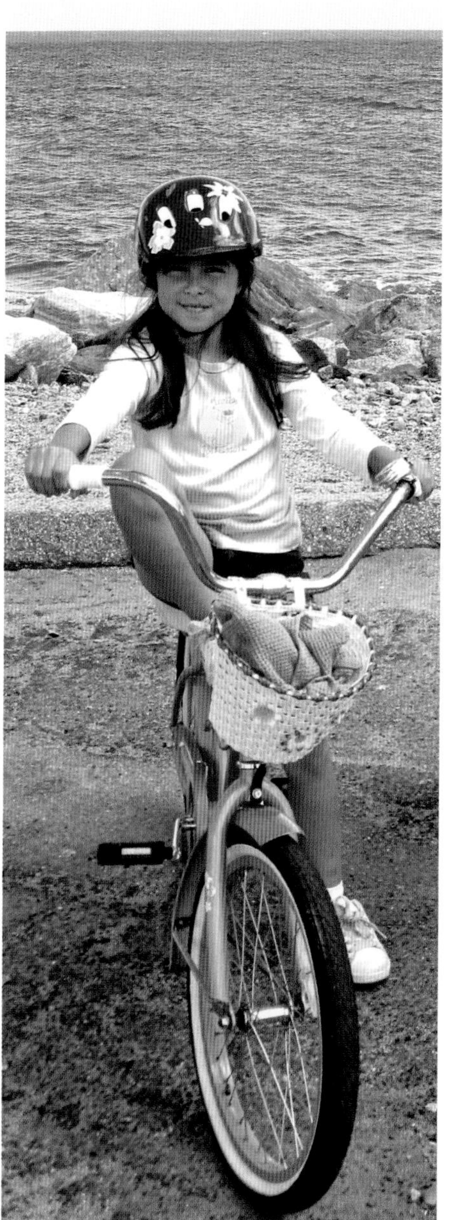

*A rider takes a breather out at the point (just off the bike path).*

**Distance** 1.2 miles

## Terrain

Entirely car-free, this route has both concrete and asphalt paving.

## How to Get There

From the 110 Freeway South to San Pedro, exit at Harbor Boulevard. Turn right onto Harbor, then right on 22nd Street, and left on Pacific Avenue. At Stephen White Drive, turn left and proceed to Cabrillo Beach parking area ($1.00 per hour).

## Amenities and Things to Do

Cabrillo Coastal Park has an abundance of seashore activities within easy pedaling distance, even for young kids. The offerings include two beaches (one with gentle harbor waves, the other with ocean surf), the Cabrillo Marine Aquarium and Point Fermin tidal pools.

## About

This ride begins on a paved bike path, flanked by lawns and shady picnic areas on one side and, on the other, by a flat, sandy beach with a pirate-ship-themed playground. Midway along, the ride extends out on the wide asphalt-topped breakwater between harbor and ocean. Windsurfers and boats, even cargo ships in the background, animate the scene.

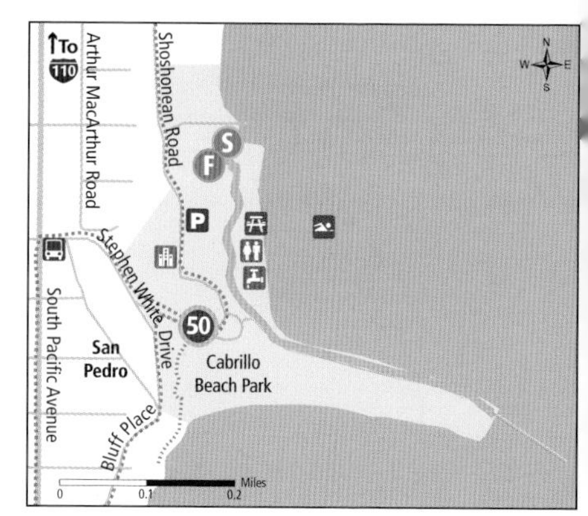

## Ride K30 - Wilmington Waterfront Park (Wilmington)

**istance** 1.9 miles

### errain

panning the length of Waterfront Park are two mooth, interconnected concrete promenades: a "low oad" at street level, and a "high road" overlooking the ark and nearby port.

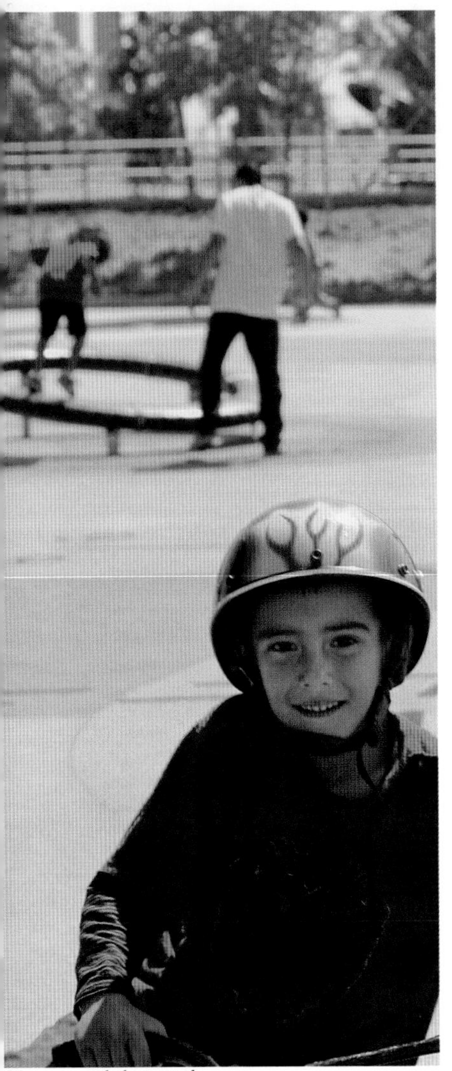

*It's a way cool playground.*

### How to Get There

From the 110 Freeway toward the Port of Los Angeles, exit onto C Street. At the ramp's end, make a left onto Figueroa Street and then, a right onto D Street. Turn right onto Wilmington Boulevard to the park.

### Amenities and Things to Do

This brand-spanking-new park—a 30-acre gem—opened in June 2011. Deft design and landscaping make this long, narrow tract feel even bigger. You'll find picnic and BBQ areas, a colorful playground, water geysers, as well as a bike-accessible observation deck with binoculars (the heavy-duty, coin-operated type, but free of charge). You can watch ships loading, or look down across the park. One aqueous feature is a matrix of holes spewing geysers from the pavement (that kids can ride through).

### About

This is a fabulous place for young cyclists. The options range from street-level spins past the playground and athletic fields to a long jaunt over and elevated pathway, across the park's four footbridges and down a short hill to the picnic area. Several short connectors between high and low ground allow kids to modify the route, improvising along the way.

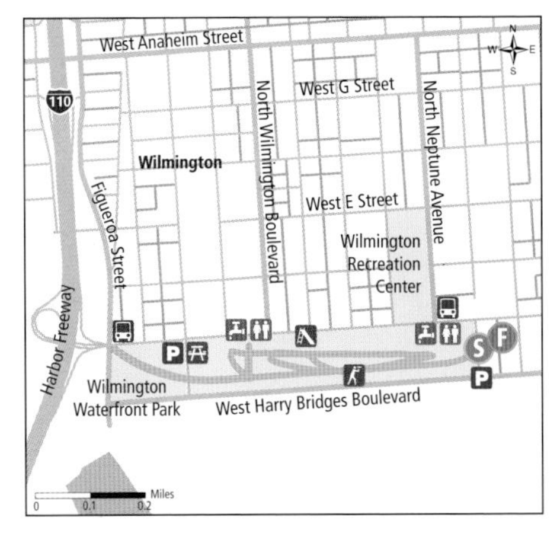

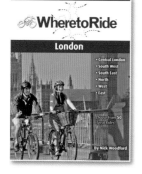

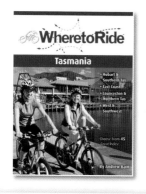

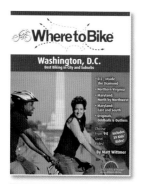

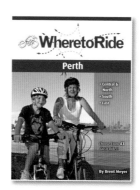

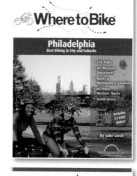

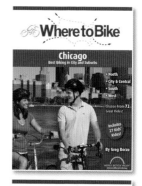

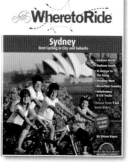

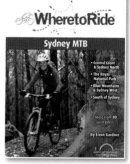

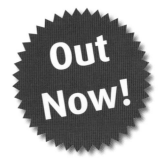

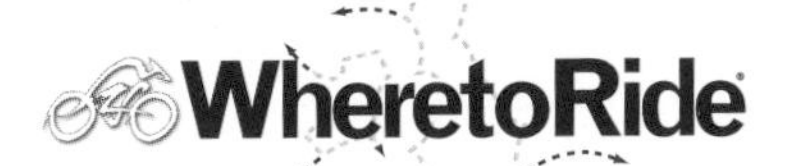

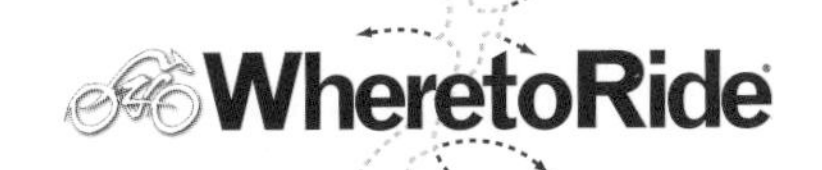


# Also in this Series!

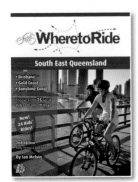

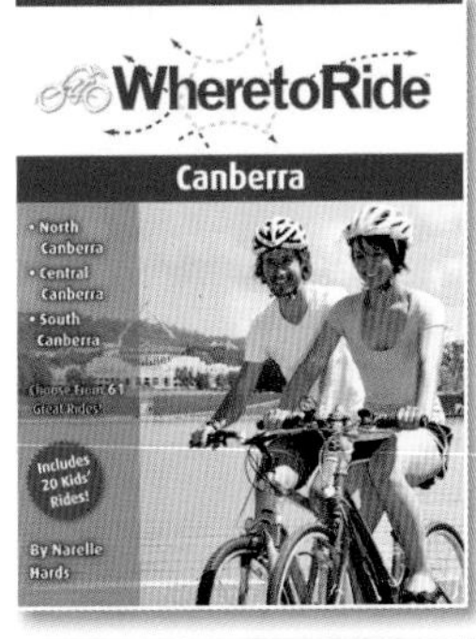


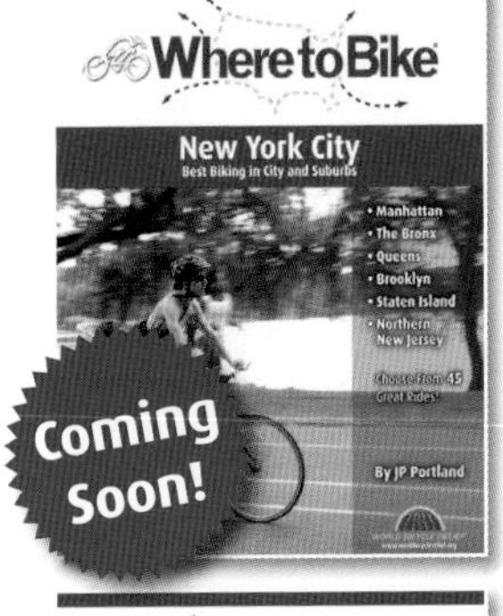


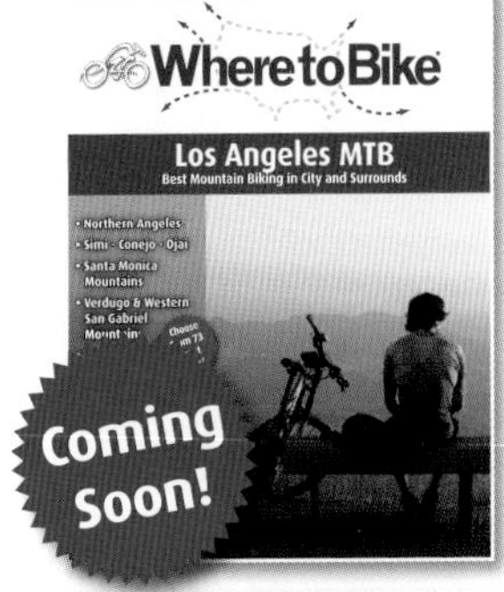

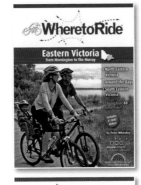


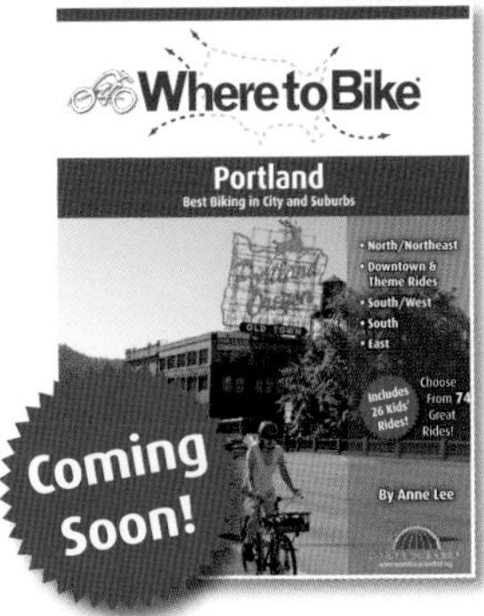


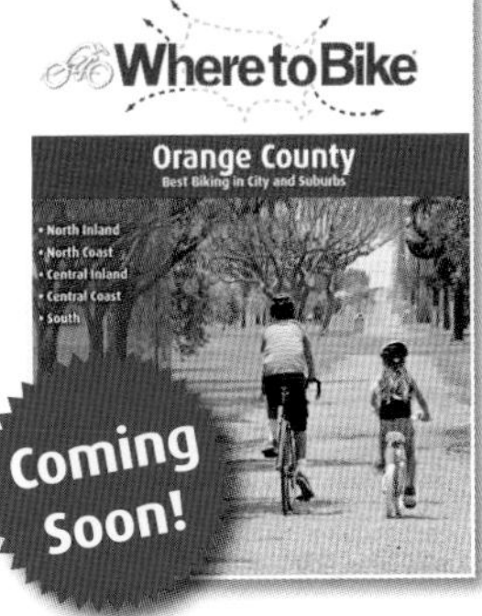


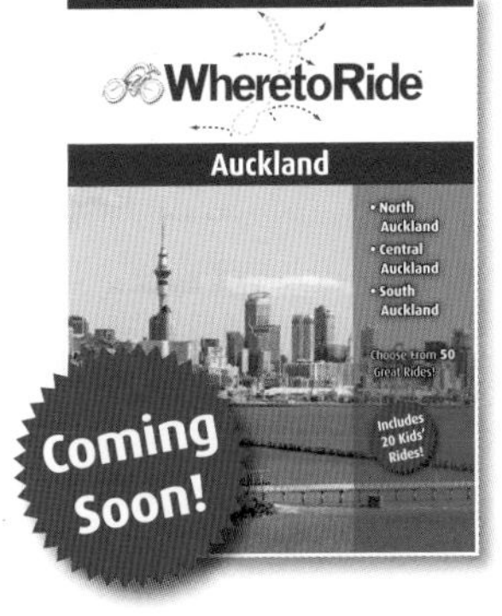

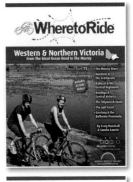


www.**WheretoBikeGuides**.com